5. 20. 77

Guide to Fitness After Fifty

Guide to Fitness After Fifty

Edited by
Raymond Harris, M.D.
Center for the Study of Aging
Albany, New York

and

Lawrence J. Frankel
Lawrence Frankel Foundation
Charleston, West Virginia

Associate editor
Sara Harris
Center for the Study of Aging
Albany, New York

Plenum Press · New York and London

Library of Congress Cataloging in Publication Data

Main entry under title:

Guide to fitness after fifty.

   Includes index.
   1. Physical fitness. 2. Exercise for the aged. 3. Physical education for the aged. 4.
Exercise—Physiological aspects. 5. Aging. I. Harris, Raymond, 1919-   II.
Frankel, Lawrence J. III. Harris, Sara, 1921-   [DNLM: 1. Physical fitness. 2.
Extertion—In old age. 3. Exercise therapy—In old age QT255 G946]
RA781.G84   613.7'04   77-2296
ISBN 0-306-30995-5

© 1977 Plenum Press, New York
A Division of Plenum Publishing Corporation
227 West 17th Street, New York, N.Y. 10011

Printed in the United States of America

Contributors

Nicholas G. Alexiou, M.D., M.P.H., Medical Director, Employee Health Service, New York State Department of Civil Service; Clinical Assistant Professor of Pediatrics, Albany Medical College, Albany, New York.

Lloyd C. Arnold, Ed.D., National Director, Health and Physical Education, National Council of YMCAs, New York, New York.

Daniel Brunner, M.D., Associate Professor, Chief, First Medical Department, Government Hospital Jaffa; Head, Donolo Institute of Physiological Hygiene, Tel Aviv University, Tel Aviv, Israel.

C. Carson Conrad, M.A., Executive Director, President's Council on Physical Fitness and Sports, Washington, D.C.

Robert H. Cress, M.D., Assistant Professor of Physical Medicine and Rehabilitation, Albany Medical College, Albany, New York.

Edward Terry Davison, M.D., Clinical Associate Professor of Medicine, State University of New York, Stony Brook, New York; Attending in Cardiology, Long Island Jewish Hospital, New Hyde Park, New York.

Herbert A. deVries, Ph.D., Professor of Physical Education and Physiology, University of Southern California; Director, Physiology of Exercise Research Laboratory, University of Southern California Gerontology Center and Mobile Laboratory, Laguna Hills, California.

Andrew A. Fischer, M.D., Ph.D., Assistant Professor of Physical Medicine and Rehabilitation, State University of New York, Stony Brook, New York; Physiatrist in charge of Department of Rehabilitation Medicine, Long Island Jewish-Hillside Medical Center and Jewish Institute for Geriatric Care, New Hyde Park, New York.

Lawrence J. Frankel, Executive Director, Lawrence Frankel Foundation, Charleston, West Virginia.

John A. Friedrich, Ph.D., Chairman, Department of Health, Physical Education, and Recreation, Duke University, Durham, North Carolina.

David Green, M.B., B.S., Clinical Associate Professor of Neurology, Department of Neurology, Albany Medical College, Albany, New York.

Paul A. L. Haber, M.D., Assistant Chief Medical Director, United States Veterans Administration; Clinical Assistant Professor of Medicine, George Washington University, Washington, D.C.

v

Raymond Harris, M.D., Clinical Associate Professor of Medicine, Albany Medical College; Chief, Subdepartment of Cardiovascular Medicine, St. Peter's Hospital; President, Center for the Study of Aging, Albany, New York.

Sara Harris, Executive Secretary, Center for the Study of Aging; Lecturer, State University of New York, Albany, New York.

Eino Matti Heikkinen, M.D., Professor of Gerontology, Department of Public Health Sciences, University of Tampere, Tampere, Finland.

Hollis S. Ingraham, M.D., M.P.H., Sc.D., Former New York State Commissioner of Health, Albany, New York; Executive Secretary, Steering Committee, Albany Medical Center, Albany, New York.

Herman L. Kamenetz, M.D., Chief, Rehabilitation Medicine, Veterans Administration Hospital; Clinical Professor of Medicine, George Washington University School of Medicine; Professorial Lecturer, Georgetown University School of Medicine, Washington, D.C.

Birgit Kayhty, M.S.C., Department of Public Health, University of Jyväskylä, Jyväskylä, Finland.

Hans Kraus, M.D., New York University Institute of Physical Medicine and Rehabilitation, New York, New York.

Maggie (Margaret B.) Lettvin, Lecturer, Department of Physical Education, Massachusetts Institute of Technology; Assistant Professor, Leslie College, Cambridge, Massachusetts.

Jana Parizkova, M.D., Ph.D., Research Worker, Research Institute of Physical Culture, Prague, Czechoslovakia.

Betty Byrd Richard, Associate Administrator, Lawrence Frankel Foundation, Charleston, West Virginia.

Manuel Rodstein, M.D., Chief of Medical Services and Director of Cardiology, The Jewish Home and Hospital for Aged; Associate Clinical Professor of Medicine, Albert Einstein College of Medicine; Associate Attending Physician, Montefiore Hospital, New York, New York.

Ernst Simonson, M.D., (deceased) Dr. rer. nat. h.c., Director of Medical Electronic Research, Mt. Sinai Hospital, Minneapolis, Minnesota; Professor of Physiological Hygiene emer., University of Minnesota, Minneapolis; Professor of Physiology emer., Johann-Wolfgang-Goethe University, Frankfurt a.M., Germany.

Ilkka M. Vuori, M.D., Associate Professor, Rehabilitation Research Center; Chief, Clinical Laboratory, Rehabilitation Research Center of Finnish Social Insurance Institution, Turku; Acting Professor of Public Health, University of Jyväskylä, Jyväskylä, Finland.

Robert E. Wear, Ph.D., Associate Professor, Department of Physical Education, University of New Hampshire, Durham, New Hampshire.

Frederick A. Whitehouse, Ed.D., Professor of Rehabilitation and Director, Rehabilitation Counseling Program, Hofstra University, Hempstead, New York.

Preface

Guide to Fitness After Fifty presents basic and applied research data, authoritative advice and tested techniques for professional workers who want to learn more about physical exercise, fitness and health for aging people and for all who seek to become more physically and mentally fit. The editors and contributors believe that physical activity and exercise following the principles and practices outlined in this interdisciplinary volume can improve the health and quality of life by increasing endurance and cardiovascular fitness, strengthening the musculoskeletal system, improving mobility, posture and appearance, and relaxing emotional tensions. Evidence at hand and discussed in this book demonstrates that properly prescribed physical activity or exercise can raise the level of physical fitness and health, both physical and mental, at any age, delay the ravages of aging, and prevent or reduce disability from musculoskeletal and circulatory disorders.

Section I, *Perspectives on Exercise and Aging*, surveys the fundamental problems and relationships of exercise to aging and health and provides historical insights and philosophic perspectives on the significance and importance of physical fitness and exercise through the centuries and in contemporary society.

Section II, *Evaluation and Physiology of Exercise*, presents objective scientific and medical evidence that reasonable improvement in fitness and other bodily functions may be achieved by people of all ages who follow well designed exercise and relaxation routines for at least 30 minutes three or more times weekly. Such programs, best begun in youth and continued throughout adulthood, but begun at any age, can improve mental and physical health and help aging people to cope better with the inevitable and too often self-inflicted emotional and physical stresses and strains of daily living. Appropriate testing of the individual before and after exercise is essential to measure improvement and progress.

Section III, *Motivation and Planning*, provides examples of tested programs and recommendations by experts with extensive experience in developing successful exercise programs for aging people at home, in community agencies, institutions, and other health and educational systems, including television.

Section IV, *Practical Exerccise and Relaxation Programs*, presents physical exercise and relaxation techniques which have helped men and women over fifty develop better physical, mental, musculoskeletal and cardiovascular fitness. These preventive and therapeutic programs include jogging, calisthenics, stretching, relaxation and other types of appropriate exercises. They add vim, vigor, vitality, health and happiness to the life of middle-aged and older people and cushion the stresses and strains of growing old. Proven by experience and practice to be safe and helpful, they will do no harm — provided proper instructions and health precautions are followed.

The editors wish to express their appreciation to the contributors, Seymour Weingarten and Stephen Dyer of Plenum Press, Raymond Newkirk, Robert Newkirk, James Blake and the staff of Newkirk Products, Inc., Mrs. Laura Campaigne of St. Peter's Hospital Library, Thomas Erskine, Nancy Bishop and Rosalie Pietrocola of the Center for the Study of Aging for their assistance.

Raymond Harris, M.D.
Lawrence Frankel
Sara Harris

Contents

Section I

PERSPECTIVES ON EXERCISE AND AGING

Section II

EVALUATION AND PHYSIOLOGY OF EXERCISE

Section III

MOTIVATION AND PLANNING

Section IV

PRACTICAL EXERCISE AND RELAXATION PROGRAMS

APPENDIX

Introduction

PHYSICAL FITNESS FOR OLDER AMERICANS –
A NATIONAL RESPONSIBILITY AND OPPORTUNITY
INTRODUCTION

A scientific and social breakthrough of great significance is the recognition that many problems historically attributed to aging are really the products of neglect, abuse, and lack of fitness. Testimony on physical fitness and its implications for older Americans before the Senate Subcommittee on Aging on April 22, 1975 led Congress to amend Titles III and VII of the Older American's Act to provide money to educate, inform, motivate and enlist support and participation of older persons in physical activities for the purpose of enhancing their general health (Conrad, 1976).*

Historically, leadership in the field of fitness was assumed by the President's Council in 1956 when it was established as the President's Council on Youth Fitness by Dwight D. Eisenhower as a result of a widely publicized study showing American youth were not as physically fit as their European counterparts. In 1963, the agency became the President's Council on Physical Fitness and the present name was adopted in 1968 to indicate the council's concern for developing mass participation sports programs. It was reorganized on September 25, 1970, by Executive Order 11562, and the Secretary of Health, Education and Welfare was charged to carry out the following seven-point national program of physical fitness and sports:

(1) Enlist the active support and assistance of individual citizens, civic groups, professional associations, amateur and professional sports groups, private enterprise, voluntary organizations and others to promote and improve physical fitness and sports participation programs for all Americans;

(2) Stimulate, improve and strengthen coordination of federal services and programs relating to physical fitness and sports participation;

(3) Encourage state and local governments to enhance physical fitness and sports participation;

(4) Seek to strengthen the physical fitness of American children, youth and adults by systematically encouraging the development of community-centered and other physical fitness and sports participation programs to encourage innovation, improve teacher participation and strengthen state and local leadership;

* Conrad, C. C. (1976) *Aging* No. 258, April, pp. 11-13.

(5) Develop cooperative programs with medical, dental and other similar professional societies to encourage and implement sound physical fitness practices;

(6) Stimulate and encourage research in the areas of physical fitness and sports performance;

(7) Improve school health and physical education programs for all pupils, including the handicapped and the physically underdeveloped, by assisting educational agencies in developing quality programs to encourage innovation, improve teacher preparation and strengthen state and local leadership.

The operational activities of the Council include:

(1) Direction of continuing public service information programs about the nature and extent of the physical fitness problem;

(2) Provision of technical and consultative services to national and state educational, recreational, fitness and health systems;

(3) Coordination of physical fitness activities of federal and state agencies;

(4) Direction of motivational and awards programs; and

(5) Promotion of support for physical fitness and mass amateur sports development programs.

As a catalyst, the Council has secured the co-sponsorship of many organizations and representatives of the private sector and government agencies, supporting more than 50 national projects which further the Council's goals. Significant progress has been made in a number of the aforementioned areas during the past year. Governors' and Mayors' Councils on Physical Fitness have increased; information and technical assistance programs have been expanded and extended to new groups; the private sector has supported a number of new participation progams developed by the Council; and the Presidential Sports Award Program for adults has been expanded.

EXERCISE PATTERNS OF AMERICAN ADULTS

A major activity of the President's Council on Physical Fitness and Sports is the study of the exercise and sports participation habits of American adults, including those over the age of 50. A National Adult Physical Fitness Survey was conducted for the Council by Opinion Research Corporation, Princeton, New Jersey, which interviewed 3,875 men and women, 22 years and over. This survey documented the extent to which Americans were involved in regular exercise and/or sports programs and dramatically emphasized the responsibility and opportunity Americans face to improve the dynamic health of all Americans.

The survey revealed:

(1) 45 percent of all American men and women (roughly 49 million of the 109 million total) do not engage in physical activity for the purpose of exercise.

These sedentary Americans tend to be older, less well-educated and less affluent than those who exercise.

(2) Of the 60 million adult Americans who exercise, nearly 44 million walk, more than 18 million ride bicycles, 14 million swim, 14 million do calisthenics and 6.5 million jog.

(3) The favorite participatory sports in order of popularity are swimming, bowling, golf, tennis, softball, volleyball, waterskiing and skiing.

(4) Concern about health, the desire to lose weight and the enjoyment one derives from sport and physical activity were the major reasons why people exercise. Only one of every five American adults has been advised to exercise by physicians.

(5) The most active adults are those who participated in two or more sports while in secondary school and/or college. More than two-thirds of these still exercise regularly as opposed to fewer than one-half of those who were not athletes.

(6) The least active Americans are those who never took physical education. Only six percent of them ride bicycles, only four percent swim and only two percent jog. The comparable percentages for adults who have taken physical education are 21 percent, 17 percent and seven percent.

For individuals over 50, the situation is even more dismal than it is for younger Americans. For example, of the 28,682,280 men and women age 50 and over, only the following percent participated in a lifetime sport on any competitive or non-competitive basis during 12 months prior to the survey:

Sport	Competitive	Non-Competitive
Bowling	8 percent	11 percent
Golf	6 percent	9 percent
Swimming	Less than ½ percent	12 percent
Tennis	Less than ½ percent	2 percent

A total of 15 percent, age 50 and over, rode a bicycle (four percent riding daily or almost every day, two percent 3-5 times a week and three percent 1-2 times a week).

Fifteen percent of those over 50 participated in calisthenics (nine percent exercising daily or almost every day, three percent 3-5 times a week and two percent 1-2 times a week). Jogging was an activity for five percent of the age 50 or older, with three percent participating daily or almost every day, and one percent 3-5 times a week. Swimming was the second most popular activity for age 50 and older, with 14 percent now participating. Of these, two percent swam daily or almost every day, two percent 3-5 times a week and four percent 1-2 times a week. In the 50-59 age group, 38 percent walked for exercise. Thirty-nine percent of adults 60 or older walked for exercise.

NEW GOALS FOR ADULT FITNESS

The findings of this survey convinced Council members and staff that a major emphasis should be placed on fitness programs for older Americans. Medical authorities supported this need.

Dr. Theodore Klumpp, a prominent New York physician and a medical consultant to the PCPFS, advised the members of the Council staff that "remaining active is the key to staying alive. Stress is necessary to keep bodies in good tone. For example, one way to stimulate the thyroid gland is through stressful exercise. However, many people won't exercise for fear it will provoke a heart attack." Dr. Klumpp does not agree with this apprehension, stating that exercise opposes the effects of stroke or heart attack. "Blood clots form when the blood flow is sluggish rather than when it is vigorous."

Through the past decade, I have questioned a number of older people, including Lowell Thomas and several centenarians, and have attempted to read all reports and articles regarding the commonalities of older people throughout the world. A classic example of a person who lived the good life is my friend Larry Lewis. Larry retired as a full-time waiter at the St. Francis Hotel in San Francisco, but continued an active regimen at 105 years of age. For many years, Larry ran six miles every morning in Golden Gate Park.

Many healthy old people do lead a very active life, involving a considerable amount of vigorous physical activity every day either in their work or through their exercise and physical activity program. Alexander Leaf, M.D., reported in the *National Geographic* magazine, January 1973, "Every Day is a Gift When You Are Over 100" that older people from Ecuador, Kashmir and Abkhaza, where people allegedly live much longer and remain more vigorous in old age than in most modern societies, engage in much physical activity. Their traditional farming and householding practices demand heavy work from males and females from early childhood to the end of their lives. Superimposed on the usual labor is the mountainous terrain. Simply traversing the hills on foot during the day's activities assisted their high degree of cardiovascular fitness and general muscular tone. When Dr. Leaf returned from his visits, is it any wonder that he took up jogging?

The Dunbar and Gallup studies on longevity to isolate the factors present in the way of life of men who have outlived their contemporaries by a generation and who have enjoyed life in good health found three major commonalities:

(1) They have a self-imposed discipline, and naturally will forego the second helping or second drink.

(2) They work hard all their lives at something they enjoy. If their work does not involve hard physical labor, they exercise regularly and vigorously. Many were great walkers, hikers and climbers and even at 100 years of age continue to walk a mile a day or more.

(3) Probably most significant of all, they have a constant cheerfulness, an optimism. They enjoy each day and look forward to tomorrow.

The exercise practitioner like myself, who has seen what oldsters can do physically, wonders just how much our conservatism has shortchanged older people. In the swimming pool at various physical fitness clinics during the past 12 years, I have had many individuals over 60 follow a 450 calorie workout lasting an hour. In Monterey, a 68-year-old man did so. In San Francisco, a woman of 66 and another of 76 did so. When I asked the 76-year-old how often she swam, she replied, "Every day except Saturday and Sunday." "Why not then?" I asked. Her answer was, "Because the YMCA is closed then." In Phoenix, an 80-year-old woman followed the clinic workout. She also swam every day.

The slow progressive build-up and regularity of participation is the key to a comfortable, safe exercise program. A few basic aspects of workouts for older people, including those in pools, should be explained. Even in group classes, the leaders should assess the exercise tolerance level of each individual and gear the intensity of the activity to that level.

In working with older people, particularly those who have been sedentary for an extended period, it is important to stress flexibility, strength and cardiorespiratory endurance in the order listed. Obviously, older people should receive clearance from their physician prior to engaging in a physical fitness program.

After a period of progression in walking, in which an individual can walk three miles in 45 minutes, the well person can move into more vigorous cardiorespiratory work. Whether such circulatory endurance is done in individual or group programs, the participant should stay away from oxygen debt or windedness thereby permitting a comfortable long workout. Remember, it is not how hard you work but how long you work.

All age groups should have physical exercise. Older Americans must exercise daily to enjoy optimum healthful living. I believe that many of the infirmities of old age can be prevented by systematized exercise earlier in life and that the elderly can improve their physical condition by regular supervised physical activity.

If oldsters can work physically to their advantage, is it not time that we launch a national emphasis for them to do so? This is a responsibility the President's Council accepts and an opportunity we welcome.

This book brings together and provides much needed information to all people who believe in the value of physical fitness and relaxation after 50, and who want not only to develop but also to participate in the sorely needed area of more effective fitness activities for older Americans.

C. Carson Conrad, Executive Director
President's Council on Physical Fitness and Sports

Section I

Perspectives on Exercise and Aging

Fitness and the Aging Process

Raymond Harris, M.D.

INTRODUCTION

One summer not too long ago, I rocked on the porch of a run-down cabin overlooking the Atlantic Ocean at Bar Harbor, Maine, and watched a grey and white adult herring gull preening itself on a craggy rock on the beach. It was high noon, and the tide was coming in. I wondered when the middle-aged bird would take off. Just as the water engulfed the rock, the gull swooped off into the sky.

Many of us, 50 years of age and over, are like this bird, perched and slumped at our desks, leading lives of inactivity, preening ourselves and taking it easy during the high noon of middle age as the unrelenting tide of life, lapping at our physical foundations, threatens our health and survival. Fortunately, in sharp contrast to this gull's world, the harsh Darwinian principle of "survival of the fittest" no longer applies to the world of man where scientific advances and medical resources support the survival of the physically unfit, the sick and the old. As a result, older people are living longer, and every 10th American is 65 years of age or over. The over-65 population alone already represents the total population of all ages of the nation's 21 smallest states. By the year 2000, if the birth rate continues to drop, 50 percent of the American population will be "over 50," indicating the potential scope and importance of better fitness after 50.

If being "over 50" is not to mean being "over the hill," more attention must be paid to physical fitness. Better physical and mental fitness is necessary not only to improve the survival, but, equally important, to improve the quality of life in aging people so they can look and feel well, carry out their daily duties and responsibilities readily and easily with enough physical reserve to enjoy their social, civic, cultural, and recreational activities and meet unusual or emergency demands. The goal of physical fitness is to develop efficiency of heart and lungs, muscular strength, endurance, balance, flexibility, coordination and agility to enable aging people at all ages to live vigorously, energetically and healthfully. Proper diet and physical exercise to

3

build physical fitness are the two props for insuring better health in old age. At least one aspect of aging, the decline of efficiency, can be inhibited by 25 years and more, provided there is systematic and lasting application of suitable physical training (deVries, 1966).

BARRIERS TO PHYSICAL FITNESS

One cause of diminished physical fitness in people over 50 years of age is that modern man, built for the stone age and constructed for activity, now lives complacently and inactively, although more comfortably, in our sofa age, no longer getting enough regular physical exercise that is so vital for optimal body functioning and good health. Much of our daily work is physically undemanding and truly unsatisfying. Although there is no proof that exercise extends life, there is sufficient evidence that physical fitness can improve the quality of life and delay or prevent some of the deteriorative changes of aging. For such effects to be obtained, muscles, heart and circulation must be exercised regularly and vigorously, as suggested in this chapter and developed in other chapters of this book.

Other major causes of poor physical condition in people 50 years of age and older are the changes due to the aging process, the neuromuscular deterioration that seems to accompany it, and hypokinetic disorders.

Changes of Aging

The changes due to the aging process affect the structure and function of the brain, central nervous system and peripheral nerves, as well as those of the musculoskeletal system. With age, a color pigment, lipofuscin, accumulates in the nerve cells. At the same time, there is a loss of peripheral neurons, cortical neurons and Nissl substance, and an increase in glial elements of the brain.

The brain weight is greatest at 20 years of age and then decreases seven to 11 percent in weight between the ages of 20 and 96 years. It is estimated that the cerebral cortex of the normal young adult brain contains about 10 to 12 billion neurons, and about 100,000 nerve cells are lost each day (Brody, 1970). This loss is most evident in the temporal gyrus, less in the precentral gyrus and visual cortex and least in the postcentral gyrus of the brain.

These aging changes in the brain and central nervous system impair sensory perception and motor responses so that the older person's coordination, motivation, ability and desire to exercise lessen and the simple, effortless responses of youth become slower and more labored in later life (Birren et al., 1959). Neuromuscular performance decreases, and simple reaction time and discrimination reaction time, reflecting central nervous system integrity, increase. Formerly, it was believed that these times were strictly a function of age, but recent evidence suggests that they may also be a function of an individual's psychological or physical fitness level (Wyrick-Spirduso, 1975). In addition, blood vessel disease may reduce the blood and oxygen supply to the brain and cause further deterioration of the brain function. These changes may produce a situation in which observed events do not register quickly enough in the consciousness of older people to permit appropriate behavior in emergency situations requiring alertness and prompt action. For example, an older person crossing a street must scan the scene, note the presence of cars, their movement and the state of the traffic signals. By the time he does this, his decision to cross the street may be antiquated and even hazardous (Birren et al., 1959) when he finally steps off the curb.

Sensory changes due to aging reduce visual, auditory and sensory perception and decrease coordination and muscular movements, involving flexibility, strength, endurance, adjustable or suitable rate of movement, stability, posture and timing, so that mobility and coordination also become limited. Flexor movements become dominant and rotation component decreases as senescent motor ability and behavior become impaired. Such changes may cause the very old person to assume a more infantile posture and limit his movement.

The range and versatility of motor responses also narrow in the older person because the tonic neck and other reflexes, which normally contribute to walking ability, become impaired as a result of faulty feedback between movement and body image. Habitually sedentary elderly subjects suffer not only muscular deterioration, but also distortion of body image. They perceive their bodies as broader and heavier and body activities as more strenuous than they actually are. Such faulty feedback is established between movement and body image so that the progressive restriction of physical exercise produces a corresponding alteration of their body image, greater clumsiness and increased fear of physical activity (Kreitler and Kreitler, 1970). Older people lose the pleasure of movement simply for the sake of moving, which children enjoy; they eventually become reluctant to move at all and may opt to remain in a chair or bed.

Neuromuscular Deterioration

Muscle disuse, due to a more sedentary way of life, and loss of muscle cells, leads to a decline in muscle strength. Between the ages of 20 and 30, a person's muscle strength is maximal and gradually declines to 80 percent by the time he reaches the age of 65. The average strength of women is about two-thirds that of men (Åstrand and Rodahl, 1970). The rate of decline in muscle strength is greater in the leg and trunk muscles. Physical training, previous physical conditioning, and the degree of engagement of muscle synergists may influence such decline.

Power output and maximal work output, measured by running or crank-turning, also deteriorate with age. Such impairment has been attributed to a reduction in coordination ability, as well as impaired heart and pulmonary function, and the failure to allow for the speed limitations in 70- and 80-year-olds (Shock and Norris, 1970). The maximum oxygen consumption and cardiovascular respiratory capacity also decrease with age, being 30 percent lower at 50 years of age and 45 percent lower at age 70 than at age 30. Aerobic (oxygen-dependent) work capacity declines about one percent per year.

Physical work capacity decreases more in sedentary people after the age of 20. It decreases at a slower rate and to a lesser degree in trained, physically fit and active older persons. As a result, a trained 65-year-old man may actually have a better physical work capacity than an untrained 35-year-old person. Such data suggest that physiologic rather than chronologic age and physical fitness influence the capacity for physical work and that changes in physical capacity are not inevitably a result of aging, but rather a result of physical disuse and inactivity which exercise and training can improve.

Mental and physical ability need not necessarily decline with age so that an individual's value comes to an end when he retires or grows old. Training can be used to improve specific neuromuscular coordination and skills, and exercise to strengthen muscles, divert one's mind from problems and reduce neuromuscular tension. Such exercise and training can increase endurance and cardiovascular fitness, eliminate fatigue and stimulate metabolism, at least up to age 65. Over the age of 70, the ability to train and improve the cardiorespiratory system by proper exercise appears possible but needs further research to assess methods and results.

Changes Due to Hypokinetic Disorders

Many physical changes in older people are mistakenly attributed to aging when they actually result from hypokinetic disease, poor physical fitness or lack of proper conditioning. As people age and become physically inactive and more unfit, their flexor muscles shorten; antigravity muscles supporting the head, body and joints weaken. Weakness of the back and shoulder muscles causes poor posture and leads to a humpbacked appearance. These postural changes, together with poor expansion of the chest and diaphragm, further restrict breathing and reduce the volume of oxygen older people can inhale, thereby limiting their maximal level of physical activity. Arthritis and other neck deformities may impinge on the arteries and further interfere with blood flow to the brain. Such decrease of blood flow may aggravate the already reduced oxygen supply and decreased cardiac output that occur with age.

Mobility may be limited by incoordination and adaptive shortening of muscles, and/or immobility of joints, muscle spasms, muscle spasticity, as well as muscular changes due to the aging process. Many elderly individuals find it progressively more difficult to stand up after sitting and to go up and down stairs because of weakness of their back and hip muscles as a result of poor muscular tone due to disuse and lack of proper exercise. In addition, musculoskeletal, vascular and neurological disease may further limit mobility. *Marche à petits pas* type of gait may be noted in patients with diffuse cerebral disturbances, especially cerebral arteriosclerosis, as well as in patients with paralysis agitans. Locomotion is slow with this type of gait and the patient walks with short, mincing, shuffling footsteps and a loss of associated movements. Occasionally, bizarre dancing movements on the balls of the feet, hopping walking movements, pronounced heel to toe movements, irregular steps, generalized weakness of the lower extremities or the entire body and easy fatigability may be noted. The Parkinsonian gait is caused by extrapyramidal conditions while the gait of spastic hemiplegia may be caused by any lesion that interrupts the pyramidal innervation to one-half of the body. A spastic ataxic gait may occur in diffuse disease of the nervous system, including posterolateral sclerosis of pernicious anemia and multiple sclerosis involving both the pyramidal and proprioceptive pathways.

THERAPEUTIC MEASURES

Preventive Measures

Proper physical exercise, as described in this and other chapters of this book, should be prescribed at all ages to maintain and improve physical fitness, mobility, joint flexibility, muscular strength, neuromuscular coordination and cardiovascular fitness. Such improved physical fitness activity can prolong normal walking patterns into old age and reduce the hazards of falls, loss of equilibrium and other accidents. Even when the musculoskeletal, respiratory, cardiovascular and central nervous systems have already deteriorated due to lack of physical conditioning and/or disease, properly prescribed and adequately supervised exercise, followed for an extended period of time, can be expected to partially improve fitness and other functions. The direct effect of physical activity stimulation upon the central nervous system may delay aging changes. Nerve cells, which fail to receive and process stimuli, involute and atrophy. Physical activity generates impinging stimuli and excitation which affects the entire chain of neurons. The continued reaction in speed decision-making in response to continually changing unpredictable stimuli may enhance neuronal longevity and efficiency. Exercise stimulating metabolism, respiration, blood circulation, digestion and glands of external secretion may protect against senile involution of brain cells (Harris, 1975).

Medical Measures

With normal aging, vigor may diminish slightly, but the normal elderly person in good health and good physical fitness enjoys and radiates vigor. Many middle-aged and older people who consult physicians often lack such vigor and suffer from symptoms and signs of poor physical fitness, including undue breathlessness, excessive worry, tension, fatigue, insomnia, backache and muscular aches and pains. Since these functional complaints simulate those of organic disease, a complete medical checkup should be the cornerstone of any program to improve physical fitness after 50. Once organic disease has been ruled out, individual programs for physical fitness can be designed according to the kind of life one wishes to lead and enjoys doing.

In some elderly people, undue fatigue, decreased muscle strength, lack of endurance, loss of weight, emotional disturbances and depression may result from a drop in the level of androgen, thyroid or other hormones in the body. Appropriate hormone substitution therapy may dramatically restore their health and vigor. If nutritional deficiency is responsible for the decrease in vigor and vitality, proper nutrition can usually reverse the process.

Elderly people with diminished visual and auditory perception should be given proper aids and retrained to improve their ability to be independent, useful and needed. Poor eyesight, poor hearing, loss of balance or equilibrium and dizziness interfere with mobility and independence. Good vision is important to the elderly and proper glasses should be prescribed when necessary to provide good vision for the specific seeing jobs that they must accomplish. Even simple walking becomes a problem to the patient with marked presbyopia whose leg or hip conditions make it essential for him to watch carefully where he steps. Bifocal glasses may correct his presbyopia, but walking for the patient with regular bifocals may be impossible unless the patient awkwardly tilts his head down to look through the top part of his glasses. Eye glasses with very small, low-set segments for close vision or lenses that are not bifocal may be a better remedy. Poor hearing should also be corrected with appropriate hearing aids whenever possible.

Older people can also be helped to become independent and useful by delegating to them household responsibilities which they can perform, or by involving them in group activities where they can contribute their talents. The older person, particularly the one with some brain impairment, should not be forced to do tasks requiring abstract thinking. Simple programs with physical activity are preferable for most older people. However, some older persons are still capable of performing creative and imaginative work and should be encouraged to do so.

Minor foot injuries or other discomforts in the lower extremities should never be minimized, downgraded or overlooked. Such injuries often prove more disabling to an older person than to a younger one and should be corrected properly and promptly before permanent injury ensues.

Conditions producing unsteadiness, diminished sensory perception, dizziness and/or lightheadedness should be diagnosed properly and corrected before the elderly patient falls and injures himself. When these conditions cannot be corrected, supportive devices, canes or walkers, should be prescribed as preventive measures to avoid permanent disability.

Physical Exercise

In people of any age without disease, impaired vigor, undue fatigue and various muscular aches and pains must be attributed to poor physical fitness, poor emotional health or the neuromuscular change of age which impair coordination and reduce the capacity for physical exertion. In such patients, properly supervised and prescribed therapeutic physical exercise on land or in water can develop better endurance and cardiovascular fitness, reduce fatigue, stimulate metabolism, aid digestion, reduce constipation, improve vigor and flexibility of joints, and develop better neuromuscular coordination and skills. Such physical activity, providing an outlet for the tensions and worries of daily life, improves well-being and sleep patterns. Appropriately designed muscular exercise will reduce free-floating tensions, channel inhibited aggression, release kinesthetic stimuli and provide profound emotional satisfaction. It consumes "free-floating energies," prevents internalization of aggressive tendencies, breaks the faulty feedback pattern between movement and distortions of body image due to prolonged inactivity and reestablishes a feeling of security. Muscular movements initiate stimuli in muscle spindles which are essential for optimal functioning of the central nervous system. There appears to be a relationship between an individual's mood and his muscle condition and posture. The gamma motor system appears involved in this relationship. It is a feedback servomechanism which is involved in the coordination of muscle movements. In this system, the muscle spindles act as the sensors and the hypothalmic centers in the midbrain constitute an important relay center in facilitating and coordinating proper functioning of the stretch mechanisms of muscles. Any feeling of happiness, alertness or attention may increase the gamma motor system activity. Unhappiness, drowsiness or lack of attention may decrease the activity in these fibers (Åstrand and Rodahl, 1970).

Although the best way to improve the muscular strength and physical condition of young and middle-aged people is to increase gradually the amount of exercise performed or the speed at which it is performed, exercise as a therapeutic or prophylactic modality for older people must be approached more systematically and cautiously. Therapeutic exercise must be prescribed according to age, sex, physical fitness level, intensity, duration, frequency and variety. In general, it is safe for older people with or without heart disease to start simply with nontaxing mobility exercises to limber up their muscles and joints. Static stretching exercises and calisthenics to improve muscular strength, endurance and flexibility can be safely performed by most reasonably healthy people even up to 79 years of age, provided they are done with slow cadences. Such exercise can generally be prescribed without subjecting the patient to ergometric testing. Later, additional exercises can be added as necessary and practical to improve cardiovascular fitness and muscle strength (deVries, 1974).

Walking is undoubtedly the safest and best exercise for most ambulatory patients with or without heart disease. It is sometimes helpful to know that men 60-65 years of age tend to walk with a significantly shorter step and stride length, and wider foot angle than younger men. There is also a progressive decrease in cadence in subjects between 40-65 years of age (Murray et al., 1964). Patients may be instructed to walk a few blocks daily at a prescribed rate and gradually increase the distance and rate so that in several months they can walk four miles an hour if no untoward effects are observed in heart rate, blood pressure, shortness of breath, chest pain or other adverse cardiovascular signs.

Running-jogging exercise, brisk walking, hiking, bicycling and swimming, which use the major muscles of the body, exert much greater demands on the cardiovascular system and should be carefully monitored with regard to heart rate. It is preferable to assess with reasonable accuracy the older patient's maximal work capacity during submaximal work stress, using a bicycle ergometer, or treadmill, as discussed in Chapter 11. Such testing should be done prior to writing the exercise prescription. For the elderly person, a bicycle calibrated for ergometric testing is easier than a treadmill. During such testing, the blood pressure, heart rate and serial electrocardiograms should be taken every minute to determine changes in contour or rhythm. The development of shortness of breath, chest pain, dizziness, prolonged fatigue, a heart rate over 120 beats per minute or a systolic or diastolic blood pressure rise of more than 20 and 10 mm Hg respectively suggests that the exercise may be too strenuous and should be stopped. The development of ST-T wave depression and inversion of T-waves, widening of QRS complex or cardiac arrhythmias should also terminate the testing procedure. A significant drop in blood pressure or other untoward complaints are also warning signals to reduce the amount of exercise or to stop it.

Once these testing results have been achieved, the exercise can be prescribed with the help of appropriate equivalent activity charts.

Physical exercise should also be used to strengthen the muscles that keep and support the spine in normal condition and alignment. Well-developed abdominal muscles protect and prevent damage to the spinal cord. Walking or running upstairs or uphill develops leg and trunk muscles and helps protect the back against injury. Stretching and limbering up exercises improve joint movements, counteract stiffness and improve metabolism of the joint cartilages. All joints should be gently moved every day without force as far as they will go. A prolonged static load on a joint compromises the articular cartilage while movement in the joint increases thickness of the cartilage and facilitates exchange of nutriments.

Better physical fitness also appears to reduce the risk of death from cardiovascular disease, such risk of death being two or three times greater in inactive persons than in active people. The probability of surviving the first heart attack is also two or three times greater in physically active men than in inactive men.

Aquatic Exercise

The physiological effects of exercise in water are similar to those on dry land. The blood supply to the working muscle increases, heat is evoked during muscular contraction and muscle temperature rises. The increased muscle metabolism raises the demand for oxygen and more carbon dioxide is released.

Aquatic exercises utilizing the resistance and bouyancy of water enable many people to move muscles and joints in a nontaxing way that may be impossible for them to move out of the water. The body is 22 times lighter in the water and many exercises can be done with less effort in water. Turbulence permits adjustable resistance and the amount of work and overload of an exercise can be augmented by increasing the speed at which the movement is done, turbulence and resistance increasing with the speed of the movement in the water.

Calisthenics in water stimulate circulation, strengthen muscles and aid flexibility and balance. They are excellent as an initial conditioning program to help the individual build up sufficient physical strength and fitness in order to progress later to the more vigorous effort necessary to improve cardiovascular fitness. Older people performing these exercises in a group setting often get more enjoyment out of such exercise and are more motivated to continue their exercising efforts. Such exercises are particularly good for out-of-condition people to help limber up their muscles, improve joint action and circulation, relieve fatigue and stress, and facilitate relaxation.

Swimming and other water sport exercises involve many muscle groups and can easily be graded for progressive conditioning. Many handicapped individuals unable to move easily on dry land become more mobile and relaxed in the pool where the warmth of the water relieves pain and muscle spasm and induces greater relaxation. With relief of pain, the elderly patient can move in greater comfort and increase his range of motion. Elderly patients performing exercise in pools should be cautioned to hold on to ladders or other objects when they get in or out of the pool. A hypertensive patient should be advised to enter the pool slowly in order to minimize a momentary rise in blood pressure, which may occur as he enters the pool. In the water, his blood pressure may fall, falling still more when he rests afterwards. Such patients should be advised to get out of the water slowly and to hold on to a ladder since they may feel giddy or faint upon assuming an upright position or getting out of the pool too quickly.

CONCLUSION

Lack of adequate exercise and the neuromuscular deterioration resulting from the aging process and hypokinetic disorders are the two major causes of poor physical condition in people over the age of 50 without disease. Properly supervised and prescribed therapeutic physical exercises on land or in water can restore and improve the general physical condition of such people by developing in them better muscular endurance and cardiovascular fitness, improved vigor and enhanced neuromuscular coordination and skills. Walking, running-jogging exercises, hiking, bicycling and swimming, utilizing the major muscles of the body, are the most beneficial. Aquatic exercises, making use of the resistance and buoyancy of the water, enable many elderly people to move muscles and joints in a nontaxing way that is impossible out of water.

Physical activity and exercise at all ages is essential to preserve the health of aging people and to retard the changes produced by the aging process and disuse as people grow old. Before any exercise is prescribed, a complete medical checkup should be the cornerstone of any program to improve physical fitness in people over the age of 50. Persons with diminished visual and auditory perception should be provided with proper glasses and hearing aids to improve their sensory deficits.

REFERENCES

Astrand, P.-O. and Rodahl, K. (1970) *Textbook of Work Physiology,* Chapter 4, McGraw-Hill Book Co., New York.

Birren, J.E., Imus, H.A., and Windle, W.F., (Eds.) (1959) *The Process of Aging on the Nervous System*, Charles C Thomas, Springfield, p. 144.

Brody, H. (1970) In *Interdisciplinary Topics in Gerontology*, Vol. 7 (H.T. Blumenthal, ed.), S. Karger, New York, p. 9.

de Vries, H.A. (1966) *Physiology of Exercise for Physical Education and Athletics*, William C. Brown, Dubuque.

de Vries, H.A. (1974) *Vigor Regained*, Prentice-Hall, Englewood Cliffs.

Harris, R. (1970) *The Management of Geriatric Cardiovascular Disease*, J.B. Lippincott Company, Philadelphia.

Harris, R. (1974) *NY State J Med* 74, 972.

Harris, R. (1975) In *Physical Exercise & Activity for the Aging* (U. Simri, ed.), Proceedings of an International Seminar, Wingate Institute for Physical Education and Sport, Wingate, Israel.

Kreitler, H., and Kreitler, S.H. (1970) In *Medicine and Sport, Vol. 4: Physical Activity and Aging* (D. Brunner and E. Jokl, eds.), Karger, Basel, p. 302.

Murray, M.P., Drought, A.B., and Kory, R.C. (1964) *J Bone Joint Surg* 46-A:335.

Shock, N.W. and Norris, A.H. (1970) In *Medicine and Sport, Vol. 4: Physical Activity and Aging* (D. Brunner and E. Jokl, eds.), Karger, Basel, p. 92.

Wyrick-Spirduso, W. (1975) (in preparation).

History of Exercises for the Elderly

Herman L. Kamenetz, M.D.

INTRODUCTION

The history of exercise has been written many times from various perspectives but with little emphasis on exercise for older people. The present chapter may well be the first such attempt to depict the changing fads and fashions in exercise for the elderly over the centuries.

Certainly, greater suppleness of muscles, better circulation in the extremities, increased amplitude in pulmonary ventilation, greater freedom in motion and a feeling of well-being are experiences an older person appreciates just as much as a younger one, possibly even more as these qualities may have gradually decreased over the years.

But it was probably always an old-fashioned philosophical attitude that taught every person's individual concern was to do what he thought was good for himself. Only in the 20th century did all this change, and much more so in the second half. But, then, there were never before 20 million Americans over 65 years, a full 10 percent of the United States' population. In this age of senior citizens and White House Conferences on Aging, of Medicare and Golden Age Clubs, of gray power and gerontology, exercise for the elderly has come of age and has at last been duly acknowledged a place in its own right in the medical armamentarium.

ANCIENT CHINA

In ancient China, exercises, although not necessarily reserved for older people, were probably practiced by them. These exercises might represent the oldest known, dating back to mythical times in which hygienic practices were inseparable from religious precepts. When it became known to French Jesuits in the 18th century, the system was being taught by Chinese Taoist bonzes. Returning from Peking, the missionaries Father Amiot and others reported on the Kung Fu in the fourth volume of their *Memoirs on the History, Arts, Sciences and Customs of China* (1776-1789).

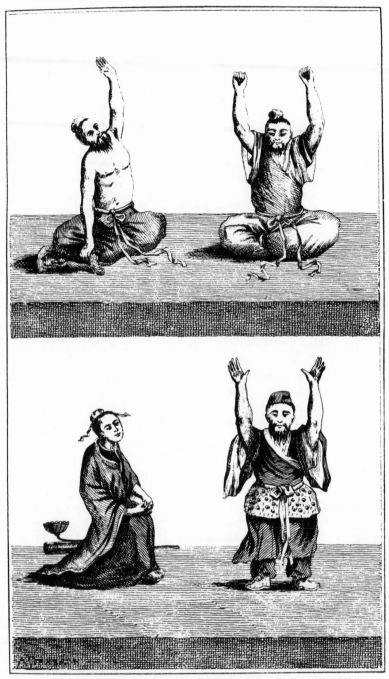

Fig. 1.   Exercises from the Kung Fu system. After Amiot *et al.*, vol. 4, 1779.
(Courtesy of National Library of Medicine, Bethesda, Maryland.)

The Kung Fu consisted of postures, breathing and other exercises with apparently little motion. According to the Chinese priests the system was practiced centuries before the Christian era. Some authors believe the Kung Fu to be even more ancient. Although it was reported that the system was elaborated by disciples of Lao-tzu, the philosopher and founder of Taoism who lived in the sixth century B.C., its age is indeed difficult to establish.

These postures and exercises were transmitted over the centuries by priests. Their paucity of motion and their ritualistic nature lead us to assume that they were practiced as much by the old as by the young. The 18th century report on the Kung Fu, consisting of 11 pages, includes 20 figures which, primitive as they be, clearly show the classic postures and motions demonstrated by older persons (Fig. 1).

The most important book of medicine in ancient China is probably the *Nei Ching*, long attributed to Huang-Ti, the Yellow Emperor (Veith, 1949), who is assumed to have died in 2598 B.C. But, as in the Kung Fu, there is much controversy about the date. To ascribe a work to Huang-Ti is a matter of honoring the Emperor and not necessarily indicating its authorship or age (Kamenetz, 1960). Pollak (1968) considers it a well-established fact that the *Huang-Ti Nei Ching* (The Book of Medicine of the Yellow Emperor) was written by unknown authors in the first century B.C. He believes that Huang-Ti lived sometime between 2200 and 1080 B.C., and that it was one of the emperor's teachers, the legendary Ch'ih Sung-tzu, who founded medical gymnastics. His system, used prophylactically and for the treatment of diseases, may well have been related to Kung Fu. It included breathing exercises, rubbing the abdomen, tapping the thorax and motion of all segments of the body, including the eyes, mouth and tongue.

From these beginnings may have developed the system of Tai Chi Chuan, sometimes translated as shadow-boxing, believed to have been founded by Chang Sen-Feng, a philosopher who lived during the Sung Dynasty (960-1279). Characterized by slow, circular motions of all segments of the body, it is admirably fitted for the elderly and can be seen practiced by old men in the streets of present-day China.

ANCIENT GREECE

In the early days of Greece, as in other ancient cultures, procedures for health and recovery from disease were directed by priests. These priest-physicians were attached to asclepia or temples of healing, which are the predecessors of hospitals. Asclepia were dedicated to Asklepios (later to become Aesculapius in Rome), the god of medicine and son of Apollo. Hygienic exercises were part of the regimen and were prescribed for individuals of all ages. These exercises were different from those practiced by the younger generations as part of their education, their games, their preparation for war and athletic competition. The Olympian games date back to 776 B.C.

Herodicus, born in 480 B.C. and tutor of Hippocrates, was the first to establish medical gymnastics, separating it from the athletic and the military (Cocchi, 1824). His *Ars Gymnastica*, an elaborate system of exercises, drew much criticism for being too strenuous. Plato at times praised him (Cocchi, 1824) and at other times criticized him. His criticism was, however, also directed against his successes. Wrote Hufeland: "To such an extent did he carry his ideas that he compelled his patients to exercise and to have their bodies rubbed, and by this method he had the good fortune to lengthen for several years the lives of so many enfeebled persons that Plato reproached him for protracting that existence of which they would have less and less enjoyment" (Graham, 1902).

Although Hippocrates, Herodicus' most famous disciple, also criticized his master for the physical overexertion he forced upon his patients, there are many instances throughout the books ascribed to the Father of Medicine in which exercises are recommended. "Speaking generally, all parts of the body, which have a function, if used in moderation and exercised in labours to which each is accustomed, become thereby healthy and well-developed, and age slowly; but if unused and left idle, they become liable to disease, defective in growth, and age quickly" (Hippocrates, Withington, trans., 1927).

The Greek philosophers all recognized gymnastics as a means to preserve health. Socrates (470-399 B.C.) in the words of Montaigne two thousand years later (after Xenophon, Banquet II), "old as he was, found time to make himself taught dancing and playing upon instruments and thought it time well spent" (Montaigne). Plato (427?-347 B.C.), his disciple, and the latter's disciple, Aristotle (384-322 B.C.), saw great value in temperate exercises as conducive to good health. Mendez, a physician of the 16th century, quoted Aristotle's views from the eighth book of *Ethics*, the fourth book of *Metaphysics*, and his *Categories* (Mendez, 1553).

ANCIENT ROME

Roman medicine was mostly practiced by Greek physicians. Outstanding among them was Asclepiades of Bithynia (124-56 B.C.). The most famous physician since Hippocrates and called by some the "Hippocrates of chronic disease" (Guthrie, 1958), Asclepiades disagreed in many ways with the Father of Medicine. He maintained that nature can do not only good but also harm and, to combat the harm, he recommended diet, massage, bathing and exercise. Because of his insistence that the physician study and treat chronic disease, Major (1954) described Asclepiades as the Father of Geriatrics. Except for a few extant fragments, we know Asclepiades only through other writers. From Pliny we know that walking was among the rules for preserving health, together with the judicious use of food and wine, as recommended by Asclepiades (1955) in his book *On Common Aids*. This and other exercises, which he always prescribed in moderation, might well have been practiced by his patients of advanced age.

But what these must have particularly enjoyed was a therapy which seems admirably fitting for the aged — be they healthy or weak — and which became very fashionable under Asclepiades. First known under the Greek term *aiora* (balancing), later called gestation in Rome, from the Latin *gestare* (to carry), this therapy consisted in the transportation of the individual in a sedan chair, a litter, a carriage, on horseback or in a boat. Depending upon the type and speed of the vehicle, the nature of the road or the motion of the water, various degrees of vibration or

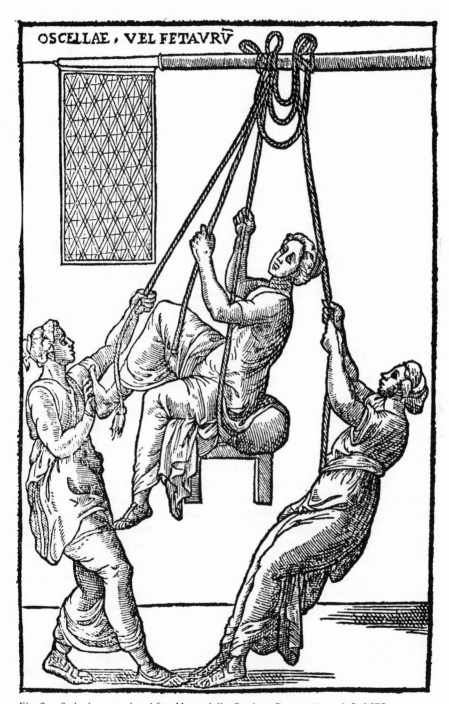

Fig. 2.   Swinging exercise. After Mercurialis, *De Arte Gymnastica*, ed. 2, 1573.

shaking were achieved with the expectation of beneficial effects on physical and mental disturbances.

An 18th century writer (Gumpert, 1794), having collected fragments concerning Asclepiades, has the following to say about therapeutic transportation:

> "Of all the exercises which have been devised for the treatment of diseases, assuredly the easiest, and by far the most convenient, is transportation, which the patient can use, even if he is so infirm that he cannot move himself. He can be busy in the fields, outdoors, enjoy the sunshine, be restored by fresh air: he can be moved in a quiet and pleasant way, as long as he pleases.

> " 'But several kinds of transportation are available: which are in accordance both with the strength and with the means of the patient, that they may not be too fatiguing for the weakest nor too expensive for the lowly. The gentlest of transportations is by boat, either in harbor or on a river: more strenuous in a ship on the deep sea, or by litter or bench: rougher by vehicle. And these themselves can be lessened and mitigated.' Most physicians think transportation is not to be employed except in the remission of fever, and in terminal disease. But Asclepiades says it should be used also in recent and severe and burning fever, and especially for dispelling it.

> "The effect which transportation exerts on the body is this, that the passages are made more open. Doubtless fever arises, according to Asclepiades, from obstruction of the pores and impeded removal of the corpuscles. Therefore, in order to treat it, he devised remedies which should dissolve the stagnations and restore the interrupted flow of corpuscles; and to this end especially he designated transportation, which, by its gentle, passive motion removes obstructions, impels the lagging corpuscles, and restores their removal. Hence we can also understand what it is, moved by which Asclepiades praised transportation in recent and severe fever, and especially in dispelling burning fever."

A variation of therapeutic transportation was hanging beds in which the patient was gently balanced. Asclepiades is credited with their invention but there is no precise information about this device. Gumpert (1794), who found fragmentary descriptions in Celsus, Pliny and Mercurialis (1569) on what he calls hanging couches (Fig. 2), wrote this:

> "Mercurialis thinks that these were attached at their four corners by ropes to the roofs of beds in such a way that they are raised a little from the ground, as if they seemed to be hanging in the air. Celsus informs us of the twofold way of using them: the couch ought either to be suspended and moved, or at least a small rope placed under one foot of the bed, and so the couch moved this way and that by hand.

> "The effect, for the sake of which Asclepiades used hanging couches, was no other than what we have already seen derive from transportation. Hence Pliny says: he also devised other comforts by also suspending couches, by whose swaying he either mitigated diseases or allured sleep."

Such passive exercise was no doubt particularly prescribed for the weak and the old and advocated over many centuries, even as late as the end of the eighteenth century (Tissot, 1780). It is often mentioned in medical writings of ancient Rome as an important part of the metasyncritic treatment of the Methodist school of medicine, founded by Asclepiades (Aurelianus, 1950).

Celsus, born about 25 B.C., was probably not a physician but he wrote an important medical treatise, *De Medicina*, and advocated exercise as a hygienic measure.

The Roman preoccupation with old age was quite evident, and discussions on means to reach it and prolong life are found in many places. Likewise it was generally believed that physical exercise is one of the means to prepare for old age. Yet, it seemed understood that such preparation is restricted to the younger years. Except for modern times, discourses on exercises ignored old age, and those on old age did not mention exercise.

Cicero's speech *De Senectute* (On Old Age), completed in 44 A.D. at the age of 62, a year before his death, provides a good harvest for our purpose by a man who knew Asclepiades and who composed his numerous speeches while walking, dictating to his secretaries who had to walk along with him (Licht, 1961). He asserts that "it is possible for a man by exercise and self-control (*exercitatio et temperantia*), even in old age, to preserve some of his original vigour." Exercise in moderation as a means to fight against old age is again mentioned when he recommends to his young friends (XI. 36) "to adopt a regimen of health, to practice moderate exercise (*utendum exercitationibus modicis*)." He speaks of the possibility of continued physical labor into a high age (XVII. 60), giving the example of a Valerius Corvinus who, "after passing the ordinary span of life, lived on his farm and cultivated it and continued his pursuit of agriculture to his hundredth year." Elsewhere (XVI.56), he exclaims: "Well, then, was there cause to pity the old age of these men who delighted in the cultivation of the soil?" But to this tilling of a farm, so proper for the elderly, Cicero adds only sedentary games which markedly contrast with the sports of younger generations (XVI. 58): "Let others, then, have their weapons, their horses and their spears, their fencing-foils, and games of ball, their swimming contests and foot-races, and out of many sports leave us old fellows our dice and knuckle-bones. Or take away the dice-box, too, if you will, since old age can be happy without it" (Cicero, Falconer, trans., 1964).

Martial (c.40 - c.104 A.D.) tells us much about the customs of his times when he advises: *"Folle decet pueros ludere, folle senes"* ("It is befitting the old as well as the young to play the follis," a little air-filled ball).

Antyllus, as early as the second century, spoke out against too much bedrest, as we learn from Oribasius (326-403 A.D.) who 200 years later preserved much of previous writings. Antyllus discriminated between the acutely and the chronically ill and allowed the latter to stay in bed only during exacerbations. "During the intervals nothing should prevent them from moving about, because they require movement and varied stimuli" (Oribasius, Bussemaker and Daremberg, trans., 1851-1876).

Galen (130-200 A.D.), the most famous of all physicians in Rome and, after Hippocrates, the outstanding authority for more than a millenium, wrote about 500 books, possibly 16 on exercise and massage (Jüthner, 1909). In the few extant fragments he, like many others, decried the exaggerations of exercises and preached principles of well-fitting exercises for the old. "The best exercises of all are those which can not only train the body but also delight the mind. . . . So, not to incur danger would be the best qualification of all exercises taken for the benefit of the body" (Licht, 1961).

Flavius Philostratos, who lived about 250 A.D., wrote a treatise on gymnastics which was discovered in the 19th century and translated in 1858 by Daremberg into French. The best information about Philostratos and a good picture of exercise in the Greco-Roman civilization are given in Jüthner's book (1909) on Philostratos.

Much of the medical knowledge of ancient Rome has been preserved only in compilation, either by encyclopedists such as Celsus or by other physicians. Most authors accepted exercises in the medical armamentarium, notwithstanding differences in their medical opinions.

Caelius Aurelianus, who lived in the fifth century A.D., like Antyllus, separated acute and chronic conditions by presenting his compilations in two books, *On Acute Diseases* and *On Chronic Diseases*, frequently mentioning exercise. He was the last of the great compilers of the Roman period. The medical writings of the following centuries only reflect, if not flatly repeat, what was previously said by the great physicians in Greece and Rome, and particularly by Galen. For more than a millenium Galen's word was law and medicine stood still.

MIDDLE AGES

During the Middle Ages, physical fitness and care of the body were neglected. Possibly, because hygienic practices in the fashion of the day were intertwined with heathenism, or public spectacles reminded people of the tragedies of early Christendom, or physical education of the young was practiced — at some time at least — in the nude, as indicated by the term gymnastics (the training took place in gymnasia), all physical culture fell in disrepute, and even physical well-being was less appreciated with the development of Christianity. However, physical work became part of the monastic life in the Order of Saint Benedict, founded in 529 A.D. (Joseph, 1949).

Arabic writings by Syrian, Persian, Jewish and Christian physicians living between the present Near East and France and representing Arabic medicine, sparsely bridge the gap of a millenium between the period of medical culture in Greece, Rome and Alexandria, and the Renaissance of medicine.

One of the earlier physicians of this period (850-950 A.D.) was Isaac Judaeus, a Jew born in Egypt who said "Nothing is more harmful to the regulation of health than idleness," as Licht (1961) found in Gazius (1491).

Avicenna (980-1037 A.D.), the most famous of the Arabian physicians and called the Prince of Physicians, used exercises and adapted them to the age of the person, healthy or sick.

Maimonides (1135-1204 A.D.), the foremost Jewish philosopher and physician of the Middle Ages, complained about the little recognition exercise had in his era: "One does not consider exercise, though it is the main principle in keeping one's health and in the repulsion of most illnesses" (Maimonides, Gordon, trans., 1958).

Referring specifically to the elderly, he recommends in *Regimen Sanitatis V*, Chapters 17 and 18, ". . .massage with oil in the morning, after sleep, followed by walk or slow riding." And again: "Elderly people require that their bodies move, because the constitution of their bodies needs warmth. No single elderly person should rest and repose without having done some exercise. On the other hand, he does not need to do strenuous exercise, because exertional athletics cools [body] warmth that is weak, and extinguishes it" (Maimonides, Rosner and Muntner, trans., 1970-1971).

What was known in medicine by Galen's time was preserved to a large extent over several centuries, either in the original or in translations. The hygienic value of exercise is mentioned twice in the *Regimen Sanitatis Salernitanum* "the first medieval health book and the only expression of Greek medical tradition in the early Middle Ages" (Joseph, 1949).

RENAISSANCE

With the rediscovery of all things Greek and Roman, the educative, hygienic and therapeutic values of exercise surged again to the fore. With the invention of the printing press in the middle of the 15th century the Greek and Latin classics, hidden and forgotten in libraries for centuries, started to reappear, stimulating philosophers, educators and physicians among many others to recognize the benefits of exercise.

Throughout the entire history of therapeutic exercise, massage or what might be called transportation or traveling (the gestation of Roman times) has been referred to as passive exercise or passive gymnastics. In many ancient writings (e.g. Galen) and others as recently as the 19th century (e.g. Ling), massage is discussed as a passive form of exercise. Occasionally a clear distinction is made between the two.

Leone Battista Alberti (1404-1472), an architect and hygienist, wrote an education work, *Of the Family*, in which he calls special attention to physical exercise even in early infancy and as becoming still more important with increasing age (Joseph, 1949).

Various games were played in those days including medieval soccer, a game depicted in a fresco by Giovanni Stradano (1536-1605) in the Palazzo Vecchio of Florence (Joseph, 1949). The players of this game, called Florentine football or Calcio, may have included some between the ages of 18 and 45, according to a detailed description in 1688 (Bardi, 1902).

Of particular fame among the enthusiastic renovators of ancient Greece and Rome are Gazius and Champier. Antonius Gazius of Padua (c1449-1528) published his *Florida Corona* (1491), a "crown of flowers" gathered from Hippocrates, Galen and other ancient writings. Symphorien Champier (1472-c1539), a French physician, published *Rosa Gallica* 21 years later (1512). Both wrote about the hygienic virtue of exercise but without always clearly distinguishing between active and passive movements.

This period also saw the beginning of a movement destined to flower in our own age. *Gerentocomia*, the first book on geriatrics, was published in 1489, more than four centuries before the term was coined, by Gabriele Zerbi (c1450-1505), professor of philosophy at Padua and later professor of medicine at Rome (Zeman, 1944; Zerbi, 1489).

SIXTEENTH CENTURY

The earliest printed book on exercise written by a physician was published in 1553 in Seville, Spain, and translated into English in 1960. In this *Book of Bodily Exercise*, Christobal Mendez, in contrast to many of his contemporaries, neither wrote in Latin nor restricted himself to previous writers. He drew much from his own information and experience.

Like Aristotle whom he quotes in his Prologue, he writes: "Only exercise (which is movement) is an easy way to preserve health. It is the most profitable and includes and replaces all other treatment." Two types of exercise range particularly high in Mendez' esteem: walking and ball playing. ". . . I do not believe there is a lady who is not in a position to close the door of a room and to stroll for two hours before meals in one of those halls. I swear that although your ladyships pass your lives without doing this, you could live longer and better without troubles by doing so." And elsewhere: "In walking all the animal faculties are exercised." Speaking of ball playing he says that ". . . it has the proper conditions required of exercise," and ". . . there are many benefits in the ball game . . . ."

Mendez specified exercise for each of the six ages. "The fifth age is old age, which is past forty or more years, and in this one the proper exercise is to ride a mule or to walk for a while on foot. If one had the habit of doing [a more strenuous exercise which] preserved his health well, it is good to keep doing it in moderation. . . . Furthermore men very well regulated in adolescence and youth, in becoming old benefit from very few exercises in keeping themselves healthy. The proper exercise for this and the sixth age, which is decrepitude from seventy years on, is gentle movement and use of temperance in everything he has been used to. . . . Also it is good to rock old men very gently in cradles because as they return to the age of children we have to give them the same kind of exercise."

Sixteen years later, in 1569, another physician published a book on exercise, which was to remain the most important work on the subject for centuries to come. In *The Art of Gymnastics among the Ancients*, a treatise of 308 pages in quarto, written in Latin and beautifully illustrated, Hieronymus Mercurialis (1530-1606), professor of medicine at Padua, Bologna and Pisa, presented a compilation of the subject since Hippocrates' times, listing not less than 96 authors (Kilgour, 1960). Mercurialis discussed the medical value of exercises, sports and games, and established guidelines for their indications and contraindications which have served as the basis for medical gymnastics for a long time thereafter. He recommended exercise for "every period of our existence, from the beginning unto the end."

His advice sounded very different from that of Girolamo Cardanus, his predecessor at the University of Padua (1501-1576). Although practicing gymnastics himself daily, Cardanus did not recommend them to older men (Cardanus, 1562).

"With the ancients, as it should be with ourselves," says Mercurialis in Blundell's words (1864), "age was obviously held to be a relative thing. . . . Men of mature years in those times exercised to 'ward off old age'." He preaches "moderation in all things, by which human life is prolonged," recommending walking and dancing that could "strengthen the weak bodies of boys, women and old men," and ball games of various types, some played with a large ball, others with a small one, but good for the health of the old and the young.

It is regrettable that Mercurialis does not tell us more about a few games, particularly the troque, named after the instrument used in this game. Says he: "The troque was more among slack exercises, suitable rather for old than young persons and, affecting gently the arms and legs, was more serviceable to those who were not able to join in the greater exercises."

Persons who lead a sedentary life urgently need gymnastics, said Mercurialis, and older persons should have special exercises (Joseph, 1949). As many before him, and with special reference to Galen, he extols the virtues of walking, the most universal of all exercises, recommending slow walking even to the weak and to sickly old men (Blundell, 1864).

Among the exercises discussed by Mercurialis were loud reading and speaking (vociferation), laughing, weeping and holding the breath. Such and similar vocal and respiratory exercises had been practiced for health reasons in ancient India and China and in Greco-Roman times. Revived during the Renaissance, they waxed and waned in importance throughout history and were often mentioned in relation to health during the 16th century (Finney, 1968). The French physician, André du Laurens, in his discussion *Of Old Age* says that "exercise preserveth our youthfulnes long and many yeares," and mentions vocal exercise for "old folke" (1599).

SEVENTEENTH CENTURY

Mercurialis established the basis for medical gymnastics and his masterpiece, the *Gymnastic Art*, soon became widely known in many lands. New editions were issued in the 17th century and reprinted as late as 1672 in Amsterdam. Many authors referred to him, with or without due credit, among them Richard Mulcaster, a London headmaster, who in 1581 borrowed extensively from him without attribution (Finney, 1968), and Blundell (1864), a London physician, who almost three centuries later translated "the whole text of Mercurialis", simplifying the wordy Latin of the sixteenth century but adding his own observations and experience without always clearly distinguishing between the old and the new.

One of Mercurialis' commentators during his lifetime (he died in 1606) was Marsilius Cagnatus in Verona (1605). In the second book of his *Preservation of Health*, he "insisted that the middle-aged particularly need regular exercises because in this period many ailments may be latent, which appear later and shorten life. On the other hand, old age requires and desires repose" (Joseph, 1949). Cagnatus included laughing and weeping among exercises, as did many others at the threshold of the seventeenth century.

Joseph Duchesne, also called Quercetanus (1544-1609), court physician to Henry IV of France, recommended singing to old men, together with reading, playing instrumental music and other light exercises among which he included card-playing. For old persons who were formerly accustomed to more strenuous exercises he particularly recommended walking (Duchesne, 1648).

The English philosopher Thomas Hobbes (1588-1679), Francis Bacon's most famous disciple, also practiced vocal exercises in the mid 17th century. As told by Aubrey (1957): "...he sang aloud (not that he had a very good voice) but for his health's Sake: he did beleeve it did his Lunges good, and conduced much to prolong his life." He lived to the age of 91.

In the course of the century, however, "ancient ideas of the value of vocal and respiratory exercises for the preservation of health, which had persisted throughout the Renaissance, gradually receded" (Finney, 1971). While misunderstood "physiology", mostly under the influence of the iatromechanical school, was one reason for this rejection (Finney, 1971), this same school of thought and the unprecedented interest and progress in physiology led to a general gain in the acceptance of medical gymnastics.

Numerous books of the 17th century document the growing scientific understanding of physiologic functions. Many are characteristically entitled "On the motion of...", from Fabricio d'Acquapendente's *De Motu Animalium* in 1614, studying animals to better understand human anatomy; to William Harvey's *De Motu Cordis* in 1628, exposing the circulation of the blood; to Borelli's *De Motu Animalium* in 1680, discussing muscle mechanics in the doctrine of iatrophysicists.

While there was great controversy between the iatrophysical (or iatromechanical) and the iatrochemical schools, advances achieved during this period did much to establish a solid foundation for medical gymnastics. Support came from still another direction. Strongly reacting against both prevailing schools, Thomas Sydenham (1624-1689), like Hippocrates, believed in the healing power of nature and warmly advocated exercise to help nature. His strong influence on many of his contemporaries continued into the following century. Many of the most famous physicians rallied to his views. So great was his fame that he was called the "English Hippocrates", and Herman Boerhaave, one of his most famous followers, the "Dutch Sydenham".

EIGHTEENTH CENTURY

This century, characterized by Garrison (1960) as the "age of theories and systems," saw important contributions to the fields of exercise and aging. Francis Fuller, one of Sydenham's followers, published his *Medicina Gymnastica* in 1705, a popular work which went through nine editions and was translated into German.

Outstanding in the early 1700s was Friedrich Hoffmann (1660-1742) who, much influenced by Borelli's school, contributed a great deal to establish a solid foundation for medical gymnastics. In the first of his 12 *Dissertationes Physico-Medicae*, on longevity, published in 1708, he declared mental and bodily exercises to be among the most reliable means to assure a long life without invalidism. He emphasized the importance of regular active exercises. In the sixth dissertation, entitled "On movement considered as the best medicine for the body", he wrote: "Old persons must neither rest all the time, nor do heavy physical activities; moderate movements suffice for their maintenance, comparable to a light breeze maintaining a small flame. We must always pay attention to the degree of their strength. The weakest will be contented with a promenade by litter or carriage. The stronger will do good with a moderate walk. We must always take into consideration the influence of the habit" (Hoffmann, 1708).

Hoffmann's classification of occupational movements as exercise deserves, as Licht (1961) points out, our particular attention. "We shall place among the exercises the occupational movements of workers and farmers — such work as threshing wheat, cutting wood, harvesting and other agricultural tasks. The strength and good health which peasants enjoy prove to us how much these occupations contribute to prolong life and to protect health."

Similar to Hoffmann in Germany, Nicolas Andry in France (1658-1742) spoke highly of exercise. In 1723, when he was dean of the Paris school of medicine, he presented an essay on the value of moderate exercise in the preservation of health. He described walking as an example of moderate exercise recommended to all, but of particular value in two periods of life, childhood and old age.*

So fond was Andry of this thesis that he presented it again 18 years later, in 1741. In the same year he gave a new name to an old specialty in his book, *Orthopedics or the Art to Prevent and Correct Deformities in Children*, in which he recognized exercise as the best means to prepare children for a healthier and longer life. He was 83 when the book was published.

Another outstanding contribution to medical literature and another "first", this time addressed directly to old age, was published a few years earlier. The author, Sir John Floyer (1649-1734), had a long life as a practicing physician behind him over which he had acquired a great reputation as a proponent of hydrotherapy when he published, at the age of 74 or 75, the first book in English on geriatrics, *Medicina Gerocomica* (Floyer, 1724; Neuburger, 1948). He was only the first in a long line of physicians interested in the care of the old, a new field which developed during the 18th century primarily in Great Britain before spreading to other countries.

In the same city and in the same year (London, 1724), George Cheyne of Aberdeen (1671-1743) published and saw three printings of his *Essay on Health and Long Life*. (By the end of the following year seven editions had appeared.) He had a personal interest in the subject; at one time his weight was 445 pounds and he suffered from great shortness of breath. For this he recommended talking much and aloud (Major, 1954). But "of all the exercises that are, or may be used for health, walking is the most natural" (Licht, 1961).

This was also the opinion of Giuseppe Nenci, professor of medicine at Siena, who in his *Discussions on Gymnastics* (1766) advocated light daily exercises for

---

*His explanation was still reminiscent of Galen: walking improved the dissipation of pituite.

older persons and who mentioned walking and riding as the most natural exercises, beneficial to both body and mind.

Benefit to both body and mind ranked high in the scale of values in this century of enlightenment and of the movement for a return to nature. Educators and philosophers agreed with physicians to place walking in fresh air among the first of all physical activities for young and old alike. In America, as told by Betts (1971), Benjamin Franklin (1706-1790) sprinkled his writings with comments on exercise, and Benjamin Rush (1745-1813), who as a young physician had delivered his *Sermon on Exercise*, recommended gentle exercise even in old age (1772).

What Licht (1961) describes as "the first book on therapeutic exercise as we know it today," *Medicinal and Surgical Gymnastics*, by Joseph-Clément Tissot (1747-1826), appeared in 1780.* Tissot wanted exercise to be adapted in type, intensity and duration to the age, sex and temperament of the patient and to the work he was used to doing. Thus, ". . .an old man may support more easily an intense exercise than a man in the midst of maturity not accustomed to motion and work. Yet, . . .old people must exercise less vigorously and for shorter periods than fully developed men." Except for exercises which would be specifically contraindicated in the patient's special case, Tissot has a rule for the elderly person, namely to continue the exercises to which he is accustomed. Indeed, as habit has rendered them easier, they can only be the more agreeable to him, and he would expose himself to harm if all of a sudden he would replace his exercises by others to which he is not used."

Concluding his advices to the elderly for the choice of their physical activities, Tissot writes in delightful terms which seem to span two millennia, reminding us as much of Virgil 18 centuries before as of the ecologists two centuries after the publication of his book: "Finally, physical activities of the old must be gentle and moderate, they must neither fatigue their solids nor stir their blood too much; examples are walking on foot, games, moderate exercises, the pleasures of the country, and above all those of life in the country, surrounding their bodies with the fragrant parts of plants and making them breathe a pure and healthful air."

The 18th century, which had produced such a great number of writings on geriatrics (Müller, 1966) since Hoffmann's concern for a long and healthy life, closed with the book that probably had the greatest impact of all. So great was the interest in the subject that Christoph Wilhelm Hufeland (1762-1836), a German physician, wrote a book on the *Art of Prolonging Life* (1796) when he was in his early 30s. *Macrobiotik*, as the author named it in its later editions, was soon translated in all European languages and Chinese. A book mostly of preventive medicine and general hygiene, Hufeland wrote it for doctors as well as the general public. Much of its advice is still as valuable as it was in 1796. Hufeland lists 10 ways of living that shorten life and 18 ways to lengthen it. Among the latter he mentions a reasonable physical education, physical activities and cultivation of mental and physical forces. He recommends older persons get "sufficient exercise, yet to avoid violent jolting" (Müller, 1966).

---

*By 1797, there were translations in German, Italian and Swedish. An English translation was published in 1964.

NINETEENTH CENTURY

After Floyer's Britain and Hufeland's Germany, France developed as the center in the care and maintenance of the aged. Such interest was most concentrated in two Parisian hospitals, Salpêtrière and Bicêtre. These institutions became the two focal points of geriatric care and research, to which physicians from France and other countries turned for leadership throughout the 19th century and later. One great medical leader at this time was Philippe Pinel (1745-1826), hygienist and psychiatrist. Just as the American colonies fought for their freedom from England and the French proletariat for their freedom from the ruling classes, Pinel fought for the freedom of the insane from their chains. With his fight for a more humane treatment for the mentally sick and the old, Pinel obtained immortal fame. By 1823, the Salpêtrière had no more prison-like rooms and was used exclusively as a hospital; the number of its "patients" was reduced by half from 8000 to 4000 and each had his own bed. It became the hospital for old female patients; old men were hospitalized at Bicêtre. Between 1802 and 1830, 15 doctoral theses were presented at the Paris school of medicine on geriatric subjects (Geller, 1965). Among the important books on geriatrics were those published by Prus in 1840, by Durand-Fardel in 1854, by Charcot in 1867, all in France, and by Canstatt in 1839, in Germany.

If interest for the later years of life came mainly from Paris, appreciation of the value of exercises in the preservation of health came mainly from Stockholm. Although physical exercise had become recognized as an important factor in the promotion and preservation of good health in the previous century and Pinel ordered physical activities for his patients now freed from the emptiness of institutional life, the greatest stimulus to systematized exercise came from Per Henrik Ling (1776-1839), a Swedish fencing master, who deserves credit for most of the fame of Swedish gymnastics and Swedish massage. The creation of the Central Institute of Gymnastics in 1814 by the Swedish government for the teaching of Ling's system can be considered the point of departure of modern kinesitherapy, a term created by Georgii, one of Ling's disciples, and comprising medical gymnastics and massage. From Sweden the idea spread rapidly to all European countries and America.

At the same time, Franz Nachtegall invented a system of gymnastics in neighboring Denmark and Friedrich Ludwig Jahn (1778-1852) developed the method known as *Turnen* in Germany. Although these systems were aimed mostly at youth, the movement extended to all ages. Jahn's method was practiced for its health benefits by many old men in many a *Turnverein* founded by German immigrants in the United States.

Among the followers of Ling were two American physicians, the brothers George and Charles Taylor. Each published a book on the *Swedish movement-cure*. The first one with 896 pages in 1860 by George Taylor saw several editions and was followed by more books, all on the same subject. George also invented therapeutic devices for the American public, similar to those that made Gustav Zander, a Swedish physician, famous. These instruments, replacing physical therapists, were featured in numerous Zander institutes in Europe and America. They can still be seen, albeit in some modified forms, in many physical therapy departments and health centers.

Exercises were also practiced in conjunction with hydrotherapy, a method used by mature and elderly people throughout the centuries for the cure and prevention of disease. Gerontologists such as Floyer and Hufeland extolled the wholesome virtues of water used externally, and under the influence of lay healers, notably the Silesian peasant Vinzenz Priessnitz and the Bavarian priest Sebastian Kneipp, hydropathic establishments flourished in the United States in the 19th century. They bloomed together with American spas particularly during the second and third quarters, and faded with them toward the end of the century.

Among the numerous other popular activities at spas that appealed to the older generation were dancing and promenades in well-kept parks. In 1884 White Sulphur Springs in Virginia opened the first golf course in the United States to provide outstanding physical exercise for people of any age. Ten years later, this queen of the Virginia springs closed her doors (Reniers, 1941). In many spas, exercise was part of the water-cure, and although most visitors cared less about the water than about the social life, many older people relied upon the waters for their health.

Older persons were also the most enthusiastic followers of certain health apostles who presented exercise as one of the means to preserve youth or prolong life. We will name only two, both physicians. Outstanding in the first half of the 19th century was Sylvester Graham (1794-1851). In addition to Graham flour, Graham bread, Graham crackers and Graham boarding houses, Dr. Graham advocated exercise as exhilarating, horseback riding to forestall pulmonary consumption and regular activity to deter infirmity in old age (1839). Unfortunately Graham could not follow the advice given in his *Graham Journal of Health and Longevity* and in his *Lectures on the Science of Human Life*, for he died at the age of 57.

A few months later John Harvey Kellogg (1852-1943) was born. A proponent of similar principles of healthy living among which exercises played a major role, he became physician-in-chief of the Battle Creek Sanitarium in 1876. Stimulated by a visit to the Zander Institute in Stockholm, he simplified gymnastics for the patient by mechanotherapy, inventing many apparatuses himself. As recounted by Schwarz (1970), Kellogg at the age of 70 in the early 1920s prepared physical fitness exercises for a company and was able to perform them repeatedly at a good pace himself, after having exhausted his secretary. A shining example of successful aging and undefatigability, he was 91 when he died.

Although exercise was accepted as a means to maintain body and mind in good health and to prevent some diseases, the concept that exercise may also be of curative value in the treatment of disease was more controversial. Nevertheless, some physicians treating older patients felt that exercise may ward off the effects of diseases of long standing, a thought that had been expressed in Greco-Roman times. It was well expressed by Dr. William H. Byford in 1858 who wrote, "There is probably no chronic disease in which exercise may not be employed as a remedy, and I think it is the principal curative means in many of them". In the same year, Dr. Augustus Willard, president of the Medical Society of the State of New York, spoke on the prevention and cure of chronic diseases by air, exercise and sunlight (1858).

Recommendations of exercise in the prevention and treatment of chronic diseases in general soon became quite specific in certain diseases. By the end of the 19th century, exercise therapy had made great advances in the treatment of deficiencies of the locomotor apparatus, most frequently encountered in persons of middle or advanced age. It was a natural sequence to developments in physiology during the century (DuBois-Reymond, 1881). Heinrich Frenkel's system of exercises in locomotor ataxia became quickly known after his first communication in 1890 and was soon applied to other chronic diseases.

Of particular interest is the application of exercise in cardiovascular disease as the latter may manifest itself in minor deficiencies often considered the result of normal aging processes. William Stokes of Ireland, in a treatise on the heart in 1854, had already said, "The symptoms of debility of the heart are often removable by a well-regulated course of gymnastics, or by pedestrian exercise, . . ." although he reminded his colleagues to be more cautious in those advanced in life. The brothers August (1839-1886) and Theodor Schott (1852-1921), physicians in Nauheim, a German spa, combined carbon dioxide baths, resistance exercises and graduated walks to treat cardiac insufficiencies (1916).

Max Joseph Oertel (1835-1897), laryngologist in Munich, developed graduated walking into a therapeutic system known as terrain-cure (1885). In a given spa, trails were laid out which were marked in numbers and colors according to a scale of increasing difficulties depending upon the length and the slope of the walk. The physician prescribed the walks according to the progress of the patient in his cardio-pulmonary reserve. Max Herz in Vienna (1865-1936) combined the methods of Schott and Oertel and added mechanotherapy à la Zander. The terrain treatment and related methods, first developed as a therapy for cardiovascular disease, either isolated or associated with pulmonary insufficiency or obesity (particularly in the system of Oertel who treated himself in this manner), were used with benefit by many persons who visited spas or their private physicians in their search for a regimen that counteracted the effects of aging.

By now, the therapy of old age was an accepted part of medicine. With the increasing interest in this field differentiations developed. In 1873, Foissac distinguished three periods of old age: the first, which is a continuation of virility, spanning the years between 70 and 85; the second, of confirmed old age, between the ages of 85 and 100; and the third, of exceptional old age, the age of centenarians. Clinical medicine had come a long way since the playwright Molière (1622-1673), a fellow Frenchman, only two centuries earlier, presented a character called *Géronte*, who was referred to as "old man of forty" (1666).

TWENTIETH CENTURY

The history of exercises for the elderly in this century is still in the making and will have to be completed at a later date. Many contributors to this book have participated in the making of this history and parts of it are to be found in each·of the chapters of this book. However, a few far-reaching events deserve to be recorded.

Early in the century, a special name was still missing for the new branch of medicine that deals with advanced age. It was supplied in 1914, together with a basic textbook, by Ignatz L. Nascher who wrote *Geriatrics: The Diseases of Old Age and Their Treatment*. This volume of 517 pages was followed by a second edition in 1916 and by other books on the same subject, most notably *Geriatrics* by Malford Thewlis in 1919, with several later editions, all dedicated to I.L. Nascher, the Father of Geriatrics.

Yet, Nascher did not go very far in the use of exercises for his geriatric patients. Although he recognized the need for "mental and physical exercise and recreation," he wrote: "Active athletics are naturally out of the question, even gymnastics cannot be undertaken, but calisthenics are beneficial. . . . The best form of exercises for the aged is walking up a slight incline with frequent rests."

After World War I, a more aggressive use of medical gymnastics in the restoration after injuries was extended to chronic diseases and other conditions, and old age was no disqualification. Coughlin, reporting in 1919 on the benefits of exercise he had observed among old people including his own patients, observed, "Sir Herman Weber, who has recently died in his ninety-fifth year, attributed his longevity in great part to physical exercise."

Continuing investigations in the physiology of muscular exercise throughout the 20th century led to more changes in medicine and surgery. The years immediately following World War II saw a great impetus in the use of medical gymnastics which became an outstanding part in the newly developing medical specialty of physical medicine and rehabilitation. Such advances in turn favored the development of new interest in the care of geriatric patients.

In the course of the general movement for greater physical activity by the healthy and the sick, surgeons started to question the advisability of keeping their patients so long in bed after surgery. The strongest advocate against the "abuse of bedrest", Daniel Leithauser, published in 1946 his book on *Early Ambulation* which included a history of the subject and 126 references since 1899.

Beginning about 1950, cardiology has shown increasing departure from the previously unquestioned regimen of complete bedrest after myocardial infarction to greater and earlier activity. At the same time sports medicine was sanctioned by the establishment of chairs in several European schools of medicine. Greater interest in sports medicine also developed in the United States after the early 1960s.

The recognition that persons physically active even in the later years are healthier than sedentary persons has given new impetus to physical exercises and sports for older people, as this book well documents. While this idea is not new, modern research has supplied supportive data which add a scientific basis. The advisability of exercises for people in their 70s and 80s, provided precautions are taken, is no longer a serious question. Guidelines for tests before, during and after physical exertion have been published by individual authors and organizations, but publications on appropriate exercises themselves and specific guidelines for older people are still too few and incomplete (Nörenberg, 1969; Scharll, 1969; Kamenetz, 1971;

Ellfeldt and Lowman, 1973). This volume will help to narrow the gap of what needs to be done and how to do it.

REFERENCES

Alberti, Leone Battista. *Della Famiglia*. In Joseph (1949).

Amiot, Joseph-Marie, Bourgeois, Cibot, et al. *Mémoires Concernant L'Histoire, les Sciences, les Arts, les Moeurs et les Usages des Chinois*, par les Missionnaires de Pékin. 15 vol. Paris, Nyon, 1776-1789, vol. 4, pp. 441-451; vol. 13, pp. 373 ff.

Andry de Bois-Regard, Nicolas. L'exercice modéré est-il le meilleur moyen de se conserver en santé? *Thesis*, Paris, 1723 and 1741. In extenso in Dally (1857), pp. 502-517.

 − *L'Orthopédie ou l'Art de Prévenir et de Corriger dans les Enfans les Difformites du Corps.* Paris, Veuve Alix, 1741.

Asclepiades. *His Life and Writings.* Antonio Cocchi's Life of Asclepiades and Christian Gottlieb Gumpert's Fragments from Asclepiades translated by Robert Montraville Green. New Haven, Conn., Licht, 1955.

Aubrey, John. *Brief Lives.* Edited by Oliver Lawson Dick. Ann Arbor, Univ. of Michigan Press, 1957, p. 155. In Finney (1968).

Aurelianus, Caelius. *On Acute Diseases and On Chronic Diseases.* Edited and translated by I. E. Drabkin. Chicago, University of Chicago Press, 1950.

Bardi, Giovanni de. Essay on the play of Florentine football. *Badminton Magazine*, 1902. In Joseph (1949).

Betts, John R. American medical thought on exercise as the road to health, 1820-1860. *Bull. Hist. Med.*, 45 (2): 138-152, March-April 1971.

Blundell, John W. F. *The Muscles and Their Story, from the Earliest Times; including the Whole Text of Mercurialis, and the Opinions of Other Writers Ancient and Modern, On Mental and Bodily Development.* London, Chapman & Hall, 1864.

Borelli, Giovanni Alfonso, *De Motu Animalium.* Rome, 1680.

Byford, W[illiam] H. Physiology, pathology and therapeutics of muscular exercise. *Chicago Med. J., 1* (8): 359-382, 1858.

Cagnatus, Marsilius. *De Sanitate Tuenda.* Lib. II: De Arte Gymnastica. Padua, 1605. In Finney (1968), Joseph (1949).

Canstatt, Karl Friedrich. *Die Krankheiten des Höheren Alters und ihre Heilung.* Erlangen, Enke, 1839.

Cardanus, Hieronymus. *De Subtilitate et de Rerum Varietate.* Venice, 1562. In Joseph (1949).

Champier, Symphorien. *Rosa Gallica.* Nancy, 1512.

Charcot, Jean Martin. *Leçons Cliniques sur les Maladies des Vieillards et les Maladies Chroniques.* Paris, 1867.

Cheyne, George. *An Essay on Health and Long Life.* London, Strahan, 1724.

Cicero, Marcus Tullius. *De Senectute.* Translated by W. A. Falconer. Cambridge, Mass., Harvard, 1964.

Cocchi, Antonio. *Life of Asclepiades.* Milan, 1824. In Asclepiades (1955).

Coughlin, Robert E. Physical exercise in later life. *Medical Record (N.Y.)*, 95: 558-561, 1919.

Dally, N[icolas]. *Cinésiologie ou Science du Mouvement dans ses Rapports avec l'Education, l'Hygiene et la Thérapie.* Paris, Librairie Centrale des Sciences, 1857.

DuBois-Reymond, Emil. *Über die Übung.* Berlin, Hirschwald, 1881.

Duchesne, Joseph (Quercetanus). *Ars Medica Dogmatica-Hermetica.* Frankfurt, 1648. In Joseph (1949).

Durand-Fardel, Charles Louis-Maxime. *Traité Pratique des Maladies des Vieillards.* 1854. In Geller (1965).

Ellfeldt, Lois, and Lowman, Charles Leroy. *Exercises for the Mature Adult.* Springfield, Ill., Thomas, 1973.

Fabricio d'Acquapendente, Girolamo. *De Motu Animalium.* Venice, 1614.

Finney, Gretchen [Ludke]. Vocal exercise in the sixteenth century related to theories of physiology and disease. *Bull. Hist. Med., 42*(5):422-449, Sep.-Oct. 1968.

 − Fear of exercising the lungs related to iatro-mechanics 1675-1750. *Bull. Hist. Med.*, 45(4): 341-366, Jul.-Aug. 1971.

Floyer, Sir John. *Medicina Gerocomica, or The Galenic Art of Preserving Old Men's Healths.* London, Isted, 1724.

Foissac, Pierre. *La Longévité Humaine ou l'Art de Conserver la Santé et de Prolonger la Vie.* Paris, Baillière et Fils, 1873.

Frenkel, Heinrich S. Die Therapie atactischer Bewegungsstörungen. *Munch. med. Wschr.,* 37:917-920, 30 Dec. 1890.

Fuller, Francis. *Medicina Gymnastica: or, A Treatise Concerning the Power of Exercise, ...* London, Knaplock, 1705.

Garrison, Fielding H. *An Introduction to the History of Medicine.* Ed. 4. Philadelphia, Saunders, 1960.

Gazius, Antonius. *Florida Corona.* First published under the title: De Conservatione Sanitatis. Venice, 1491.

Geller, Guido. Die Geriatrie an der Salpêtrière von Pinel bis Charcot. *Thesis*, Zurich. Wil, Meyerhans, 1965.

Graham, Douglas. *A Treatise on Massage*. Philadelphia, Lippincott, 1902.

Graham, Sylvester. *Lectures on the Science of Human Life*. Boston, Marsh, Capen, Lyon & Webb, 1839, pp. 658-659. See also Shryock, Richard H. Sylvester Graham and the popular health movement, 1830-1870. *Mississippi Valley Hist. Rev., 18*: 172-183, 1931. In Betts (1971).

Gumpert, Christian Gottlieb. *Fragments from Asclepiades of Bithynia*. Weimar, 1794. In Asclepiades (1955).

Guthrie, Douglas. *A History of Medicine*. London, Nelson, 1958.

Hippocrates with an English translation by E. T. Withington. New York, Putnam, 1927, Vol. 3, p. 339. On joints, LVIII.

Hoffmann, Friedrich Wilhelm. *Dissertationes Physico-Medicae.* . . . The Hague, 1708. In Dally (1857), pp. 206, 233-240.

Hufeland, Christoph Wilhelm. *Die Kunst das Menschliche Leben zu Verlängern*. Vienna, Franz Haas, 1796.

Joseph, Ludwig H. Gymnastics from the middle ages to the 18th century. *Ciba Symposia 10*(5): 1030-1060, March-April 1949.

Jüthner, J. *Philostratòs über Gymnastik*. Leipzig, 1909.

Kamenetz, Herman L. History of massage. In Licht, Sidney. *Massage, Manipulation and Traction*. New Haven, Licht, 1960.

–*Exercises for the Elderly*. Phoenix, Arizona, Armour Pharmaceutical Company, 1971.

Kilgour, Frederick G. Introduction. In Mendez (1960).

Laurentius, Andreas (André du Laurens). *A Discourse of the Preservation of the Sight; of Melancholike Diseases; of Rheumes, and of Old Age*. Transl. Richard Surphlet (London 1599), introd. by Sanford V. Larkey. Oxford, Univ. Press, 1938. In Finney (1968).

Leithauser, Daniel J. *Early Ambulation and Related Procedures in Surgical Management*. Springfield, Ill., Thomas, 1946.

Licht, Sidney. History. In Licht, Sidney. *Therapeutic Exercise*. Ed. 2. New Haven, Licht, 1961.

Mac-Auliffe, Léon. *La Thérapeutique Physique d'Autrefois*. Paris, Masson, 1904.

Maimonides, Moses. *The Preservation of Youth: Essays on Health*. Translated from the Original Arabic by Hirsch L. Gordon. New York, Philosophical Library, 1958.

– The Medical Aphorisms. Translated and edited by Fred Rosner and Suessman Muntner. New York, Yeshiva University Press, 2 vols., 1970-1971.

Major, Ralph H. *A History of Medicine*. Springfield, Ill., Thomas, 1954.

Mendez, Christobal. *Libro del Exercicio Corporal*. Seville, Torre, 1553. *Book of Bodily Exercise*. Translated by Francisco Guerra. New Haven, Licht, 1960.

Mercurialis, Hieronymus. *De Arte Gymnastica*. Venice, Giunta Press, 1569.

Molière. *Le Médecin Malgré Lui*. (The Doctor in Spite of Himself.) 1666. *Les Fourberies de Scapin*. (The Rogueries of Scapin.) 1671.

Montaigne, Michel de. *Essais*. Book III, Ch. XIII. Paris, Garnier, 1962, p. 569. *Essays*. Translated by Charles Cotton. Garden City, N.Y., Doubleday, 1947, p. 465.

Müller, Karl. Die Entwicklung der Geriatrie im 18. Jahrhundert. *Thesis*, Zurich. Zurich, Juris, 1966.

Nascher, Ignatz Leo. *Geriatrics: The Diseases of Old Age and Their Treatment*. Philadelphia, Blakiston, 1914.

Nenci, Giuseppe. *Discorsi sopra la Ginnastica e sopra l'Utilità dell'Osservazione nella Medicina Pratica.* . . . Lucca, Giusti, 1766. In Joseph (1949).

Neuburger, Max. John Floyer's pioneer work. *Bull. Hist. Med.*, 22:208-212, 1948.

Nörenberg, Ruth. Krankengymanstische Betreuung alter Patienten. *Krankengymnastik* 21: 374-379, Aug. 1969.

Oertel, Max Joseph. *Therapie der Kreislaufstörungen*. Leipzig, 1885.

Oeuvres d'Oribase. Translated by Bussemaker and Daremberg. Paris, 1851-1876. In Licht (1961).

Pollak, Kurt. *Wissen and Weisheit der Alten Ärzte: Die Heilkunst der Frühen Hochkulturne*. Düsseldorf, Econ-Verlag, 1968.

Prus, Clovis-René. Recherches sur les maladies de la vieillesse. *Mém. acad. roy. méd.*, 1840. In Geller (1965).

Reniers, Perceval. *The Springs of Virginia; Life, Love, and Death at the Waters*. 1775-1900. Chapel Hill, Univ. of North Carolina Press, 1941.

Reveillé-Parise, Joseph Henri. *Traité de la Vieillesse Hygiénique, Médical et Philosophique*, Paris, Baillière, 1853.

Rush, Benjamin. *Sermons to the Rich and Studious, on Temperance and Exercise*. London, 1772. Reprinted Litchfield, Conn., 1791. *Medical Miscellanies*. Philadelphia, 1809, vol. I, pp. 196, 395, 429, vol. II, pp. 82-93. *Selected Writings*, edited by Dagobert D. Runes. New York, Philos. Lib., 1947, pp. 103, 358-372.

Scharll, Martha. *Altersgymnastik*. Stuttgart, Thieme, 1969.

Schott, Theodor. *Physikalische Behandlung der Chronischen Herzkrankheiten*. Berlin, Springer, 1916.

Schwarz, Richard W. *John Harvey Kellogg, M.D.* Nashville, Southern Publishing Association, 1970.

Stokes, William. *The Diseases of the Heart and the Aorta*. Philadelphia, Lindsay & Blakiston, 1854, p. 357 ff.

Taylor, Charles F. *Theory and Practice of the Movement-Cure.* . . . Philadelphia, Lindsay, 1861.

Taylor, George H. *An Exposition of the Swedish Movement-Cure.* . . . New York, Fowler & Wells, 1860.

Thewlis, Malford W. *Geriatrics, A Treatise on Senile Conditions, Diseases of Advanced Life, and Care of the Aged.* St. Louis, Mosby, 1919. (Ed. 6: *The Care of the Aged,* 1954).

Tissot, [Joseph-Clement]. *Gymnastique Médicinale et Chirurgicale.* Paris, Bastien, 1780. Tissot's *Medicinal and Surgical Gymnastics*, translated by Elizabeth and Sidney Licht. New Haven, Licht, 1964.

Veith, Ilza. *The Yellow Emperor's Classic of Internal Medicine.* Translated from the Chinese. Baltimore, Williams & Wilkins, 1949. Berkeley, Univ. of California Press, 1966.

Willard, Augustus. Air, exercise and sunlight. Annual address delivered before the Medical Society. *Transactions Med. Soc. State of New York*, pp. 3-22, 1858.

Zeman, Frederic D. The Gerontocomia of Gabriele Zerbi. *J. Mount Sinai Hosp., 10*(5): 710-716, Jan.-Feb. 1944.
– Life's later years: Studies in the medical history of old age. Part 10: the eighteenth century. *J. Mount Sinai Hosp., 12*(4):939-953, Nov.-Dec. 1945.

Zerbi, Gabriele. *Gerentocomia, Scilicet de Senum Aura atque Victu.* Rome, 1489.

Preservation of Physical Fitness

Hans Kraus, M.D.

INTRODUCTION

The past 50 years have dramatically changed our way of life. As we become more sedentary and subjected to increased strain, our lack of sufficient exercise leads to reduced muscular strength and flexibility, decreased cardiovascular and pulmonary function and a deleterious tension syndrome. Such overstress and underexercise causing "hypokinetic disease" can accelerate premature aging. On the other hand, proper exercise contributes to longevity and preserves function in old age (Karvonen, 1959).

FITNESS PROBLEMS OF AGING

Strength and flexibility decrease with aging, but if they decrease from a high level obtained by proper physical fitness during childhood and youth, they will not drop so readily to the abysmally low level so often seen in relatively young people and particularly in middle age and older people. It is commonly accepted that an otherwise normal 50-year-old or even a 40-year-old may experience trouble climbing a couple of flights of stairs because of a lack of cardiovascular and muscular fitness, but this response is by no means natural or inevitable. The fact that one's heart is unable to cope with a relatively small strain like climbing stairs may explain why this same heart may fail even worse under excessive mental or physical stress. The physically inactive individual shows signs of aging earlier in life, exists physiologically at a lower potential, and is less well equipped to maintain homeostasis and to meet the daily stresses of life. Such a low level of function combined with forced suppression of "fight and fight" response enhances the incidence of disease (Kraus, 1976).

The best way to preserve physical fitness in old age is by starting physical fitness programs in early childhood. Quite appropriately, our interest in the fitness of the aging began in a posture clinic at Babies Hospital, Columbia-Presbyterian Hospital, where Dr. Sonia Weber and I for several years ran a series of tests to determine basic strength and flexibility of key posture muscles in conjunction with other postural tests. We established some basic values for strength and flexibility of these key posture muscles which then were tested in a low back clinic in Columbia-Presbyterian Hospital. A team of specialists, under the direction of Dr. Barbara Stimson, examined back patients to determine the cause of the increasing incidence of back problems. At this clinic and later at New York University, we saw a total of approximately 5,000 patients. More than 80 percent of these back patients were deficient in one or more of the key posture muscle groups shown as the cause of underexercise and overstress in the production of back pain (Kraus and Weber, 1962).

Later, tests of 5,000 school children between the ages of six and 16 revealed a very high percentage (57.9 percent) had similar shortcomings (Kraus et al., 1954). At intervals, tests taken in Europe, which at the time had a less mechanized and more physically active population, showed much better results. The failure rate never exceeded 10 percent (Kraus and Hirschland, 1954; Kraus, 1957).

We soon realized that underexercise and overstress were also factors in the production of other disease, including myocardial infarction (Kraus, 1957; Morris and Crawford, 1959), hypertension, overweight (Johnson et al., 1956), nervous tension (Sainsbury and Gibson, 1954), musculoskeletal pain, headache, and so forth (Appleton, 1956; Kraus and Hirschland, 1953; Kraus et al., 1959). Dr. William Raab and I compiled our observations in a book, *Hypokinetic Disease* (disease produced by lack of exercise). Our impression was that underexercise and overstress, both inherent in our present civilization, combine to produce this disease (Fig. 1) (Kraus, 1964).

PREVENTIVE PROGRAMS

From the start, we were interested in prevention and treatment (Kraus, 1964; Kraus and Raab, 1961). Much had been done in reconditioning at the Beckmann Clinic in Ohlstadt, Germany, where people showing signs of losing the battle against tension and underexercise mainly due to overweight, musculoskeletal pain and elevated blood pressure, improved considerably under a program of gradually increasing physical activity and dietary management, and equally important, their separation from family and work, the sources of tension. Their incidence of sickness dropped 50 percent after only one month of reconditioning (Brusis, 1961). Similar reconditioning centers exist in East Germany, Switzerland and Austria, and there are more than 3,000 in Russia (Kraus and Raab, 1961).

Over the intervening years we found that just as important as the reconditioning of the hypokinetic adult was the prevention of the underexercised and overtense state through fitness programs started in early childhood. Good fitness programs in school, starting in the first grade and continuing throughout elementary school, high school and college (Jokl, 1959), are essential to prevent deterioration in fitness and health arising from hypokinetic disorders and aging. Such programs should not only attempt to develop muscular fitness and flexibility but also teach children and adolescents to take better care of their own bodies and to be more responsible for their own health.

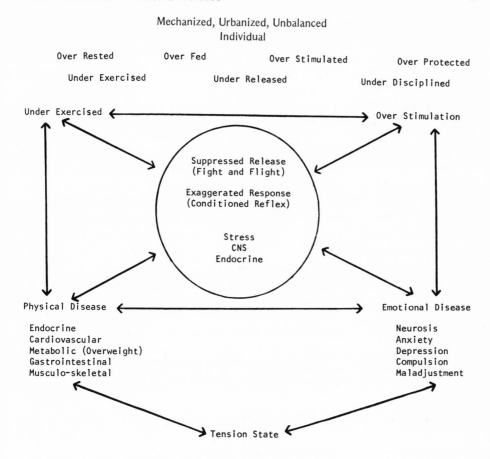

Fig. 1. Mechanisms of hypokinetic disease
Reproduced with permission from *Hypokinetic Disease*, Kraus and Raab, Charles C Thomas, Publisher.

Many programs in prevention can be usefully directed towards exercise and relaxation. Such programs started in early childhood could easily attempt to teach discipline and responsibility for one's own health, including the avoidance of health hazards such as alcohol, cigarettes, reckless driving and abuse of one's body.

Such school programs exist in Germany and Switzerland, but unfortunately, little has been done on our own country. This is why the Frankel Preventicare program for older people described in this book is so important as an example of what can be done to reclaim lost physical fitness at any age. Programs like this should become available on a national basis and tie in with our whole working population. It would be essential not only to refer people for three to four weeks of reconditioning, but to stimulate them to conduct their own fitness programs while working. Every company or factory should make available room for reconditioning exercises for their employees. There are too few such programs in this country and these are still far from being generally used.

CONCLUSION

Fitness programs in all schools from elementary through college levels and national reconditioning programs for adults are long overdue in this country. Good physical work starting in childhood and continuing throughout the whole school and academic life should include daily exercise classes of at least an hour. Business and industry should allot time for exercise breaks rather than for coffee breaks.

Reconditioning centers should be established where people who are getting "deconditioned" and more susceptible to one or more of the chronic degenerative diseases have an opportunity to rest, get reconditioned and return to work with healthier bodies and a more placid frame of mind. There must also be health education programs for these persons to understand their need for regular physical activity and motivation for them to want to be active (Kraus, 1976). Forthcoming legislation in health care must include the fundamental need for exercise in the prevention and treatment of disease and aging.

REFERENCES

Appleton, L. (1956) *Study on Fitness or Performance of West Point Cadets,* New York University Press, New York.

Brusis, O.T. (1961) Ueber die Indikation von Fruehheil-Verfahren mit Terrainkuren bei Sozialversicherten mit Kreislaufschaeden und ueber die Pruefung des Kurerfolges. Inaugural-Dissertation, Munich 1961.

Johnson, M.L., Burke B.S., and Mayer, J. (1956) *Am J Clin Nutr* 4, 231.

Jokl, E. (1959) *JAMA* 169, 97.

Karvonen, M.J. (1959) Effects of Vigorous Exercise on the Heart, in *Work and the Heart* (F.F. Rosenbaum and E.L. Belknap, eds.), Paul B. Hoeber, New York, p. 199.

Kraus, H. and Hirschland, R.P. (1953) *J Amer Assn Health Phys Ed Recreation* 24, 17.

Kraus, H. and Hirschland, R.P. (1954) *Research Quart* 25, 178.

Kraus, H., Nagler, W., and Weber, S. (1959) *G P* 20, 121.

Kraus, H. and Hirschland, R.P. (1954) *N Y State J Med* 54, 212.

Kraus, H. (1957) *Physical Fitness News Letter*, Sept.

Kraus, H. and Raab, W. (1961) *Hypokinetic Disease – Diseases Produced by Lack of Exercise*, Charles C Thomas, Springfield, Ill.

Kraus, H. (1964) *N Y State J Med* 64, 1182.

Kraus, H. and Weber, S. (1962) *Arch Environ Health* 4, 408.

Kraus, H. (1976) in Keelor, R. *Aging* 258 (April) 6.

Morris, J.N. and Crawford, M.D. (1959) *JAMA* 169, 1389.

Sainsbury, P. and Gibson, J.G. (1954) *J Neurol Neuro Surg & Psychiatry* 17, 216.

Public Health and Fitness–The Outdoor Life and Other Antidotes to Enemies of Fitness

Hollis S. Ingraham, M.D.

INTRODUCTION

Physical fitness, a state which can be evaluated easily in the trained athlete, is more difficult either to measure or define in the average citizen. It is a condition which includes a sense of well-being, a joy of living, an ability to perform well on the daily job and, lastly, staying alive. The last is the easiest to quantify for an individual or a nation and, on the whole, survival is perhaps the best single criterion of fitness. In any event, each of the advanced countries has good data on life expectancy which can be used for comparative purposes. Comparative mortality statistics are admittedly rough indices, but they illustrate what can be achieved and serve as guides to short term health goals.

It is now general knowledge that length of life in the United States lagged seriously behind that of many other nations in the 25 years after World War II. In the age period of 45-64, the American male has survived less well than in any other comparable area of the world. After age 65, his life expectancy has been about average, but well below the best. The American female has had an average life expectancy in the age period 45-64 and has been close to the best at ages beyond 65 (Statistical Bulletin, 1971). In the very recent past, there was some indication that female rates in the United States were losing ground. The American male at middle age is clearly at a disadvantage as far as life expectancy is concerned and requires help to improve his fitness and longevity. The measures to be discussed are also applicable to the female with only a quantitative difference.

ANTI-FITNESS FACTORS

Fitness or the lack thereof doubtless depends on many factors. The five most important factors in our society at this time are all basically under the control of the individual and depend little on new initiatives by government.

Cigarette Smoking

At the top of the list is cigarette smoking. The cigarette is the single most lethal agent in America today. Every year in this country, several hundred thousand people die needlessly from diseases induced by cigarette smoking. Three out of four victims are in their prime productive years, most of them men in otherwise vigorous health. Cigarette smoking produces many chronic changes in its victims, but its most lethal effects are lung cancer, coronary heart disease and emphysema. While pipe and cigar smoking are also deleterious to health, their impact on mortality is so much less than that of cigarettes that, for all practical purposes, they may be almost disregarded. Men, as a group, are heavier smokers than women and, in addition, are apparently much more sensitive to the toxic action of tobacco. It is notable, however, that the lung cancer death rate among women is now rising sharply (American Cancer Society, 1976).

Alcohol

Second on the list of enemies of fitness is the overuse of alcohol. Alcohol is responsible for most cirrhosis of the liver, which has been rising as a cause of death in this country. Alcohol contributes to overeating and provides nothing but empty calories. It is an accessory factor in several diseases and disorders. The disastrous social consequences of chronic alcoholism are well-known and need not be elaborated here. Combined drinking and driving constitute a major cause of death and disfigurement on our highways. Careful studies have verified through autopsy what most veteran police officers knew from personal observation – in most single car accidents, the driver had been drinking to excess (Haddon and Bradess, 1959). Many victims are young people in their teens and early twenties, which is especially tragic. It is somewhat surprising to learn that the drunken pedestrian forms a large segment of highway deaths (Haddon et al., 1961). In addition to being a grave threat to himself, the drunken driver is a menace to all other drivers, passengers and pedestrians on the highways.

Overeating

Third on our list is overeating, which ranks high as a deadly enemy of the American people. Almost three decades ago, a study at Cornell University of the effects of the quantity of food eaten by laboratory animals on their survival was published in one of the better lay periodicals under the title "The Thin Rats Bury The Fat Rats."

This situation is also true of people, as life insurance statistics have long shown. Americans are among the best fed people in the world. Not only do we consume greater quantities of food generally, but we also eat an excess of fats. It is not merely a coincidence that the United States ranks high in the rates of death due to hypertension, coronary heart disease and diabetes. There is a long list of diseases more common in the obese, but these three are major threats to the survival of the overweight.

Late Diagnosis

The fourth enemy is the failure to seek medical advice at the early appearance of symptoms of illness or at any change in bodily condition or function. The example that comes instantly to mind is cancer. Many forms of cancer can be treated successfully if treatment is begun early. Most people know this, but too many fail to act quickly enough, with tragic consequences. There are, of course, other conditions in which early treatment can halt progression of a disease. Hypertension is a good example of a major cause of death, which is now largely amenable to modern therapy. Again, early treatment is most efficacious. But even relatively late therapy can be valuable. In the meantime, however, the disease may have produced irremediable damage.

Underexertion

The fifth enemy of fitness is underexertion of the muscular system, which can contribute to obesity and to other morbid changes. In an interesting study made about 10 years ago, investigators compared Irishmen who had come to this country with their own brothers who had stayed in Ireland (Trulson et al., 1964). The brothers in the United States ate more, weighed more and had a higher death rate from coronary heart disease than their brothers in Ireland, who walked more. Numerous other studies have shown an association between lack of physical exertion and higher death rates from cardiovascular disease. The nature of the protective effect of exercise has not been elucidated but appears to be a reality.

PUBLIC HEALTH CONSIDERATIONS

In my judgment, the preceding five factors are the principal enemies of fitness. There are others, of course, but, at this time and under conditions existing in this country, they are less important. Far down the list are the deteriorating environment and the deficiencies of our medical care system. These matters concern the public and Congress far out of proportion to their present effect on our survival and fitness, but in no way should one denigrate the desirability, indeed the necessity, of cleaning up the environment or the fact that health will eventually be seriously imperiled if we fail so to do. However, the impact on mortality figures from a deteriorated environment has, to date, been scarcely discernible (Statistical Bulletin, 1973), except for certain work environments which have proved dangerous. Even in some of these, deaths have been largely limited to cigarette smokers (Selikoff et al., 1968). Similarly, there can be no question of the need to give great attention to the availability, cost and quality of medical care. However, if we were to provide the best medical care system that present knowledge can assure without at the same time changing people's habits and attitudes, we could add only a fraction of a year to the expectation of life in this country. On the other hand, if, without any change in our medical care system, we could educate the American public to change its habits of self-care, approximately five years would be added to the life expectancy of the American male and about another year to the life expectancy of the American female.

Although a rather gloomy picture of the state of health in the United States has been given, it must be admitted that some very recent reports have been more favorable. The most striking is the decline in deaths in all forms of heart disease, which has now become a nationwide phenomenon (King, 1973). Peculiarly, the drop has been somewhat greater among males. Also it is reported that the expectation of life for both males and females has surged to a new high. These facts, together with the considerable and sustained lowering of the infant mortality rate, do offer encouragement. The reasons for the post-war lag in mortality reduction in the United States and the very recent spurt are surely multitudinous and may never be fully understood. The modern treatment of hypertension has certainly contributed to reductions in death from that form of heart disease, and it is reasonable to believe that the many years of health education in the schools and by voluntary and official agencies are now showing results. This belief should provide encouragement for redoubling of efforts to stimulate more self-help in the area of health care.

ANTIDOTES TO ENEMIES OF FITNESS

What can be done about our five worst enemies? It appears that mankind has not yet found the means by which an affluent society can protect many of its members from themselves, but certain measures must be tried.

Public Health Education

The large amount of money spent on research and health education on the cigarette peril has so far had little obvious effect on cigarette consumption. Young people appear to be taking up the habit with unabated enthusiasm. However, there are indications that the middle-aged male, who is the most vulnerable, is smoking less as a result of publicity on the cigarette danger. This reduction is most obvious among male physicians. Efforts must be continued on this most serious problem, with hopes that education may have a cumulative effect.

Similarly the consumption of alcohol remains high, and drunken drivers proliferate. The American public, to protect itself, must eventually be aroused to deal harshly and uncompromisingly with the drunken driver. Interest in alcoholism itself seems to be increasing. In time, this may be translated into practical results.

There have been hopeful signs that the public is increasingly interested in the subject of diet. The health food fad, despite its many laughable aspects, is one indication that a growing number of people appreciate the close relationship of food and health. The obvious lesser extent of gross obesity among the well-educated is another optimistic portent, as is the current interest in books on diet and the increased use of unsaturated fats. Although food quackery is obviously prevalent, it seems that sound health education on the subject of food is making remarkable progress.

There is little question that Americans are utilizing medical services to a greater extent than previously. Blue Cross, Blue Shield, commercial insurance, Medicare and Medicaid have all helped, but have not always sufficiently encouraged early diagnosis and treatment. The figures on early discovery of cancer with concomitant improved survival offer the best evidence of increased awareness of the need for and value of early medical consultation. The continuing drop of deaths from hypertension and the sharp decline in infant mortality are further good indices of an aroused public interest in proper medical care.

The Outdoor Life

The renewed participation in the outdoor life is one of the most striking trends of our time. This phenomenon became apparent shortly after World War II and appears to be accelerating rather than diminishing. It affects both sexes of all ages and includes a wide variety of activities, most of which involve active exercise. Bicycling, jogging and tennis are the three that are most obvious to the general public as being vastly more popular within the last decade. Others include skiing, boating, back packing, swimming, hiking, birdwatching, snowshoeing, mountain climbing, fishing, gardening, woodcutting and just plain walking. Hunting has held its own, but has not increased as rapidly as most of the previously listed. Golf has been steadily increasing in popularity for many decades.

In view of the recognized health benefits that accrue from regular exercise, this growing interest in the outdoor life should be encouraged in every way with only one caution: each person should check with his physician before undertaking any new and vigorous form of physical exertion and should, henceforth, exercise his common sense as well as his muscle. In any form of vigorous activity, it is wise to practice moderation, to start slowly and increase one's load gradually. It isn't possible to make a general statement about which kind of outdoor sport is preferable from a health standpoint. There are many varieties of exercise as the other chapters in this book describe, and which one a person chooses must depend on his circumstances and his individual preference, except when prescribed as part of a therapeutic regimen. Certainly a person will get more benefit if he chooses a form that gives him enjoyment.

Walking may be the best form of outdoor enjoyment for many people, particularly for those beyond middle life. It doesn't need special equipment and can be done almost anywhere for as long or as short a period as desired, and one can set his own pace. Some people like to hunt and walk; others prefer fishing and walking. Some are birdwatchers. There are many varieties of walking, including walking for walking's sake, but whatever the reason, the result can be and usually is beneficial.

Cycling is currently popular. Here again one can set his own pace and enjoy the countryside while toning up leg muscles and improving circulation.

Jogging is enjoying a tremendous vogue. This again can be as vigorous and prolonged as fancy dictates.

For those who have a woodlot, the ax and the saw are excellent tools for work, relaxation and even profit in these energy-short times. One can also say a good word for gardening, which can be more exercise than the tyro might think. Tremendous competitive effort is involved in racing with the weeds. Gardening, of course, is doubly valuable today in our era of galloping food prices.

Winter is always just around the corner and with it in much of the United States comes a special form of exertion — snow shovelling. Many of us are very dubious of the purported ill effects of shovelling snow, and, in particular, the belief that snow shovelling is a very potent cause of myocardial infarction. This is mostly a newspaper myth. It is quite probable that more people have heart attacks while in bed during snowstorms than while shovelling. Of course it's true that each winter some individuals have heart attacks while working in the snow, or just after, but whether the association is causative and whether they might have survived longer had they been otherwise engaged is problematical. The advice often quoted in newspapers, "get a snowshovel with a long handle and give it to your wife," would seem to be perpetuated by female chauvinists in the newspaper industry. It is designed more to create healthy, long-lived widows than to prolong the life of the poor benighted male over 50.

CONCLUSION

To sum up, fitness and survival depend on many circumstances, of which several of the most important can be influenced strongly by the individual's life style. Public acceptance of the necessary steps to improve fitness through individual initiative seems to be increasing, although almost imperceptible in certain aspects such as the use of cigarettes. However, public enthusiasm for outdoor activity seems boundless, and such interest will ideally create greater health consciousness in respect to the other enemies of fitness.

The tremendous upsurge of outdoor activity seems to indicate a general belief that man, to live fully, must be a well-tuned physical being. Whatever the final verdict on the extent to which exercise by itself protects physical health, two conclusions seem certain: (1) most persons experience a greater sense of well-being after exercise and (2) such exertion is helpful in combatting obesity. It is also true that nearly everyone, regardless of age or sex, can use his muscles vigorously with safety. It is the task of all health workers to encourage such use within the bounds outlined in this book.

Golf, tennis, boating, swimming, hiking, jogging, walking, gardening, lumbering, skiing, hunting, fishing, birdwatching and others — there are so many kinds of pleasant exercise that the individual should have no trouble choosing one that suits him best and is readily available to him.

The outdoor life is truly an antidote to the enemies of fitness.

REFERENCES

American Cancer Society (1976) '76 Cancer Facts & Figures.
Haddon, W., Jr. and Bradess, V.A. (1959) *JAMA* 169, 1587.
Haddon, W., Jr., Valien, P., McCarroll, J.R., and Umberger, C.J. (1961) *J Chronic Dis* 14, 655.
King, P. (1973) NYS Dept of Health *Vital Stat Rev* 7, 13.
Statistical Bulletin (1971) Metropolitan Life 52, 7.
Statistical Bulletin (1973) Metropolitan Life 54, 9.
Selikoff, I.J., Hammond, E.C., and Churg, J. (1968) *JAMA* 204, 106.
Trulson, M.F., Clancy, R.E., Jessop, W.J., Childers, R.W., and Stare, F.J. (1964) *J Am Diet Assoc* 45, 225.

Section II

Evaluation and Physiology of Exercise

Physiology of Physical Conditioning for the Elderly

Herbert A. deVries, Ph.D.

INTRODUCTION

Over the last five years several hundred older people were studied in our physiology of exercise laboratory with the following threefold purposes:

1. To determine the level of trainability in people age 50-90 years of age;

2. To learn more about the dose-response characteristics, how much exercise is enough and how much is too much;

3. To evaluate the health benefits and the expected improvement in physical vigor in older people participating in supervised exercise.

Some of the physiological changes accompanying the aging process have been discussed in some other chapters and, therefore, this discussion will be limited to those physiological aspects of aging that relate to physical working capacity or vigor. First of all, with respect to the cardiovascular system, it is known that the maximum heart rate goes down with increasing age and cardiac output decreases about one percent per year, probably as the result of a lessening of power in the heart muscle. The ability to breathe — to move air in and out of our lungs — also decreases markedly. The strength of muscles and their ability to endure long exercise bouts (muscular endurance) also decline with age, but less dramatically than the cardiovascular parameters. Physical working capacity, best measured as maximal oxygen consumption or "aerobic capacity", goes down reasonably predictably, and body composition changes. Approximately three to five percent of active body tissue is lost per decade. In practical terms, this means the fortunate few who have held their weight down to what it was at age 20 or 25 still become fatter by three to five percent per decade because active tissue has been replaced with nothing but fat.

However, three weeks of bedrest will also bring about these changes in well-conditioned young subjects, as has been demonstrated repeatedly and most clearly by Saltin et al. (1968). This, then, leads to the question of what really brings about the loss of vigor with increasing age, since there are unquestionably other factors involved than just true aging itself. We have attempted to define the problem as a multi-factorial one which considers the loss of function, or the loss of physical work capacity, due to age as being composed of at least three components: (1) a true aging factor, (2) unrecognized disease processes which contribute to loss of vigor and (3) the factor which is the result of what Kraus and Raab call "hypokinetic disease" (1961). In many cases, we suspect the last factor may be the largest of the three, although we don't yet have definitive evidence for that. But in any event, it is the only one of the three over which we can exert any control.

METHODS OF STUDY

We found it difficult to get large numbers of older subjects to come to the university to participate in an exercise experiment with the necessary physiological testing, especially since we are in an urban area. Consequently, we took our mobile laboratory right to the heart of a retirement community where we had access to 14,000 people over 50 years of age. We solicited volunteers and medically cleared 112 subjects who could participate in an exercise program designed to improve (1) aerobic capacity, (2) muscular fitness and (3) flexibility. Basically, there was nothing new or miraculous about the exercise program. Good sense and systematic progression were basic conditions in determining the important parameters and applying them in a fashion that would motivate the individual. In general, the first part of our program consisted of warm-up calisthenics. At the heart of the second phase, the jog-walk program, was a concept that the Boy Scouts of America developed many years ago, the Boy Scout Pace. We added a little progression to it and found this worked extremely well. We began with an easy 50 steps running, 50 steps walking, starting with five sets the first day, six sets the second until we got to 10 sets. At that point, we cut down the rest interval to 40 steps walking and went back to the five sets again and so on until the ultimate goal of continuous jogging for one mile was achieved.

The third phase was a technique of static stretching which improves flexibility and is useful to prevent muscle soreness. No more than a five percent incidence of any muscle problems occurred in the group whose mean age was 70. The details of our exercise program have been described elsewhere (deVries, 1974).

A series of physiological tests were conducted on each individual after he was medically cleared. It is important to emphasize that all the participants in the program were, to the best of our determinations, "healthy, normal", older men and women.

The first experiment was on men (deVries, 1970). All Ss were pretested and 66 were retested at six weeks, 26 at 18 weeks and eight at 42 weeks on the following parameters: (a) blood pressure, (b) percentage of body fat, (c) resting neuromuscular activation by electromyography (relaxation), (d) arm muscle strength and girth, (e) maximal O_2 consumption, (f) O_2 pulse at heart rate = 145, (g) pulmonary function and (h) physical work capacity on the bicycle ergometer. A subgroup of 35 was also tested before and after six weeks of training for (a) cardiac output, (b) stroke volume, (c) total peripheral resistance and (d) work of the heart, at a workload of 75 watts on the bicycle ergometer.

RESULTS

The most significant findings were related to oxygen transport capacity. O_2 pulse and minute ventilation at heart rate 145 improved by 29.4 and 35.2 percent, respectively. Vital capacity improved by 19.6 percent.

Significant improvement was also found in percentage of body fat, physical work capacity and both systolic and diastolic blood pressure for the large six-week group (N = 66). But with the smaller group which exercised for 42 weeks (N = 8), statistical significance was not achieved although the same trends were observed. Controls did not improve upon any of the above measures. No significant changes were seen in any of the hemodynamic variables tested.

A group of seven men was placed in a modified exercise program because of various cardiovascular problems. This group exercised in the same manner except that they substituted a progressive walking program for the jogging and were restricted to a maximum heart rate of 120 instead of 145. This group exercised for six weeks at the end of which time their improvement showed a similar pattern to that of the harder working normal Ss at six weeks.

Life history of physical activity was evaluated in a subgroup of 53. Neither the mean of high and low years of activity nor the peak level of activity engaged in for a period of six weeks or more correlated positively with physiological improvement found.

DISCUSSION

The trainability of older men with respect to physical work capacity is probably considerably greater than has been suspected and does not depend upon having trained vigorously in youth. Improvement in muscular function at this age level probably occurs largely by improvement of central nervous system activation and only very slightly, if at all, by muscular hypertrophy. Since no untoward incidents occurred during the 18-month tenure of our exercise program, and in view of the improvements in function demonstrated, the exercise regimen as developed was both safe and effective for a normal population of older men in the presence of medical and physiological monitoring.

In a subsequent study, 17 older women (age 52-79) from the same community participated in a vigorous three-month exercise program and again physical fitness was significantly improved although the women did not show as large an improvement in the respiratory system as men (Adams and deVries, 1973).

On the basis of these studies, we concluded that the older organism is very definitely trainable and that the percentage of improvement is similar to that of the young.

Since earlier electromyographic investigations showed that vigorous exercise has a well-defined tranquilizing effect (both immediate and long term) upon young and middle-aged men (deVries, 1968), we decided to evaluate this effect of exercise in our older population. Toward this end, the tranquilizing effects of single doses of exercise and meprobamate (a commonly used tranquilizer pill supplied on prescription as either "Miltown" or "Equanil") were compared with respect to reduction of muscle action potentials in 10 elderly, anxious subjects (deVries and Adams, 1972). Thirty-six observations were made of each subject before and after (immediately, 30 min. and one hour after) each of the five following treatment conditions: (1) meprobamate, 400 mg (2) placebo, 400 mg lactose, (3) 15 min. of walking type exercise at a heart rate of 100 (4) 15 min. of walking type exercise at heart rate of 120 and (5) resting control. Conditions 1 and 2 were adminsitered double-blind. It was found that exercise at a heart rate of 100 lowered electrical activity in the musculature by 20, 23 and 20 percent at the first, second and third post tests respectively. These changes were significantly different from controls at the one percent confidence level. Neither meprobamate nor placebo treatment was significantly different from control. Exercise at the higher heart rate was only slightly less effective, but the data were more variable and approached but did not achieve significance.

Our data suggested that the exercise modality should not be overlooked when a tranquilizer effect is desired since, in a single dose at least, exercise has a significantly greater effect, without any undesirable side effects, than meprobamate, a frequently prescribed tranquilizer. This response is especially important for the older individual in that the exercise approach can avoid the further impairment of motor coordination, reaction time and driving performance which may occur with any tranquilizer. A 15-minute walk at a moderate rate (enough to raise heart rate to 100 beats per minute) is sufficient stimulus to bring about the desired effect which persists for at least one hour afterward.

CONCLUSION

It seems then that vigorous physical conditioning of the healthy older organism can significantly improve (1) the cardiovascular system (2) the respiratory system (at least in men), (3) the musculature, and (4) body composition and generally produce a more vigorous individual who can relax better.

How Much Exercise Is Enough?

In one of our studies (deVries, 1971), 52 asymptomatic male volunteers from the Laguna Hills retirement community participated in a six-week jogging program which constituted a varying level of stress for the participants, depending upon their physical fitness level. They were tested before and after the exercise regimen with the Åstrand bicycle ergometer test for prediction of their maximal oxygen consumption. During the six-week exercise regimen, they kept daily records of the heart rate elicited by each of the five to 10 run phases and the daily peak heart rate was used in calculating the mean exercise heart rate for the six-week period. This mean peak heart rate was then used in calculating the percentate of heart rate range at which each subject worked.

It was found that:

1) Improvement in cardiovascular-respiratory function (aerobic capacity) varied directly with the percentage of heart rate range at which the subject worked.

2) Improvement in the aerobic capacity varied inversely with the physical fitness

level (Åstrand score) at the start of the program.

3) The exercise intensity threshold for older men appears to be about 40 percent of heart rate range compared with about 60 percent found by others for young men.

4) Normalizing the percent heart rate range (%HRR) for physical fitness level furnishes the best estimate of the exercise intensity threshold. On this basis, men in this age bracket need to raise their heart rate slightly above that percent HRR represented by their aerobic capacity in milliliters per kilogram per minute to achieve the intensity threshold necessary for a training effect.

5) On the basis of the data, men in their 60s and 70s, of average physical fitness, need only raise their heart rates above 98 and 95, respectively, to provide a training stimulus to the cardiovascular system. Even well-conditioned men in these age brackets need only exceed 106 and 103, respectively (when heart rate is taken immediately *after* exercise).

6) It was concluded that for all but the highly conditioned older men, vigorous walking, which raises heart rate to 100 to 120 beats per minute for 30-60 minutes daily, constitutes a sufficient stimulus to bring about some, though possibly not optimal, improvement in cardiovascular-respiratory function.

Type of Exercise (Isotonic vs. Isometric, etc.)

So far we have discussed exercise in general terms and what we have said applies only to rhythmic exercise of large body segments such as occurs in walking, jogging, running or swimming.

For any given workload that the body as a whole is subjected to, the work of the heart is greater under conditions of (1) static (isometric) muscular contraction or (2) high activation levels of small muscle masses (Åstrand, Gunary and Wahren, 1968; Lind and McNicol, 1968). This is so because the blood pressure response to exercise loading is set not by the total body work accomplished, but by the arterial blood pressure required to perfuse that muscle which requires the greatest perfusion pressure. Thus, even a small muscle working at 90-100 percent of its maximum strength occludes muscle blood flow and can raise the systemic blood pressure significantly (Lind and McNicol, 1967a and b). Isometric exercise would be undesirable because not only are high levels of muscle contraction attained, but they are also maintained without the relaxation pauses provided by rhythmic activity during which blood flow is unresisted. Thus, we may conclude that exercise programs for older people should maximize the rhythmic activity of large muscle masses and minimize (1) high activation levels of small muscle masses and (2) static (or isometric) contractions. The natural activities of walking, jogging, running and swimming seem to be best suited to this purpose. Calisthenics, if properly designed to conform to these principles, can also be very beneficial.

Prevention of Muscular Soreness

Unaccustomed exercise in sedentary older people often results in moderate to severe soreness which presents itself in 24-48 hours after the exercise. Electromyographic evidence (deVries, 1966) indicates this pain is the result of a vicious cycle of which the end result is tonic local muscle spasm in the "overused" muscles. The vicious cycle probably develops as follows: (1) overuse of the muscle produces fatigue, (2) muscle fatigue results in incomplete relaxation which causes (3) ischemia by virtue of the partial occlusion, (4) ischemia causes pain and (5) the pain causes further contraction (splinting reaction). This cycle is easily broken by application of static stretching principles (deVries, 1966). This approach resulted in less than five percent incidence of muscle soreness in our older subject population, indicating it is as effective in older participants as we have found it to be for the young in our laboratory experiments.

Finally, although our interest has been to establish guidelines to better physical fitness in the elderly, it is important to realize that physical fitness must begin in childhood to realize maximum benefits. However, when this ideal situation has not been realized, the available data suggest that the trainability of the older organism is not greatly different from that of the young. Ideally, physical fitness should be achieved in youth, pursued throughout adulthood and never relinquished insofar as is humanly possible.

REFERENCES

Adams, G. M., and deVries, H. A. (1973) *J Gerontol* 28, 50.
Åstrand, I., Guharay, A., and Wahren, J. (1968) *J Appl Physiol* 25, 528.
deVries, H. A. (1966), *Am J Phy Med* 45, 119.
deVries, H. A. (1968) *J Sports Med* 8, 1.
deVries, H. A. (1970) *J Gerontol* 25, 325.
deVries, H. A. (1971) *Geriatrics* 26, 94.
deVries, H. A. (1974) *Vigor Regained*, Prentice-Hall, Englewood Cliffs.
deVries, H. A. and Adams, G. M. (1972) *Am J Phys Med* 51, 130.
Kraus, H., and Raab, W. (1961) *Hypokinetic Disease*, Charles C Thomas, Springfield, Ill.
Lind, A. R. and McNicol, G. W. (1967a) *Can Med Assoc J* 96, 706.
Lind, A. R. and McNicol, G. W. (1967b) *J Physiol* 192, 595.
Lind, A. R. and McNicol, G. W. (1968) *J Appl Physiol* 25, 261.
Saltin, B., Blomquist, G., Mitchell, J.H., et al. (1968) *Response to Exercise after Bed Rest and After Training,* American Heart Association. *Monograph No. 23,* New York.

Effect of Age on Work and Fatigue—Cardiovascular Aspects

Ernst Simonson M.D.

Nearly all physiological functions are involved in work performance but are affected differently by age depending on type, severity and duration of work performance.

Fig. 1 schematically illustrates the involvement of the five fundamental fatigue processes (middle row) (Simonson, 1971) in the various types of work, listed in decreasing severity in the top row from anaerobic (100% max. V_{O_2}) to partially aerobic (80-100% and 50-80% max. V_{O_2}). Work below 50% max. V_{O_2}, which can be performed at a steady state of V_{O_2}, and related functions are not included because endurance is limited not by any of the five fundamental fatigue processes alone but also by psychological functions. Endurance in isometric work (last block, row 1) depends mainly on peripheral circulation as well as central nervous system reactions and subjective sensations (see chapter 11, Simonson, 1971). In the bottom row, complicating mechanisms are listed with symbols inserted in the blocks of the first row.

The inserted letter "A" means that an effect of age is well documented. Regarding hormonal depletion, it may be added that there is also a relationship between depletion of gonadal hormones with age and various types of work performance (Simonson, Kearns and Enzer, 1944). "A-" means that no effect of age on performance could be experimentally documented (isometric work, increase of body and skin temperature). In a wealth of literature related to disturbance of regulations as one of the most important fatigue processes, information on the effect of age is scanty. There is also no information on the effect of age on transmission fatigue.

---

* In part reproduced, with permission from Ernst Simonson: "Einfluss des Alters auf Arbeit und Ermudung-in physiologischer Hinsicht." H. Schmidtke (ed.) Handbuch der Ergonomie.

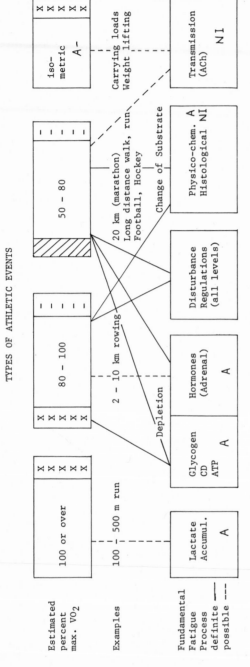
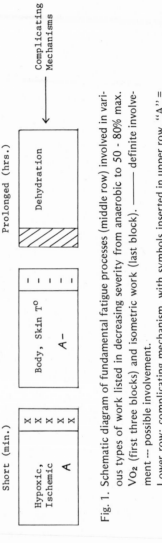

Fig. 1. Schematic diagram of fundamental fatigue processes (middle row) involved in various types of work listed in decreasing severity from anaerobic to 50 - 80% max. VO₂ (first three blocks) and isometric work (last block). ── definite involvement --- possible involvement.
Lower row: complicating mechanism, with symbols inserted in upper row. "A" = well documented effect of age. "A⁻" = no effect of age.

Pronounced degenerative histological changes in muscle, heart and central nervous system (CNS) have been found after severe, prolonged exercise in animal experiments (Simonson, 1971). But the effect of age was not investigated. It may be expected that histological changes may be more pronounced in older animals (or men) and may occur at a lower level of work.

Since comprehensive discussion of the effect of age on the various physiological and some psychological functions in work and fatigue was recently presented (Simonson, 1971), this chapter is limited mainly to cardiovascular aspects (including some results published after 1971) and to the effect of age on anaerobic power.

Anaerobic power (i.e., performance in strenuous work exceeding max. V_{O_2} which can be maintained at this high intensity for only a few minutes) depends mainly on the energy stores (mainly glycogen) in the muscles, not so much on the absolute amount (concentration) as on the speed with which the stored energy can be liberated. The endurance time of a few minutes in anaerobic work is too short to deplete the stores of glycogen and other energy yielding substances (ATP, CP).

Robinson (1938) found in his classical, cross-sectional study that maximum lactate accumulations and maximum O_2 debt decreased with age. Similar results were obtained in women by I. Åstrand (1960). Some of Robinson's subjects could be retested after an interval of 20 to 25 years; in one of these subjects, the maximum lactate accumulation decreased from 110 to 36 mg% (D.B. Dill, 1963). D.B. Dill and B. Sacktor (1962) estimate that Dill's blood lactate exceeded 100 mg% running as a junior in high school. Twenty years later, in the Harvard Fatigue Laboratory, he could push his blood lactate to 80 mg% running on the treadmill. In 1962, at the age of 68, he could attain a high of about 40 mg%. We agree with D.B. Dill and B. Sacktor (1962) "that there is not a simple relation between the phenomena of fatigue, recovery and lactic acid accumulation and removal." The results on lactate accumulation discussed so far have been obtained in systemic blood, mostly cubital venous or capillary blood. Since during leg exercise lactate is given off by the legs and taken up by inactive muscles (arms) and splanchnic region (Harris, Bateman and Gloster, 1962), the systemic blood may not reflect the accumulation of lactate in the working legs. The crucial question of maximum lactate accumulation in the legs can be answered only by muscle biopsy (Hultman, 1967). This information is not yet available.

The upper part of Fig. 2 shows a schematic sketch of maximum lactate accumulation (in venous blood) and maximum O_2 debt and V_{O_2}. The lower part shows the increase in the maximum level of oxygen attained in a young trained man, an untrained man, an older man and a cardiac patient, typical for these categories on the basis of research of various investigators. Although the effect of age (decrease) and of training (increase) on O_2 debt and lactate are parallel, there is little correlation between these two processes. Rowell et al. (1966) found no significant correlation between the concentration of blood lactate and the size of the oxygen debt. Similar results were obtained by Bang (1936) and by Knuttgen (1962), to mention but a few of numerous studies (reviewed in Simonson, 1971). However, the decrease of maximum accumulation of both lactate and O_2 debt shows the decrease of anaerobic power with age.

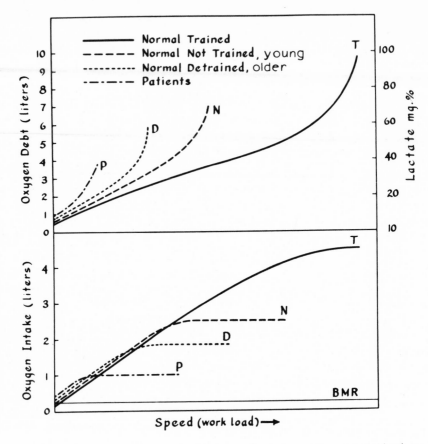

Fig. 2. Lower part: Schematic diagram of increase of oxygen and its maximum level attained in trained young men (T), average healthy young men (N), detrained or
older men (D), and heart patients (P) with increasing work load — absolute and
with reference to the basal metabolic rate (BMR). Upper part: Concomitant increase of oxygen debt (left ordinate) and blood lactate (right ordinate).

Hypothetically, this could be due to:

1. A decrease of energy stored in the muscles with age. There is no experimental
evidence for this hypothesis. The experiments with muscle biopsies of the Stockholm group (Hultman) were performed in young men. We suggested earlier that the
decrease of anaerobic power is probably not due to the absolute concentration of
glycogen and other substances in muscle.

2. A change of muscular enzyme processes with age. To our knowledge, no
experimental information for this possibility is available.

3. The inability to activate a maximum number of muscle fibers, possibly due to
central inhibition.

4. A decrease of motivation for severe exertion with age has been noted by all investigators. "It is possible to persuade almost any high school or college student to
participate...After youth, the degree of resistance increases with age. Among men in

TABLE 1

Effect Of Older Age and Heart Disease On Various Type of Performance and Related Physiologic Functions

Performance, Physiologic Functions	Age	Cardiovascular Disease
Max O_2 intake	Decreased (8)	Decreased (9)
Speed of initial increase of O_2 cons. in work	Delayed (8)	Delayed (9), (10)
Oxidative recovery	Delayed (8), (11), (26)	Delayed (9), (10)
Mechanical efficiency	Unchanged or moderately decreased at higher age (8), (12)	Unchanged or moderately decreased dependent on degree of decompensation and load (9)
Respiratory efficiency	Decreased (8), (12), (26)	Decreased (9)
Cardiac stroke volume	Decreased (13)	Decreased (9), (13)
Pulse rate recovery	Delayed (8), (26)	Delayed (9)
Endurance, moderately heavy work	Decreased (14), (15)	Decreased (9)
Endurance, static work	Unchanged (16)	Probably little change
Muscle strength	Decreased (17, (18), (19)	Unchanged or slightly decreased
Speed repet. Movements, small muscles	Slightly decreased (20)	Moderately decreased (21)
Motor coordination, small muscles	Unchanged (20), (22), (23), (24)	Probably unchanged
larger muscles	Well maintained (25), (26)	Probably little changed

(8) S. Robinson, 1938
(9) Reviewed in Simonson and Enzer, 1942
(10) Meakins and Long, 1927
(11) König et al., 1962
(12) Durnin and Mikulicic, 1956
(13) Landowne et al., 1955
(14) Dawson and Hellebrandt, 1945

(15) Burke et al., 1953
(16) Simonson et al., 1943
(17) Quetelet, 1836
(18) Rejs, 1921
(19) Fisher and Birren, 1947
(20) Kossoris, 1940
(21) Simonson and Enzer, 1941

(22) Ascher and Baumgarten, 1925
(23) Berg, 1947
(24) Stieglitz, 1941
(25) Jokl, 1954
(26) Frolkis et al., 1965
(27) Smith, 1938

Reproduced by permission from E. Simonson (1971) *Physiology of Work Capacity and Fatigue*, Charles C Thomas, Springfield, Ill.

the 7th and 8th decades, those who can be persuaded to walk, let alone run, on the treadmill are exceptional." (D.B. Dill, 1963).

These possible mechanisms are speculative. We do not know the true physiological background for the decrease of the maximum anaerobic power. Perhaps, it is a combination of these four processes.

In Table 1, the effects of age and heart disease on various types of performance and related physiological functions are compared, based on representative publications of various authors. There is a striking parallelism between the effects of older age and cardiac disease. It may be concluded that decrease of cardiovascular capacity is a major factor in the decrease of work capacity with age.

Maximum oxygen intake (max. $\dot{V}_{O_2}$) has been in the foreground of physiological research over the past two decades. It is considered to be the most fundamental determinant of maximum work capacity and, to a large degree, of the work capacity for moderately heavy work (i.e., at work loads of about 40-60 percent of max. $\dot{V}_{O_2}$). This is schematically shown in Fig. 3, based on available information (Simonson, 1965; Åstrand and Rodahl, 1970). The top of the columns indicate the level of max. $\dot{V}_{O_2}$ in trained and untrained young men, in older men and in cardiac patients. The black columns indicate "anaerobic performance" (i.e., work of such intensity that oxygen requirement exceeds the oxygen supply, limiting the endurance to only a few minutes). The energy for anaerobic work is supplied from the energy stores in the muscles (mainly glycogen), resulting in massive lactic acid accumulation. The blank columns represent moderate aerobic work levels (40% max. $\dot{V}_{O_2}$) which can be performed at a steady state of $\dot{V}_{O_2}$ and insignificant lactic acid accumulation for many hours. The stippled part of the columns represents a transi-

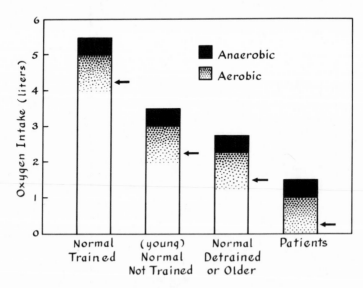

Fig. 3. Working capacity in terms of maximum oxygen intake depending on physical condition. Stippled areas show transition from aerobic to anaerobic condition. (Reproduced from Simonson, (1958) *J. Gerontol.*, Suppl. No. 2:18, "Fig. 6").

tional zone between aerobic and anaerobic work, with only partially adequate O_2 supply and endurance time of about 10 to 60 min., dependent on the level of $\dot{V}_{O_2}$ in percent of max. $\dot{V}_{O_2}$. The max. $\dot{V}_{O_2}$ increases with training and decreases with age, together with the maximum level for moderately heavy work (arrows) and for "aerobic" prolonged work. The max. $\dot{V}_{O_2}$ is lowest in a typical cardiac patient with inadequate O_2 supply even at very low work loads.

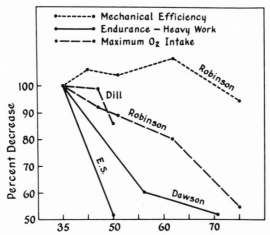

Fig. 4. Effect of age on endurance in heavy aerobic work (Dawson & Hellebrandt, 1945; Simonson, Enzer, Benton, 1943) maximum $\dot{V}_{O_2}$ (Robinson, 1938) and mechanical efficiency in moderate aerobic work (Robinson, 1938) in percent of peak performance between 30 and 40 years. (Reproduced from E. Simonson, *J. Gerontol.*, Suppl. No. 2: 13, 1958, "Fig. 5").

The decrease of max. $\dot{V}_{O_2}$ with age was first shown in the classical study by Robinson (1938) and confirmed in all later investigations. In Fig. 4, it is compared with the age trend of mechanical efficiency in moderate work and with the endurance of exhaustive work (bicycle ergometer: Dawson and Hellebrandt, 1945; running: Simonson et al., 1943). The drop of endurance in exhaustive work exceeds that of max. $\dot{V}_{O_2}$, probably because of the superimposed effect of motivation. All investigators noted that motivation to indulge in maximum effort declines with age. In contrast, mechanical efficiency in moderate work is not affected by age; even at age 75 years, the decrease of mechanical efficiency is slight.

In Fig. 5, the decrease of max. $\dot{V}_{O_2}$ with age is compared in samples with different training condition, as assembled by Hodgson (1971). While max. $\dot{V}_{O_2}$ is higher at all ages in trained subjects, the slope of the decline is not affected by training. $\dot{V}_{O_2}$ (oxygen transport) is the product of stroke volume (SV), heart rate (HR) and the arterio-venous difference of O_2 content ($\Delta A\text{-}V_{O_2}$). The $\Delta A\text{-}V_{O_2}$ in moderate and strenuous exercise does not change with age (Saltin et al., 1968). The maximum attainable SV and HR declines with age (Åstrand, 1968). Of these two functions, the drop of the max. attainable HR is functionally more important because the SV increases, with increasing work load, only up to a level of approximately 40 percent of max. $\dot{V}_{O_2}$ while HR continues to increase up to the max. $\dot{V}_{O_2}$ (Åstrand et al., 1964). Consequently, the decrease of the max. HR with age is the main reason for the decrease of max. $\dot{V}_{O_2}$ with age. There is a high correlation between max. $\dot{V}_{O_2}$ and

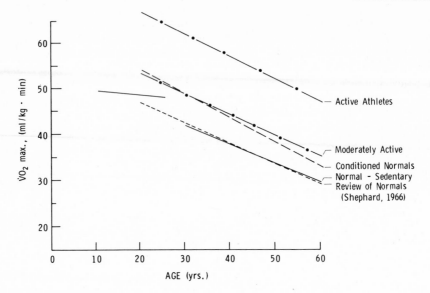

Fig. 5. Decrease of maximum $\dot{V}_{O_2}$ with age in samples with different training condition (compiled from eight studies by J. L. Hodgson, 1971).

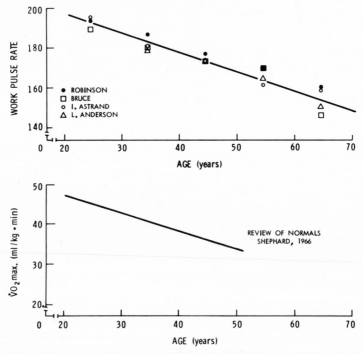

Fig. 6. Effect of age on maximum attainable work pulse rate and maximum $\dot{V}_{O_2}$ (ml/kg/min.), (compiled from results of various authors).

heart rate (see Fig. 100 in Simonson, 1971) so that max. $\dot{V}_{O_2}$ can be predicted with age correction from the heart rate with an error of about ± 15 percent (Astrand, 1969). Fig. 6 shows decrease of max. HR and max. $\dot{V}_{O_2}$ plotted from results of various authors. The reason for the decrease of the max. HR attainable in exercise is not known. It may be due to a limitation of adrenalin or noradrenalin output and corresponding sympathetic stimulation with age. Recent results by Dodek et al. (1973) suggest that a decrease of coronary blood flow with age may be involved. Aortic-coronary bypass surgery increased the max. HR attainable in a progressive exercise test from 110 before to 128 after surgery (p < 0.001) in patients with coronary insufficiency. Coronary atherosclerosis increasing with age is widespread in the majority of the population even in the absence of clinical coronary heart disease, as shown by autopsy material (Clawson, 1941; Lober, 1953).

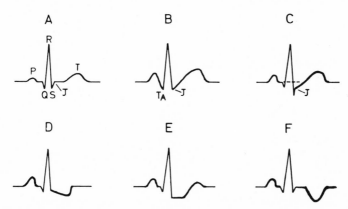

Fig. 7. Types of ST-T changes. A: normal ECG, at rest; B: false junctional ST depression resulting from atrial T wave Ta; C: true junctional ST depression. D and E: ischemic ST depression; F: isolated T wave inversion. (From Simonson, E. *Electrocardiographic stress tolerance tests.* Progress in Cardiovascular Disease, 13: 269, 1970).

The best available method for demonstration of myocardial ischemia in exercise is the "ischemic" ST segment depression in exercise, as shown in type D and E of Fig. 7. Increase of the frequency of significant "ischemic" ST depression with age in clinically healthy people was shown by various authors (Simonson, 1972). Even in moderate exercise (bicycle ergometer), the incidence increased from four percent at age 30-39 to 39 percent at age 70-79 (Strandell, 1963) and, in I. Astrand's (1969) sample of healthy men, from 10 percent below age 40 to 35 percent at age 60. Of particular interest is the comparison of ischemic-type ST depression in U.S. rail clerks (sedentary) with Italian and Yugoslavian farmers (high level of physical activity) in Table 2 (Blackburn, 1969). The absolute level as well as the age difference is most pronounced in the sedentary sample, least pronounced in the physically most active sample of Yugoslavian farmers. The incidence of coronary heart disease and presumably clinically silent atherosclerosis of coronary arteries follows this pattern.

TABLE 2

Prevalence Rates of Ischemic-type ST-T Depression
(Minn. Codes 11.1, 2, 3) in the Postexercise ECG
(None at Rest) by Age and Area
(Rates Per 1000 Men)

	Total N	Ages 40-49	Total N	Ages 50-59
U.S. rail clerks	349	59.5	498	120.1
Italian farmers (M)	369	52.5	347	65.3
Yugoslavian farmers (S)	284	28.9	415	43.2

Note: *The Ernst Simonson Conference: Measurement in Exercise Electrocardiography* (H. Blackburn, ed.)
(1969) Charles C Thomas, Springfield, Ill.

There is a high correlation between the incidence of ischemic ST depression in moderate exercise and coronary risk factors (skinfold, blood pressure, serum cholesterol) in clinically healthy men (Blackburn, 1969).

According to Gleser and Vogel (1973), the endurance (t) in work performance from 60 to 90 percent max. $\dot{V}_{O_2}$ can be predicted in young men by the equation:

$\log t = A \cdot L_r + B$, where L_r is the workload (kgm/min. bicycle ergometer) divided by max. $\dot{V}_{O_2}$

Parameters A and B are constants describing the individual's "endurance capacity" (i.e., endurance is related to the percent of max. $\dot{V}_{O_2}$). At 57 percent max. $\dot{V}_{O_2}$, the endurance time is 300 min. but is reduced to 160 min. at 62 percent max. $\dot{V}_{O_2}$ and to 55 min. at 76 percent max. $\dot{V}_{O_2}$.

An apparently high linear correlation between max. $\dot{V}_{O_2}$ and endurance (work performance) was found in middle-aged healthy women by Bruce et al. (1973), in a progressive exercise test (treadmill with progressively increasing grade and speed). Since max. $\dot{V}_{O_2}$ is reduced by age, $\dot{V}_{O_2}$ at a given moderate work level corresponds to a higher percent of max. $\dot{V}_{O_2}$. Thus, in coal miners of a body weight of 65-77 kg. at a moderate work rate of 75W (bicycle ergometer), the $\dot{V}_{O_2}$ in percent of predicted max. $\dot{V}_{O_2}$ was 38 under 40 years, increasing to 43 percent over 50 years (Henschel, 1969). Thus, the older individual worker works closer to his max. $\dot{V}_{O_2}$ (i.e., at decreased reserve capacity).

For an estimate of the allowable (that is, without undue fatigue) energy expenditure for prolonged work up to 1800 min., Bink, Bonjer and Van der Sluys (1961) proposed the equation $A_t = \log 5700 - \log t \times A_1$, where A_1 is Kcal/min. corresponding to max. $\dot{V}_{O_2}$ and A_t energy expenditure for t minutes.

At work loads under 40 percent max. $\dot{V}_{O_2}$, the endurance is limited by other factors than the oxygen transport. While exercise physiologists and clinicians have concentrated on max. $\dot{V}_{O_2}$, it must be kept in mind that all sedentary jobs and most industrial occupations are performed below the level of 40 percent max. $\dot{V}_{O_2}$. For moderate work, there is no effect of age on mechanical efficiency (Fig. 4) or $\dot{V}_{O_2}$

(Åstrand, 1969). In Henschel's (1969) investigations, elderly men and women (60-93 years) exhibited no more physiological strain working at 104 degrees F. than young people. Therefore, for moderate thermal stress and moderate work, age is not a restricting factor for tolerance (Henschel, 1969). On the other hand, respiratory oxygen utilization ($\dot{V}_{O_2}/\dot{V}_E$) decreases with age in all types of work (Simonson, 1971), suggestive of some increased strain in older people. Another limitation is the greater increase of blood pressure (Åstrand, 1968; Bruce et al., 1969), increasing cardiac work load and myocardial oxygen demand and contributing to the higher incidence of ST depression with age discussed earlier.

In this connection, it should be noted that a considerable proportion of average people probably go through life without ever engaging in efforts approaching the max. $\dot{V}_{O_2}$. Durnin (1966) substantiated this by a careful statistical study in a large group of men and women, subdivided in three age groups (young, middle-aged, older) and three relative body weight groups. The time spent in heavy (7.5 - 9.9 Keal/min.) and very heavy work (10.0 Keal) was negatively correlated to the relative body weight — in the older "thin" group 5 min. per day for very heavy work (occupational and nonoccupational) and 0.4 min. in the "plump" weight group. The total time for all weight groups in heavy work was 7 min/day in men over 45 years and 17 min./day in men from 17 to 45 years. It appears that for everyday life the capacity for moderate work is more important than the capacity for strenuous work. Cunningham et al. (1968) arrived at similar results in the analysis of leisure time activities.

There is evidence that asymptomatic cerebral atherosclerosis is as widespread as coronary atherosclerosis affecting the majority of older people (Simonson, 1964) with some correlation between these two localizations. Table 3 shows a striking parallelism between the fusion frequency of flicker (FFF) (tabulated from results of Brozek and Keys, 1945; Misiak, 1947; Simonson and Brozek, 1952; Coppinger, 1955) and the decrease of cerebral blood flow (Kety, 1955) with age. This is not necessarily a causal relationship, but implies that decrease of cerebral blood flow is

TABLE 3

Changes of Cerebral Blood Flow and Flicker Fusion
Frequency with Age

Function	Average* At Age					
	20	30	40	50	60	70
Cerebral blood flow (Kety, 1955)	60.0	-6	-10	-12	-14	-16
Flicker fusion frequency	46.0	-1.3	- 2.8	- 4.5	- 5.8	- 9.0

*Average of various authors. Simonson et al., 1941; Brozek and Keys, 1945; Misiak, 1947; Simonson and Brozek, 1952; Coppinger, 1955.

most likely involved in performance depending on the integrity of the CNS. The FFF has been used in numerous fatigue studies.

The FFF (flicker fusion frequency) is that rate of flashes where, with increasing flash frequency, the sensation of flicker disappears and becomes that of plain light. It is related to the time parameter of excitability of the visual center and probably that of the CNS in general. Simonson, Enzer and Benton (1943) found a significant drop of the FFF in middle-aged men after running to exhaustion. The decrease of the FFF is not specific, but since it is also depressed in hypoxia (reviewed by Simonson and Brozek, 1952), it is logical to assume it indicates cerebral ischemia. Observations of amnesia in strenuous athletic exercise (for example, running) strongly suggest cerebral ischemia. While the effect of age has not been specifically studied, cerebral ischemia in strenuous exercise is probably more pronounced in older people, due to asymptomatic cerebral atherosclerosis increasing in frequency and degree with age.

REFERENCES

Ascher, L. and Baumgarten, P. (1925) *Vëroff Med Verwalt* 19, 487.

Åstrand, I. (1969) Electrocardiographic changes in relation to the type of exercise, the work load and sex, in *The Ernst Simonson Conference: Measurement in Exercise Electrocardiography* (H. Blackburn, ed.) Charles C Thomas, Springfield, Ill.

Åstrand, I. (1960) *Acta Physiol Scand* Suppl. 169, 49, 1.

Åstrand, P.-O. (1968) *JAMA* 205, 729.

Åstrand, P.-O., Cuddy, B., Saltin, B., and Stenberg, J. (1964) *J Appl Physiol* 19, 268.

Åstrand, P.-O. and Rodahl, K. (1970) *Textbook of Work Physiology*, McGraw-Hill, New York.

Bang, O. (1936) *Scand Arch Physiol* 74 (Suppl. 10), 51.

Berg, W.E. (1947) *Am J Physiol* 149, 597.

Bink, B., Bonjer, F.H., and Van der Sluys, H. (1961) *T Eff Doc* 31, 526.

Blackburn, H. (1969) The exercise electrocardiogram. In *The Ernst Simonson Conference: Measurement in Exercise Electrocardiography* (H. Blackburn, ed.), Charles C Thomas, Springfield, Ill.

Brozek, J. and Keys, A. (1945) *J Consult Psychol* 9, 87.

Bruce, R.A., Kusami, F., and Hosmer, D. (1973) *Am Heart J* 85, 546.

Burke, W.E., Tuttle, W.W., Thompson, C.W., Janney, D.C., and Weber, R.J. (1953) *J Appl Physiol* 5, 628.

Clawson, B.J. (1941) *Am Heart J* 22, 607.

Coppinger, N.W. (1955) *J Gerontol* 10, 48.

Cunningham, D.A., Montoye, H.J., Metzner, H.L., and Keller, J.B. (1968) *J Gerontol* 23, 551.

Dawson, P.M. and Hellebrandt, F.A. (1945) *Am J Physiol* 143, 420.

Dill, D.B. (1963) *Pediatrics* 32 (Suppl.) 737.

Dill, D.B., and Sacktor, B. (1962) *J Sport Med* 2, 66.

Dodek, A., Kassebaum, D.G. and Griswold, H.E. (1973) *Am Heart J* 86, 292.

Durnin, J.V. and Mikulicic, V. (1956) *Quart J Exp Physiol* 41, 442.

Durnin, J.V. (1966) *Proc Nutr Soc* 25, 107.

Fischer, M.B., and Birren, J. (1947) *J Appl Psychol* 31, 490.

Frolkis, V.V., Golovchenko, S.F., Dukhovichnyi, S.M., and Tanin, S.A. (1962) *Klin Med* 40, 87 (Russ.).

Gleser, M.A., and Vogel, J.A. (1973) *J Appl Physiol* 34, 443.

Harris, B., Bateman, M., and Gloster, J. (1962) *Clin Sci* 23, 545.

Henschel, A. (1969) *Age and Heat Tolerance*, Report to Office of Civil Defense.

Hodgson, J.L. (1971) Age and aerobic capacity of urban midwestern males. Thesis. University of Minnesota.

Hultman, E. (1967) *Scand J Clin Lab Invest* Suppl. 94, 19, 1.

Jokl, E. (1954) *Alter and Leistung*, Springer-Verlag, Berlin.

Kety, S.S. (1955) In Waelsch, H. *Bio-chemistry of the Developing Nervous System*. Academic Press, New York.

Knuttgen, H.G. (1962) *J Appl Physiol* 17, 639.

König, K., Reindell, H., and Roskamm, H. (1962) *Arch Kreislaufforsch* 39, 143.

Kossoris, M.D. (1940) *Monthly Labor Review* 51, 789.

Lober, P.H. (1953) *Arch Path* 55, 357.

Landowne, M., Brandfonbrener, M., and Shock, N.W. (1955) *Circulation* 12, 567.

Meakins, J. and Long, C.N.A. (1927) *J Clin Invest* 4, 273.

Misiak, H. (1947) *J Exp Psychol* 37, 318.

Quetelet, A. (1836) *Sur L'Homme et le Development de ses Facultés*, L. Hauman and Cie, Brussels.

Rejs, J.H.O. (1921) *Arch Ges Physiol* 191, 234.

Robinson, S. (1938) *Arbeitsphysiol* 10, 251.

Rowell, L.B., Kraning, K.K., II, Evans, T.O., et al. (1966) *J Appl Physiol* 21, 1773.

Saltin, B., Blomquist, G., Mitchell, J., et al. (1968) *Response to Exercise After Bedrest and After Training*, Monograph No. 23, American Heart Association, New York.

Simonson, E. (1964) In Simonson, E. and McGavack, T. *Cerebral Ischemia*, Charles C Thomas, Springfield, Ill.

Simonson, E. (1965) Performance as a function of age and cardiovascular disease *Behavior, Aging and the Nervous System,* (A.T. Welford and J.E. Birren, eds.), Charles C Thomas, Springfield, Ill.

Simonson, E. (ed.) (1971) *Physiology of Work Capacity and Fatigue*, Charles C Thomas, Springfield, Ill.

Simonson, E. (1972) *Am J Cardiol* 29, 64.

Simonson, E., and Anderson, D. (1966) Effect of age and coronary heart disease on performance and physiological responses in mental work, Proceed 7th Internat Congress of Gerontol.

Simonson, E., and Brozek, J. (1952) *Physiol Rev* 32, 349.

Simonson, E., and Enzer, N. (1941) *Arch Intern Med* 68, 498.

Simonson, E., Enzer, N., and Benton, R.W. (1943) *J Lab Clin Med* 38, 1555.

Simonson, E., and Enzer, N. (1942) *Medicine* 21, 345.

Simonson, E., Enzer, N., and Blankstein, S. (1941) *J Exp Psychol* 29, 252.

Simonson, E., Kearns, W.M., and Enzer, N. (1944) *J Clin Endocrinol Metab* 4, 528.

Smith, K.R. (1938) *J Appl Psychol* 22, 295.

Strandell, T. (1963) *Acta Med Scand* 174, 479.

Steiglitz, E. J. (1941) *JAMA* 116, 1383.

A Follow-Up Study of the Effect of Physical Activity on the Decline of Working Capacity and Maximal O_2 Consumption in the Senescent Male

Andrew A. Fischer
Jana Parizkova

INTRODUCTION

In a previous paper, investigation was made into the maximum physical performance capacity and maximum oxygen consumption, as well as their relation to lean body mass and other functional parameters, in men in the seventh and eighth decade of life (Fischer et al., 1965). The effect of aging has been ascertained by comparison of results obtained in age groups of different decades. Physically active and inactive persons in the same decades have been evaluated in order to assess the influence of engagement in recreational exercises.

The present study deals with the results obtained by retesting all the subjects available from the previous investigation and covers a period of four years.

MATERIAL AND METHODS

Eighty-six sedentary males were reinvestigated. Statistical evaluation was made over a period of two years, since the second two years of the four year follow-up period rendered no statistically conclusive material, due to the decrease in the number of subjects. As in the previous study, subjects were selected who revealed no significant pathological conditions on clinical and functional examination, including lung function tests. The physically active group consisted of sedentary subjects who had been involved in systematic recreational sport activities of various types throughout their lives up to the time of the present investigation. The physically inactive group similarly included sedentary subjects without pathological findings, but who were distinguished from the physically active group only by their lack of involvement in any exercise.

A detailed description of the method used for measurement of maximum oxygen consumption was given in the previous communication (Fischer et al., 1965). The investigation was conducted under basal conditions in the morning. The difference between the oxygen and CO_2 content in the inspired and expired air was recorded continuously by an automatic analyzer, using the paramagnetic principle for O_2 and heat conduction-analyzer for CO_2. The analyzers were systematically calibrated by an interpherometer. The respiratory volume was recorded continuously and automatically from a gasometer attached to the inspiratory valve. The subject exhaled into a mixing vessel from which automatic samples of expired air were continually drawn into the analyzer. The mask worn had an inflated rubber base covering the nose and mouth; low resistent mica valves were used with a rubber tube of 12.5 mm diameter. A calibrated bicycle ergometer with an electric brake was used and the rate of cycling recorded continuously. A spirogram using pressure from the mask proved to be useful.

An electrocardiogram using a forehead electrode against the apex was monitored continuously on an oscilloscope and the pulse rate was taken twice per minute for 15 seconds. The ventilation volume and maximum oxygen consumption are expressed in STPD.

The lean body mass was determined by hydrostatic weighing (Brozek et al., 1949) in the modification of Parizkova (1965). The Duncan test has been used for evaluation of differences. The brackets denote significance at a 5 percent level and ± denotes the limits of reliability to 95 percent (i.e. = T.SX for the average of the group).

In our experience the following method proved to render the best results for maximum oxygen consumption determination in elderly subjects. After approximately five minutes of adaptation to the mask, resting values were measured over a period of five minutes while the subject remained seated on the bike. Exercise was started with a 50 watt load per minute for the first three minutes. The rate of cycling was maintained at a constant 70 rpm during the entire test. After the third minute, the resistance was increased by 30 watts every following minute, until the subject demonstrated exhaustion.

The experimental groups were designated by the letters N, denoting the nonactive subjects, and T (standing for trained), for the physically active groups. The suffixes 7 and 8 represent the decade in life respectively.

RESULTS

Table 1 and Figure 1 demonstrate the distribution of subjects in the four groups, their age, body weight and lean body mass in percentage of body weight. The N7 (i.e., non-active subjects in the seventh decade) included 31 persons and T7 (i.e., the physically active subjects in the seventh decade) included 28 men. The N8 group (i.e., non-active in the eighth decade) were represented by nine, and the T8 (i.e., physically active in the eighth decade) consisted of 18 men. Figures indicate initial values in the form of columns for each group. Changes after two years are represented as signs following each column.

The age distribution of the physically active and control groups were virtually the same for each decade. There were no differences in body weight or lean body mass in percentage of body weight between the examined groups.

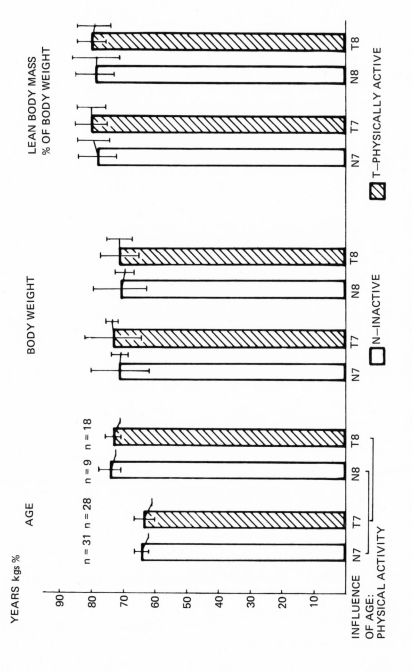

Fig. 1. Longitudinal study changes in two years.

ANDREW A. FISCHER AND JANA PARIZKOVA

TABLE 1

Distribution of Subjects According to Age, Body Weight, and Lean Body Mass in Percentage of Body Weight

Groups	Number of subjects	Age	Body weight		L.B.M. % of weight	
			Initial value	Change	Initial value	Change
N 7	31	64.13	71.32	-0.22	78.31	+1.13
σ =		±2.31	±9.23	±2.39	±5.75	±4.97
T 7	28	63.39	73.10	+0.35	80.06	-0.13
σ =		±3.09	±9.32	±1.86	±5.24	±4.53
N 8	9	73.89	70.45	-1.28	78.5	-0.16
σ =		±3.54	±8.13	±2.94	±5.7	±7.48
T 8	18	73.28	71.30	+0.398	80.29	0.61
σ =		±2.6	±6.43	±3.91	±4.57	±5.39

Figure 2 and Table 2 demonstrate well the decrease of maximum performance (expressed in watts) in the eighth decade as compared with the achievements in the seventh decade in both the N and T groups. Statistically, significantly lower values were noted in the N8 group than in the N7 group under the initial evaluation as well as after the two-year period. However, the magnitude of the decrease in maximum physical performance (expressed in watts), after two years, was practically the same in the N as well as in the T group. Otherwise, the decline in maximum physical performance ran parallel in the physically active and nonactive groups and demonstrated no statistically significant difference. The relation of maximum watts achieved to the maximum oxygen consumption can be regarded as an index of efficiency of the use of aerobically produced energy. It is evident from Figure 2 and Table 2 that the relation Max Watts/Max $\dot{V}_{O_2}$ demonstrates no significant differences in initial values of the four groups. Changes after two years are not significant either in any of the four groups.

The maximum oxygen uptake was significantly higher in the physically active groups in the seventh as well as in the eighth decade. The decline of max $\dot{V}_{O_2}$ after two years was significant in all groups except for N8 where only nine subjects were included. It is important to notice that the decline of maximum O_2 uptake runs parallel in all groups and there are no significant differences between the active and nonactive groups in the decrease of aerobic capacity in the two-year period (see Table 2.

Essentially the same picture is represented by the maximum $\dot{V}_{O_2}$ uptake related to lean body mass (Fig. 3 and Table 3). The physically active groups demonstrated again a high maximum $\dot{V}_{O_2}$/LBM. The differences in initial values are significant in the eighth decade and present but not significant in the seventh decade because of relatively higher lean body mass in the T7 group (Table 3 middle and Fig. 3). The decline in Max $\dot{V}_{O_2}$ /LBM was again significant in all groups except N8, where only nine subjects were included. No significant differences were noted between the rate of decline of this index in the four groups investigated.

The maximum O_2 pulse again demonstrated higher initial values in the physically active group of both decades, statistically significant in the eighth decade. Changes after two years in max O_2 pulse were significant only in N7 group.

Comparison of the indices investigated allows the following conclusions:

1) The difference between initial values in seventh and eighth decade and the changes in the two-year period of follow-up expresses the trends of the age changes in each function measured.

2) The change of a parameter in two years represents rate of age changes in different decades in physically active and inactive groups respectively.

3) By comparison of the results obtained in the physically active and inactive groups of corresponding age, the effect of physical activity on the investigated parameters can be established in each age group respectively.

4) Differences between the two years' changes of a parameter in the physically active and the inactive control group represent the influence of physical activity on the rate of age changes.

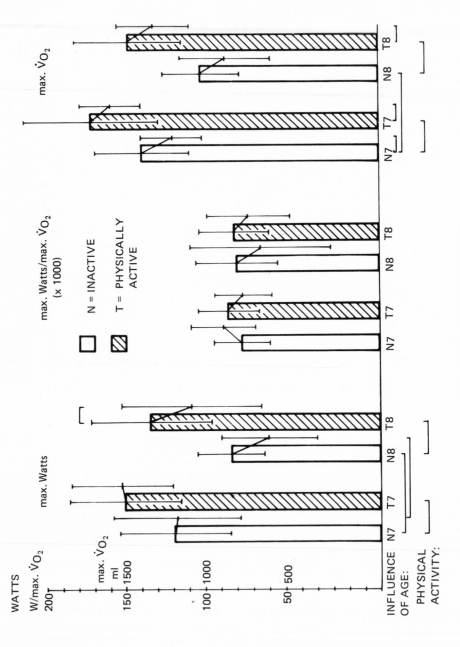

Fig. 2. Changes in maximal performance.

TABLE 2

Changes in Maximum Performance

Groups	Max. watts		Max. watts/max. V_{O_2}		Max. O_2 uptake		Max. V_{O_2} Change in %
	Initial values	Change	Initial value	Change	Initial value	Change	
N 7	129.3	-1.18	0.085	+0.011	1504	-193.7	+2.66
	±34.7	±39.5	±0.018	±0.020	±298.7	±193.7	±17.52
T 7	161.93	+1.96	0.095	-0.0095	1733	-120.2	+3.96
	±35.16	±32.92	±0.019	±0.0187	±43.51	±195.9	±0.95
N 8	94.12	-22.88	0.090	-0.015	1128	-158.86	-20.16
	94.12	-22.88	0.090	-0.015	1128	-158.86	-20.16
	±21.25	±30.73	±0.026	±0.044	±240.15	±281.20	±30.55
T 8	144.5	-26.22	0.092	-0.008	1591	-158.28	18.40
	±38.2	±29.4	±0.022	±0.026	±339.2	±226.04	±22.17

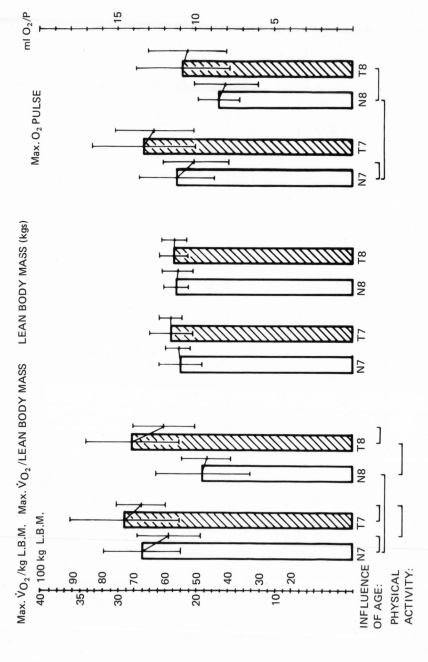

Fig. 3. Relationship of maximum $\dot{V}_{O_2}$ to lean body mass.

TABLE 3

Relationship of Maximum $\dot{V}O_2$ Uptake to Lean Body Mass

Groups	Max. $\dot{V}O_2$/LBM (kgs)		Lean Body Mass (kgs)		Max. O_2 pulse	
	Initial value	Change	Initial value	Change	Initial value	Change
N 7	27.05	-3.61	55.65	+0.70	11.23	-1.04
σ =	±5.29	±4.19	±6.78	±3.80	±2.40	±2.16
T 7	29.27	2.12	58.15	+0.4407	13.16	-0.5756
σ =	±6.97	±3.27	±6.87	±3.7391	±3.33	±2.5858
N 8	9.347	-0.698	55.01	-1.0556	8.46	-0.4088
σ =	±6.09	±3.78	±4.47	±4.75	±1.30	±2.0843
T 8	28.30	-4.094	56.85	-0.068	10.76	-0.2818
σ =	±6.14	±4.14	±4.57	±3.95	±2.96	±2.50

Figure 1 and Table 1 demonstrate clearly that all four groups are comparable, since there is no significant difference in their age, body weight and composition. Therefore, the results of functional evaluations are comparable in all four groups. There was no significant change in the body weight or LBM during the two years of follow-up.

DISCUSSION

Maximum Watts

The known decline of maximum physical performance (max. W) during aging is evident from lower values in the eighth decade as compared with the seventh decade in all groups (Fig. 2). The significantly higher performance of the physically active group in both decades investigated confirms our previous findings (Fischer et al., 1965). The rate of decrease in max. W after two years ran parallel in physically active and inactive groups and did not differ significantly.

The Mechanism of Decrease in Maximum Performance in Senescent Subjects

Two basic mechanisms can be involved in the decrease of physical performance on a bike ergometer during aging: (1) Restriction of energy production and/or (2) A decrease in conversion of energy into mechanical work. This process can be essentially estimated from the ratio between the max W to the max O_2 uptake.

No significant differences were detected in the ratio max W/max O_2 uptake. The two-year changes were not significant either, although a trend of decline can be noticed.

The conclusion can be drawn that the decrease of maximum physical performance in the age range investigated is due mainly to limitation in energy production (max O_2 uptake). This is evident also from comparison of max $\dot{V}_{O_2}$ in groups with different levels of performance. Similar to the age decrease of the max W, a significantly lower max $\dot{V}_{O_2}$ was found in N8 than in N7; the higher performance of both physically active groups is connected with a higher max $\dot{V}_{O_2}$. The two-year changes of max $\dot{V}_{O_2}$ ran parallel with decrease in max Watts.

Maximum Oxygen Uptake

The maximum O_2 uptake demonstrated the most impressive changes of all functions measured. The decrease in max V_{O_2} was statistically significant in all groups but N8, in which nine subjects were investigated.

The higher maximum V_{O_2} in physically active subjects as compared to the controls of same age is evident (Fig. 2). This confirms our previous conclusion (Fischer et al., 1965) that systematic exercise of sufficient intensity and duration can maintain aerobic capacity on a relatively higher level even in the eighth decade.

The changes in max V_{O_2} during the two-year period are of particular interest as the average decrease in the index was virtually identical in all four groups. This means that the decrease in aerobic capacity during aging ran parallel in physically active and inactive subjects. The conclusion can be drawn that the rate of age decrease in aerobic capacity in the seventh and eighth decades has not been influenced by systematic physical activity. The same applies for maximum physical working capacity. The higher physical performance and higher aerobic capacity detected in our physically active subjects as compared to inactive controls of the same age has been, therefore, achieved by proper exercising at a younger age and has been maintained only by systematic activity up to the end of this study.

A question of fundamental significance is the mechanisms of the age decrease of maximal O_2 uptake, which expresses the involution of functional capacity of the organism. The decrease of max V_{O_2} with age could be caused: 1) by loss of metabolically active (lean) body mass or 2) by decreased maximal O_2 consumption per each unit of lean body mass (LBM).

Figure 3 (in middle) shows that there are no significant differences in absolute values of LBM in kgs between the four groups and no change in LBM occurred in the course of two years. But the max V_{O_2} in relation to kg LBM (Fig. 3 left) is significantly lower in N8 than N7 and decreases significantly over a two-year period in all groups except N8 (nine subjects). This proves that the main mechanism underlying the decrease of aerobic capacity in senescence is the decreased maximum oxygen uptake of each unit of metabolically active tissue, while the loss of LBM plays no essential role in this process.

The max V_{O_2}/LBM is significantly higher in physically active subjects than in controls (see end-values after two years in the seventh decade and initial values in the eighth decade). Therefore, the higher maximum O_2 uptake and performance of physically active persons are preserved in senescence by postponing the age decrease of maximal tissue metabolism. Higher max V_{O_2}/LBM have been found in young athletes as well (Buskirk and Taylor, 1958; Sprynarova, 1960). The maximal O_2 uptake of metabolically active tissue could be limited: (1) primarily by the metabolic processes in the tissue itself or (2) secondarily by limited transport capacity of circulation.

Maximum Oxygen Pulse

The maximum O_2 pulse (max O_2 pulse), which represents the transport capacity of a heart beat for oxygen, decreases in a similar manner as the max O_2/LBM. It decreases significantly from the seventh to eighth decade in control groups, and also after two years in N7. In our previous study, a good correlation has been found between max V_{O_2}/LBM on one hand and the max O_2 pulse on the other ($r = .7$, $n = 82$). The two-year decrease of max O_2/LBM is in lower but still significant correlation with the lowering of max O_2 pulse ($r = +.3956$, $.05 > p > .01$. $y = 2.27 + .82$). The parallel decline of maximum O_2 pulse and max V_{O_2}/LBM proves that the restricted oxygen transport capacity of circulation can be a limiting factor of maximum tissue metabolism in senescent subjects. The maximum O_2 pulse was higher in the physically active groups as compared to controls and the difference was statistically significant in the eighth decade.

Functional changes in other organs precede morphological involution during aging. Age changes of the stabile component of arterial wall structure are similarly preceded by increased blood pressure (Fischer, 1966).

It can generally be concluded that morphological age changes are preceded by functional limitation in the corresponding organ. The aging process, especially the functional involution of the organism and/or special organ is, therefore, not a simple consequence of morphological loss or morphological changes of tissue. On the contrary, functional involution is a primary process and the morphological involution is a secondary one, probably a consequence of the former. Aging, therefore, represents a process of tissue change with can be postponed by preserving the functional capacity of organs and organisms on an adequate level.

CONCLUSION

Eighty-six men in the seventh and eighth decade of life who were included in our previous paper (Fischer et al., 1965), were reinvestigated after two years. All subjects were sedentary, felt healthy and failed to demonstrate significant pathological findings in clinical investigation. Thirty-six of the investigated subjects carried out systematic recreational sports and physical exercise of various types throughout their lives. The control group consisted of subjects of corresponding age and comparable body weight and composition, but who failed to engage themselves in any remarkable physical exercise. Maximum performance and maximum O_2 uptake (max V_{O_2}) were established on a bicycle ergometer, and lean body mass (LBM) ascertained.

Statistical analysis of changes during the two years of follow-up in the same subjects confirmed the conclusions on mechanisms of changes in physical performance as well as aerobic capacity, which formerly had been made by comparison of different subjects in each decade. They were:

1) The main mechanism of decrease in physical performance on cycling in the elderly is the restricted capacity of energy production. This was evident from parallel decrease in max W and max V_{O_2} while the utilization of energy expressed by the ratio max W/max V_{O_2} did not change significantly during the follow-up period.

2) Maximum O_2 uptake decreased significantly in two years but LBM was preserved without change. It is evident, therefore, that: a) the maximum metabolic rate declines with age and this leads to limitation of max V_{O_2} and b) decrease in functional capacity of the organism precedes the morphological involution of tissues. Therefore, the functional involution during aging is the primary process while morphological involution is secondary. The implication is possible that, by maintaining the functional capacity of an organ, morphological changes induced by aging and inactivity could possibly be postponed.

3) The max $\dot{V}_{O_2}$/LBM, expressing the decline of maximum metabolic rate with age, decreases parallel with max O_2 pulse. Decrease in the transport capacity of the cardiovascular system for O_2 could be, therefore, one of the limiting factors of maximum tissue metabolism in senescence.

4) Physically active subjects are characterized by a higher performance and larger max V_{O_2} in relation to weight and LBM. Systematic physical activity can maintain a higher performance capacity up to the eighth decade by preserving a greater aerobic

capacity and a higher level of maximum tissue metabolism.

5) The rate of decline in performance, max V_{O_2} and max $\dot{V}_{O_2}$/LBM in the course of two years ran parallel in both physically active and control groups. Physical activity, thus, did not influence the rate of the age decrease of performance and aerobic capacity; it preserved a higher level of these parameters, which had already been achieved at a younger age.

ACKNOWLEDGEMENT: The tests for this study were performed at the Research Institute for Physical Culture in Prague, Czechoslovakia.

REFERENCES

Brozek, J., Henschel, A., and Keys, A. (1949) *J Appl Physiol* 5, 240.

Buskirk, E., and Taylor, H. L. (1957) *J Appl Physiol* 11, 72.

Fischer, A., Parizkova, J., and Roth, Z. (1965) *Int Z Angew Physiol einschl Arbeitphysiol.* 21, 209.

Fischer, A., Parizkova, J. and Roth, Z. (1966) 7th Inter Congr of Gerontol, Vienna.

Parizkova, J. (1965) Physical activity and body composition, in *Body Composition, Proceedings of the Conference for the Study of Human Biology*, Pergamon Press Oxford, Eng., p. 161.

Sprynarova, S. (1960) *Cs Fysiol* 9, 270.

The Effect of Aging and Physical Activity on the Stabile Component of Arterial Distensibility

Andrew A. Fischer, M.D.

INTRODUCTION

Arterial distensibility can be expressed by pressure-volume (P-V) curves of the limb arteries. The P-V curves of an artery depend on two components:

1. The elastic properties of the arterial wall, which depend on its composition (i.e., on the relation of collagen to elastic fibers) (Roach and Burton, 1957).
2. The state of contraction of the musculature in the arterial wall (i.e., arterial tone) which can modify the P-V curve.

Changes in the arterial tone induce instant shifts in P-V curves, while the first component related to the structure of arterial walls is stabile (i.e., demonstrates no change unless the composition of the wall is altered).

The P-V curves of human iliac arteries in vitro demonstrate an exponential-like character (Roach and Burton, 1959) and similar curves can be obtained by in vivo measurements of extremities (Gomez, 1941; Ipser, 1935; Landowne, 1958a, 1958b; Moret, 1964; Plesch, 1947; Roach and Burton, 1957).

J. Ipser introduced the measurement of the "Damping Coefficient (D.C.) of arterial distensibility" (1960, 1935 and 1956) which expresses the curvature of the P-V relation (i.e., the decrease in distensibility of the arterial P-V curves for an increment of intra-arterial pressure by 10 mm Hg).

The D.C. has two interesting characteristics:

1. The D.C. expresses the stabile component of arterial distensibility, since neither physiologically nor pharmacologically induced short term changes in arterial tone alter its values.
2. Long term changes of blood pressure induce adoptive alteration in D.C. Hypertension increases the D.C. (i.e., decreases the stabile component of arterial distensibility). Hypotensive subjects develop a lower D.C. than normotensives. D.C. expresses, therefore, the pressure load acting upon the arterial wall to which the structure of the vessel adapts itself.

81

The present study deals with the changes of the Damping Coefficient of arterial distensibility during aging and with the effects of systematic physical activity.

METHODS

Using the method described by J. Ipser (1960, 1935 and 1956), a calibrated electronic volume oscillograph was constructed for recording of pulse volumes of the arm. A cuff served as pick-up, and a volume transducer of a strain gauge type converted the volume changes into electric current in order to record them on a polygraph. The pulse volumes were recorded at different cuff pressures which induced changes in the transmural pressure. Transmural pressure equals the difference between the intra-arterial pressure and the outside pressure encased in the cuff surrounding the limb.

A pressure-volume curve of the pulsating arteries called an oscillogram can be constructed from the known values of transmural pressures and from volume pulsations of the extremity (Gomez, 1941; Ipser, 1935, 1956; Plesch, 1947) or recorded automatically (Fig. 1).

P-V curves of arteries obtained in vivo follow an exponential trend in that the volume change (dV) can be expressed by the equation $dV = Eo. KP$, where Eo = initial distensibility (i.e., the volume change of the artery induced by an increase of intra-arterial pressure from 0 to 10 mm Hg).

"K" represents the "Damping Coefficient" of the pressure-volume curve and indicates the "damping" (i.e., decrease of distensibility (dV/dP) of the artery for an increase of intra-arterial pressure by 10 mm Hg).

Expressed in graphical presentation, the P-V curve of arteries decreases exponentially (i.e., curves toward the pressure axis) because the distensibility is decreased (damped) at higher pressures. The D.C. so expresses the curvature of the P-V curve.

Fig. 2 represents curvatures calculated for different D.C. Superimposing the oscillograms over these theoretically calculated curves, the D.C. of an individual can be established. The part of the oscillogram recorded at pressures between zero and diastolic pressure is used for this purpose, since this segment represents a mirror image of the P-V curve (Ipser, 1960, 1935).

The Duncan Test has been used for evaluation of differences. Brackets on Fig. 3 represent statistical significance on p .05 level.

MATERIAL

The first part of this study included 121 subjects. Physically active sedentary males, denoted as T (trained group), were compared with physically inactive controls, denoted as N, in the third and seventh decade of life. The suffix at each letter denoting the state of physical activity expresses the decade of life; N_{III} stands for non-active subjects in the third decade, $T_{V II}$ represents physically active (trained) persons in the seventh decade of life, etc.

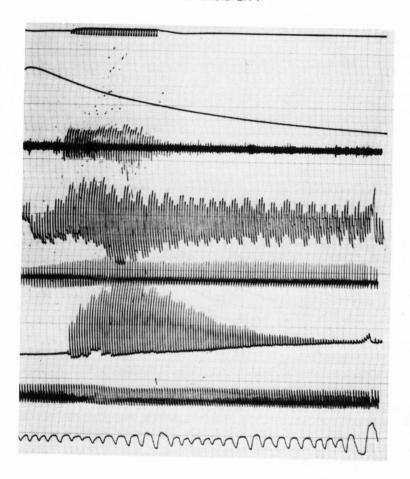

Fig. 1. Automatically recorded oscillogram and blood pressure in arm.

Channel 1. Electronically conditioned signal from a pick up in the cuff. The start of signals represents the systolic blood pressure. The signals stop at the diastolic blood pressure. Cuff pressure can be determined on channel 2.

Channel 2. Cuff pressure.

Channel 3. Korotkoff's sounds recorded by an electronic stethoscope. Note the correspondence of systolic and diastolic blood pressure with electronic signals recorded on channel 1.

Channel 4. Impedance plethysmogram of the arms.

Channel 5. First derivative (velocity) of the IPG record presented on channel 4.

Channel 6. Arterial oscillogram. Note the exponential-like decrease of volume pulsations between diastolic and 0 pressure in the cuff.

Channel 7. Second derivative of channel 4.

Channel 8. Record of respiration.

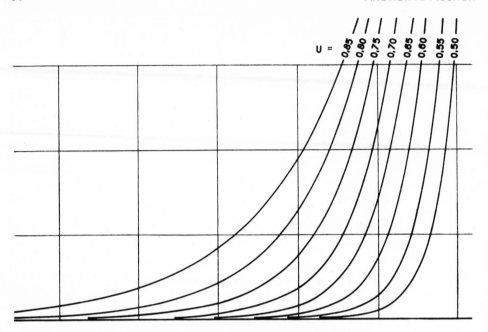

Fig. 2. Curvatures calculated for different D.C. (See text). Abscissa — pressure; ordinate — volume.

All subjects under study (except for 14 hypertensives in the third decade) felt healthy and failed to show essential pathological findings on clinical and functional evaluation. The physically active group in the third decade consisted of 27 top level athletes engaged in different types of light athletics. The physically active group in the seventh decade included 35 males who had been involved in various types of recreational sport activities throughout their lives. The N groups consisted of 30 subjects in the third decade and 29 in the seventh decade.

Table 1 demonstrates that the average age of the T and control (N) group is comparable in both the third and seventh decade.

The second part of this study deals with the diurnal changes in B.P. and pulse rate and their relation to D.C. in two groups of young athletes (16 years old). The first group consisted of nine boys who had been participants in strenuous athletic training for one year. The second group consisted of 17 boys who had two years of athletic training in the same school for young athletes.

RESULTS

Effect of Aging Upon Damping Coefficient of Arterial Distensibility

The effect of aging upon the D.C. is evaluated on Fig. 3 and Table 1.

The D.C. demonstrates a significant increase in the seventh decade, as compared with the third decade, in both control and physically active groups. The D.C. equaled $.696 \pm .013$ in N_{III} and $.57 \pm .081$ in T_{III} group, increased to $.82 \pm .027$ in

TABLE 1

Subject Groups and Hemodynamic Data

| Decade Group | Physical Activity | Age Years | Blood Pressure | | | | Damping Coefficient | Pulse Rate | Mean BP/DC |
			Systolic	Diastolic	Counted Mean			
3rd N III	Inactive 30	23.2 +2.17	118.8 ± 7.9	74.6 +9.1	88.9 ± 7.3	0.696 ± 0.013	73.5 ± 9.6	139 ±1 10.1
3rd T III	Active 27	22.8 ± 3.94	120.1 ± 10.7	76.4 ± 8.7	90.5 ± 7.8	0.57 ± 0.081	63.9 ± 9.8	168.3 ± 33
7th N VII	Inactive 29	67.3 ± 7.21	161 ± 20.4	101 ± 21.7	109.6 ± 14.4	0.82 ± 0.0272	73.3 ± 6.3	134.4 ± 20.51
7th T VII	Active 35	68.9 ± 5.65	153.7 ± 23.0	90.7 ± 12.3	111.9 ± 14.1	0.785 ± 0.064	69 ± 6.6	142.6 ± 19.97

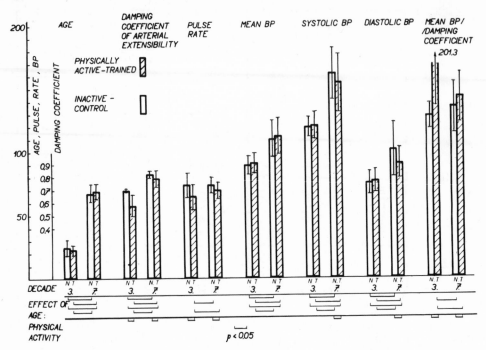

Fig. 3. Effects of aging and physical activity on Damping Coefficient (See text).

$N_{V\,II}$ and $.785 \pm .064$ in $T_{V\,II}$. The differences between third and seventh decade values are statistically significant (see Fig. 3).

The age increase in D.C. is connected with a statistically significant increase in systolic and diastolic B.P. and mean B.P. The latter has been calculated from diastolic pressure plus one-third of pulse pressure.

The ratio of mean B.P./D.C. demonstrates no significant change by aging in the control groups. The pulse rate of N groups was the same in the third and seventh decade.

Effect of Physical Activity Upon Damping Coefficient of Arterial Distensibility

The D.C. is statistically significantly lower in physically active groups in both decades of life. The lowest values for D.C. were found in physically active subjects in the third decade $(.57 \pm .081)$. The controls of same age demonstrated higher values $.696 \pm .013)$, the difference being statistically highly significant (see Fig. 6).

Similarly, the physically active group in the seventh decade was distinguished by relatively lower D.C. $(.785 \pm .064)$ as compared to the controls of the same age $(.82 \pm .027)$, $p < .001$ (see Fig. 6).

There was no significant difference between the mean blood pressure of the T and N groups. The systolic and diastolic pressures were significantly lower in the T group of the seventh decade as compared to controls, but no differences were noted in the third decade (Fig 3).

The mean B.P./D.C. ratio was significantly higher in the T groups in both decades as compared to the controls. The heart rate was significantly lower in T groups than in controls, in both decades (Fig. 3).

Analysis of individual data can be done on Fig. 4 which represents a correlation between the mean B.P. (calculated as diastolic plus one-third of pulse pressure) and the D.C. in five groups of individuals.

Since the normal value of B.P. in the third decade is 120/80, the mean B.P. is denoted by the vertical line at 93 mm Hg. The horizontal line expresses a D.C. = .7 which is the normal value in the third decade. The circled signs represent averages of groups. Circles denote subjects in the third decade and triangles denote the seventh decade. Filled-in circles and triangles represent physically active groups and open signs indicate controls.

The average of the N_{III} group falls in the middle of the cross. A shift to the right on the pressure axis represents hypertensives and increased pressure load as it is expressed by the calculated mean B.P. A shift to the left expresses hypotension.

The area above the horizontal line of normal values represents increased D.C. This is the case in physically inactive hypertensives (denoted by +) in whom the high pressure load induced an increase in D.C., shifting the values upward.

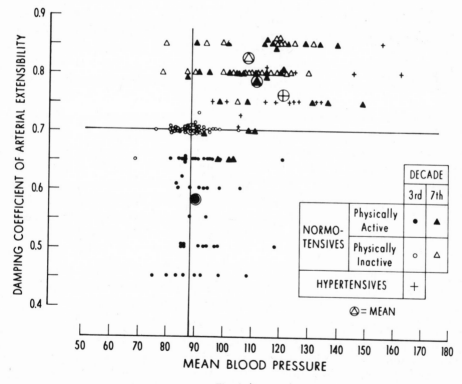

Fig. 4. (See text)

Similar changes were induced by aging, a shift to the right on the pressure axis showing an increase of mean blood pressure and a corresponding increase of D.C. (shift upward). However, it is noticeable that an average mean B.P. of 120 mm Hg induced an increase in D.C. to .76 only in young hypertensives, while an average mean B.P. of 109 mm Hg in N_{VII} group increased the D.C. relatively more, to .82.

Physically active subjects are marked by changes of opposite sense than the increase induced by aging or hypertension; the D.C. of physically active groups is significantly lower than in inactive controls of corresponding age. The difference between N_{III} and T_{III} is highly significant statistically ($p < .001$), as is the difference in the seventh decade between T_{VII} and N_{VII} ($p < .001$) (see Fig. 6).

Two other interesting facts on the effect of physical activity can be noticed on Fig. 4. Three physically active subjects in the seventh decade (T_{VII} group = black triangles) fall in the right lower quadrant, with a D.C. = .65 in spite of relatively increased mean B. P. (110-115 mm Hg). Three other subjects from T_{VII} demonstrated a D.C. = .7 which corresponds to the N_{III} group in spite of its higher mean B.P. Otherwise physically active subjects in the seventh decade maintained the D.C. on a level which is even better than in inactive persons in third decade.

Effect of Physical Activity on D.C. in Hypertensives

Another interesting relation is the effect of physical activity in young hypertensives. The few hypertensive sportsmen in the third decade who were investigated (denoted by full circles) fall in the right lower quadrant. It is surprising that relatively high mean B.P. (115-120) is connected in this group with very low D.C. values (.5, .6, .65, etc). This proves that the positive effect of physical activity upon circulation is so powerful that it can counteract even the influence of hypertension on arterial wall structure.

It can be concluded also that the decrease of D.C. in physically active subjects cannot be explained by differences in systolic or diastolic pressure.

Relation of Diurnal Changes of Blood Pressure and Heart Rate to D.C. in Young Athletes

Since a decrease in D.C. was invariably connected with lower blood pressure, two mechanisms were investigatesd by which the average blood pressure could be decreased in trained persons without changing the resting values of systolic or diastolic blood pressure:

(1) Diurnal rhythm of blood pressure changes could be different in physically active persons. Lower blood pressure at night and during the day could decrease the average blood pressure and induce lower D.C. in response to lower pressure load.

(2) Lower heart rate in physically active subjects prolongs the action of diastolic blood pressure upon the arteries, resulting in a lower average blood pressure and lower pressure load in spite of the same level of systolic and clinically measured diastolic blood pressure. In order to test this possibility, blood pressure and heart rate were measured every four hours in two groups of young athletes (16 years old)

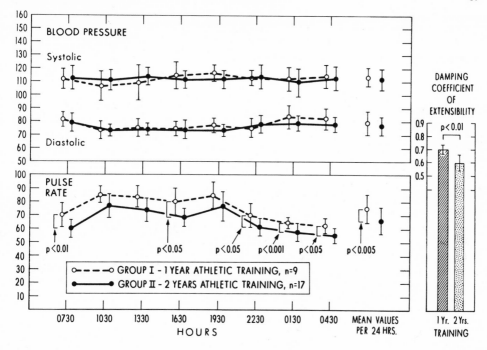

Fig. 5. Diurnal changes of blood pressure and pulse rate in young athletes.

who were involved in strenuous athletic training in the same training center. The first group (nine boys) completed one year of training while group II had had two years of the same type and intensity of light athletic training.

Fig. 5 demonstrates that the systolic and diastolic blood pressure of both groups were virtually the same during the 24 hours of measurement. However, the average heart rate was statistically significantly lower in group II which had longer training (p < .005). the lower heart rate was preserved in this group during the entire day and night.

The lower heart rates were connected with lower D.C. in group II (.6) as compared with D.C. (.7) in group I (p < .01). The conclusion can be drawn that the main mechanism by which physical training decreases the D.C. is a lowering of heart rate. Bradycardia induces prolonged diastole and decreases the average blood pressure. It is evidently this average blood pressure which represents the load acting upon arteries to which the D.C. and the arterial wall structure adapt themselves.

Hemodynamic Significance of Changes in D.C. Induced by Age and Physical Activity

Fig. 6 represents a semilogarithmic Pressure-Volume curve for the damping coefficients obtained in different groups. The transmural pressure, calculated as intraarterial blood pressure cuff pressure, is represented on abscissa. The ordinate shows

FACTORS INFLUENCING THE STABILE ELASTIC
COMPONENTS OF ARTERIAL EXTENSIBILITY

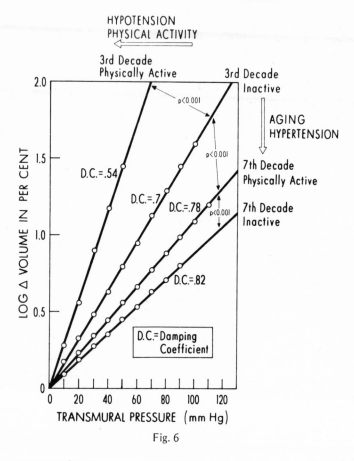

Fig. 6

the logarithm of changes in volume in percent of basic volume of the artery. The slope of the semi-logarithmic relation of P-V curves drawn for different D.C. represents the stabile component of arterial distensibility. Changes in arterial tone can shift the lines on Fig. 6 upwards and downwards, but cannot basically change the slope of the P-V relation. Therefore, Fig. 6 expresses the pulsation capacity as it is limited by the stabile component of arterial distensibility for a pulse pressure.

It is evident that the pulsation capacity limited by the stabile component of arterial distensibility decreases by aging and hypertension, shifting the line to the right. Hypotension and physical activity shift the line to the left, increasing the pulsation capacity.

Fig. 6 allows us to establish the maximum volume change of the artery at different transmural pressures. A systolic pressure of 120 mm Hg induces a corresponding volume of 1.9 percent of basic volume of the artery at D.C. = .7. A diastolic blood pressure of 80 mm Hg would induce a volume of 1.2 percent under the same conditions. The pulsation capacity would be the difference 1.9-1.2 = .7 percent of basic arterial volume. The pulsation capacity would be the difference (1.9-1.2 = .7 percent) of basic arterial volume.

The same pressure pulse would induce a pulsation volume of about .92-.65 = 2.7 percent at D.C. = .82 as was found in N_{VII} group.

The T_{VII} group lies between N_{III} and N_{VII}; its pulsation capacity with a D.C. = .78 is better than in the corresponding N_{VII} group, equaling 1.25 - .9 = 3.5 percent of basic arterial volume.

It is evident that physical activity induces changes in the stabile component of the arterial distensibility, which makes possible higher pulsation capacity. This contributes to the higher transport capacity and efficiency of the circulation in physically active persons.

DISCUSSION

Measurement of stabile component of arterial distensibility can be made by two different methods. J. Ipser used the D.C. (1960, 1935 and 1956) and demonstrated that the D.C. cannot be altered, either by physiological or pharmacologically induced changes in circulation.

S.A. Carter (1964) demonstrated that measurement of pulse wave velocity under different pressures, such as when the extremity is enclosed by a tank, allows the construction of P-V curves of the arteries. The change of V/P presented in log-log coordinates demonstrated a constant slope in the same individual. The slope of this curve failed to demonstrate any change on repeated measurements in the same person even after months. Carter, therefore, independently of Ipser and using a different method, came to the same conclusion that graphic analysis makes it possible to isolate the stabile component of arterial distensibility curves.

Using semilog coordinates, Fig. 6 represents the changes in volumes in percent of basic volume for corresponding transmural pressures. The slopes of these curves correspond to Carter's coordinates.

Both methods, measurement of volume changes by oscillometry and recording of pulse wave velocity, rendered the same conclusion, that the stabile component of arterial distensibility expressed by the slope of the curve decreases by age and hypertension. The structure of the arterial wall adapts itself evidently to the increase of blood pressure. Therefore, the Damping Coefficient (D.C.) increases, and increased damping represents a decreased distensibility.

The effect of physical activity upon D.C., expressing the stabile component of arterial distensibility, is similar to the influence of a lower blood pressure and its direction is opposite to the changes which are induced by aging or hypertension.

Athletic training, therefore, does not represent an increased load on the arterial system and circulation in the long run. On the contrary, it decreases the strain with which the blood pressure acts upon arterial walls.

The significantly smaller age increase in D.C. in T_{VII} group (.78) as compared with N_{VII} group (.82, p <.001) proves that proper systematic physical activity can maintain the stabile elastic properties of the arteries on a level corresponding to a younger age. This favorable effect of exercising is preserved in active persons even in the seventh decade and its efficacy is surprising. Some active persons in the seventh decade demonstrated a lower D.C. (better elasticity) than that seen in inactive subjects in the third decade. Hypertensive athletes demonstrated a D.C. still lower than that of the inactive controls. Thus, the effect of hypertension on arterial wall elasticity can be compensated by physical exercise. Since only a few cases of hypertensive athletes were investigated, this aspect of training deserves further study.

A peculiarity of the influence of physical activity is that the decrease of D.C. occurs without significant changes of systolic and diastolic pressures. Therefore, the calculated mean blood pressure (calculated from systolic and diastolic pressure) is on the level of that of the control groups of corresponding age. Therefore, the mechanism by which physical activity decreases the pressure load on circulation could be (1) a changed diurnal rhythm of blood pressure or (2) a decrease of actual mean pressure by prolonged diastole (i.e., prolonged action of lower diastolic B.P. induced by bradycardia).

This is also evident from comparison of active and inactive groups in the third and seventh decade. The trained group in the third decade had a significantly lower damping coefficient than the untrained group with the same level of calculated mean systolic and diastolic pressure. The lower D.C. is connected with a significantly lower pulse rate.

Measurement of blood pressure in the course of 24 hours in trained and untrained groups showed no difference in the diurnal rhythm of B.P. (Fig. 3). Therefore, the lower D.C. in trained subjects is caused mainly by a lower pulse rate.

From Fig. 6, the significance for hemodynamics of changed stabile component of arterial elasticity is evident. Changes of arterial tone shift the line of pressure-volume relation but do not change its slope. The lower slope of the lines, therefore, expresses the decreased pulsation capacity of senescent subjects, one of the factors limiting the transport capacity of their circulation.

The relation of age changes of arterial elasticity to arteriosclerosis is not clear. Abboud and Houston (1961a, b) measuring "rigidity" of the arterial system by J. Conway's method (Conway and Smith, 1956) found no relation between age changes of rigidity and clinical arteriosclerosis. There is evidence, however, that increased B.P. induces vascular lesions (Masson et al., 1959).

It is of interest that physically active subjects with a lower D.C. (higher distensibility) are marked also by lower serum cholesterol level than in physically inactive subjects of corresponding age (Fischer and Zbuzek, 1964).

CONCLUSION

1. A calibrated volume oscillograph was developed for quantitative recording of pulsation volumes of human limbs. From the volume oscillogram the pressure volume curve of the arteries of human limbs was constructed. By graphic analysis, two components of arterial distensibility can be distinguished. The "Damping Coefficient" of arterial distensibility (D.C.) expresses the decrease (damping) of the pressure-volume curve for an increment of arterial pressure by 10 mm Hg. Thus, the D.C. expresses the curvature of the arterial P-V curve in mathematical terms.

2. One component of the P-V curve expressed by the D.C. does not undergo short-term changes and, therefore, expresses the stabile elastic properties of arterial walls, bound very probably to their structure. The distensibility of arterial wall structure measured by this stabile component decreases with hypertension and aging.

3. Systematic physical activity acts on the stabile elastic properties of the arterial walls in a similar manner as does hypotension; what this means is that the long-term effects of physical exercise do not represent an overload to circulation but, on the contrary, decrease the strain by which the blood pressure acts on the arterial walls.

Systematic physical activity alters the stabile elastic properties of the arterial walls in an opposite manner than does aging: it keeps the elasticity of the arteries on a level comparable to that of the younger age groups. The changes of arterial elasticity in physically active persons contribute to the higher transport capacity of the circulation by preserving greater pulsation capactiy of the arteries in senescent persons.

4. The favorable effect of physical activity on arterial elasticity can be maintained by systematic training up to the eighth decade of life.

5. Physically active hypertensives can have a better D.C. (index of stabile component of arterial elasticity) than normotensives of corresponding age. This proves that the decrease of pressure load by physical activity (by bradycardia) is so effective that it can compensate for the influence of hypertension on arterial wall structure.

6. The main mechanism by which physical activity decreases the strain on the circulation system is bradycardia. This is evident from the correlation between the index of stabile elastic properties of arteries and pulse rate in persons with the same blood pressure.

For protection of arteries against aging changes of their stabile elastic properties (which probably express changes of arterial wall structure), physical activity which induces bradycardia must be chosen.

ACKNOWLEDGEMENT: The tests for this study were performed at the Research Institute for Physical Culture in Prague, Czechoslovakia.

REFERENCES

Abboud, F.M. and Huston, J.H. (1961a) *J Clin Invest* 40, 1915.

Abboud, F.M. and Huston, J.H. (1961b) *J Clin Invest* 40, 933.

Carter, S.A. (1964) *Canad J Physiol and Pharmacol* 42, 399.

Conway, J. and Smith, K.S. (1956) *Brit Heart J* 18, 467.

Fischer, A. and Zbuzek, V. (1964) The relation between the elasticity of brachial artery and the serum indices of lipid metabolism in aged men and the influence of physical activity on them. Proceedings of the IV Congressus Cardiologicus Europaeus, Prague.

Fischer, A. (1960) (Czech text) *Casopis lekaru ceskych* 99, 1121.

Gomez, M.D. (1941) *Hemodynamique et Angiocinetique*, Hermann & Co., Editeurs Paris.

Ipser, J. (1960) *Cor et Vasa* 2, 12.

Ipser, J. (1935) (Czech text) *Casopis lekaru ceskych* 74, 890.

Ipser, J. (1956) *Rev Czechos 1 Med* 2, 136.

Landowne, M. (1958a) *J Gerontol* 13, 153.

Landowne, M. (1958b) *J Appl Physiol* 12, 91.

Masson, G.M., Corcoran, A.C., Page, I.H. (1959) *Cleveland Clinic Quarterly* 26, 24.

Moret, P.R. (1964) *Bibl Cardiol*, 15, 40.

Plesch, J. (1947) *The Blood Pressure and Angina Pectoris*, Bailliere Tindall and Cox, London.

Roach, M.R. and Burton, A.C. (1957) *Can J Biochem Physiol* 35, 681.

Roach, M.R. and Burton, A.C. (1959) *Can J Biochem Physiol* 37, 557.

Feasibility of Long-Distance (20-90 km) Skihikes as a Mass Sport for Middle-Aged and Old People

Ilkka M. Vuori, M.D.

INTRODUCTION

Physical exercise has received increasing recognition as one of the popular forms of recreation having favourable effects on health. Consequently, appropriate forms of exercise should be developed to make the best possible advantage of its beneficial effects. The exercise program should be sufficiently attractive to maintain continual interest and participation. It should have favourable physiological effects, particularly on respiratory and circulatory systems, and participation should include a minimum risk of health complications.

A special skihike (ski marathon) institution has been established in Finland to promote active interest in physical exercise, particularly in skiing and to provide an attractive goal for continuous physical training and favourable experiences of physical activity. Skihikes are 20-70 km, occasionally even 90 km, noncompetitive skiing trips with open participation. Prolonged cross-country skiing is known to bring about exhaustion which is not regarded as a solely negative feature, owing to the resulting pleasurable experiences during and particularly after the effort. The relatively long distances prevent speed from getting too fast which obviously contributes to minimizing health risks. "It is not the length of the trip but the speed that kills." Records are kept of the departures and arrivals of the participants as well as the distances skied. Necessary food and first aid supplies are available during the hikes. Organization authorities are informed of the causes for any break-offs due to serious illness or injury, as well as of the total number of drop-outs.

Skihikes have developed into popular mass sport events. The purpose of this study is to test the correctness of certain assumptions on which organized skihikes are based:

1. Intention of participating in a hike provides a stimulus to keep up or even intensify a continuous interest in physical exercise and participation is associated with sensations of pleasure.

2. Health risks involved in skiing are relatively insignificant although the physical effort is found unusually severe by most participants and no health certificates are required.

Particular attention was paid to examining middle-aged and old people because they are likely to experience the heaviest relative loading through skiing. The most serious health complications can be expected to ensue from circulatory, and particularly cardiac, overloading. Cardiac loading caused by physical exercise is mainly applied to the aerobic energy metabolism required for proper myocardial function. Cardiac loading during physical exertion can be estimated by monitoring the factors affecting myocardial oxygen demand (e.g., heart rate) as well as the adequacy of myocardial oxygen supply with the aid of the electrocardiogram.

DESIGN AND GENERAL DESCRIPTION OF THE INVESTIGATION

The following information was gathered to attain the purpose of the study:

Object of Study	*Method*
Statistical data concerning skihikes:	
— all skihikes (1955-1970) (age and sex distributions of participants, distances, any serious complications)	— inquiries to the Central Board of Skihikes (population 1,020,706)
— skihikes in 1967-1970 (information as above plus weather conditions, break-offs and all complications)	— postal questionnaires I and II to organization committees of individual skihikes (population 62,365)
I Physical performance capacity and manner of skiing performance	
— quality and quantity of physical training as well as social background data	— postal inquiries to participants in two separate skihikes (postal questionnaire III, n = 808, response rates 91.7 and 93.7 percent)
— health and physical conditions	— health examination of all participants over 50 years of age in four separate skihikes (n = 169, representing 95 percent of total)
— food and fluid intake during skiing	— diary entries by skihikers (n = 59)
II Cardiac load during skiing	
— heart rate, ECG, blood pressure, intra-cellular enzymes	— individual biological measurements during eight skihikes and numerous corresponding skiing trips arranged for research purpose

— break-offs, causes of illness and deaths during and after skiing

— inquiries to the Central Board of Ski-hikes, postal questionnaires I-III plus information from authorities, family members, etc.

III Effects of skiing on cardiac load during short exercise at constant load:

— oxygen supply of myocardium as reflected by resting and exercise ECG

— various factors affecting myocardial oxygen consumption

— individual biological measurements during ten skihikes and three other skiing trips arranged for research purposes one to two days before the trip and 15-90 minutes after the trip, all at the same hour of the day. (population 252)

Statistical Data Concerning Skihikes and Skihikers

The number of skihikers from 1955-1970 was 1,020,706. The largest number of hikers per year was about 140,000. Organized skihikes have increased from one to 205 per year (Fig. 1).

About 44 percent of the participants have been adult males, 25 percent adult females and 31 percent boys and girls under 18 years of age. About 39 percent of the male hikers belonged to the age group 18-24 years, 54 percent to the age group 25-49 years and about eight percent were above 50 years of age. No distinct relationship could be detected between age and length of hike.

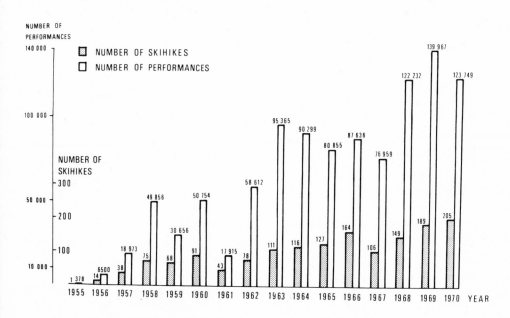

Fig. 1. Number of skihikes and registered skiing performances in 1955 - 1970.

All social classes were represented in the population but the higher layers were somewhat over-represented. Forty-five percent of the participants were manual laborers doing heavy or moderate physical work according to the classification of Saltin and Grimby (1968). Rural and urban populations were represented in roughly equal proportions to total population in the country.

Comment

The rapidly growing numbers of skihikers and skihikes indicate their importance as a prominent sport event. The distributions of age, social class and place of residence suggest that vast portions of population have accepted this form of physical exercise which seems well worth promoting and supporting. On the other hand, the present extent of skihiking requires sufficient knowledge of the physiological and possible patho-physiological effects of skiing as well as of minimizing possible health risks. The demand of relevant data is even more accentuated by the fact that such interest in other prolonged heavy exercise (e.g., jogging) is continuously increasing in many countries.

I. PHYSICAL PERFORMANCE CAPACITY OF SKIHIKERS AND SKIING PERFORMANCE

The physical capacity of the hikers is primarily dependent on their state of physical training and health. Distance, speed, weather conditions and other factors affect the demands of hike; food and fluid intake during skiing also contributes to the load caused by skiing.

Material and Methods

Postal Questionnaires

Questionnaires were sent to a representative sample of participants over 18 years of age, in one long skihike (90 km, LSH = long skihike) and one average long skihike (20-70 km, ASH = average long skihike). This was done to establish previous health and the quantity, quality and motivations of interest in physical exercise, as well as to determine certain variables describing social background. The number of responses in the LSH group was 579 persons (93.7 percent). The corresponding figures for the ASH group were 229 persons (91.7 percent). The classification of physical activity in labor and leisure was done by employing the modified method of Saltin and Grimby (1968).

Health Examination

The purpose of the examination was to establish the state of the circulatory system. The subject pool consisted of participants in four separate hikes, all above 50 years of age. They were requested by mail to be examined within one to two weeks after the hike. The population was 169 subjects (95 percent). Case histories were described by means of specially structured questionnaires, filled out by the subjects themselves and completed by doctors' interviews, including the Rose inquiry (1962) for establishing possible cases of angina pectoris. Clinical laboratory investigations (ESR, Hb, Hcr, blood sugar, urine albumin, urine sugar, urine blood, VC, FEV and body weight) were carried out using routine laboratory methods. Ergometry (mechanical bicycle ergometer, Monark) was carried out as follows: (1) three minutes of warming up was followed by (2) six minutes of submaximal load, then by (3) two to three minutes of more severe load which, according to the Åstrand-Ryhming nomogram (1954), was estimated to exceed the maximal aerobic power by about 20 percent. The aerobic power was indirectly determined by using heart rate and respective submaximal load (Åstrand and Ryhming, 1954). The obtained value was corrected for age and classified as "index of physical fitness" according to I. Åstrand (1960). The resting, exercise and post exercise ECGs were recorded for all subjects (employing at least leads CH_2, CH_5, and CH_7 at rest and, as a rule using 12 standard leads in recovery) at two-minute intervals employing the Elema Mingograph 24 B or the Hellige Simpliscriptor-device, paper speed being 50 mm/sec. Interpretations were done independently by four trained persons who, as in all other sections of the study, did not have any knowledge of the time of recording or the identities of the subjects. Even the direction of the ST segment was regarded in interpretation (Punsar et al., 1968). The combination of the interpretations was performed by the author of this study. In cases of disagreement in the interpretations of the four persons, the less pathological represented by at least two opinions was determined as the final code in order to prevent false positive interpretations.

Diary Entries

Information about food and fluid intake, rest pauses during skiing and speed was gathered by means of diaries especially designed for the purpose. Complete notes were recorded by 59 hikers. The accuracy and reliability of the method was tested by observing a few subjects' food and fluid intake without their knowledge and then by comparing the obtained results with diary entries. The agreement was confirmed as satisfactory.

Statistical Method

All computations in the study were made on an IBM 1130 or, in certain cases, on a PDP-8 computer by employing conventional statistical methods. Factor analysis and multiple regression analysis were also employed. The statistical signficance of the difference between tabulated parameters was tested by accepting paired observations only.

Results

The distribution of the hikers' interest in physical exercise is shown by Fig. 2 Health and physical fitness were among the essential subjective factors to motivate interest in physical activity (Table 1). Six factors were formed by using factor analysis on original items (Table 2). These factors explain 89.4 percent of the variance of the mean scores.

Between 65-80 percent of the LSH subjects and 35-44 percent of the ASH subjects (belonging to various age groups) reported that they had increased physical exercise when intending to participate in a skihike. The reported increase of activity was considerable and generally started several months ahead of the expected hike.

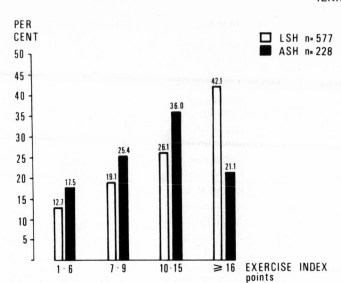

Fig. 2. Recreational physical activity of LSH- and ASH-skier populations in 1969 expressed as "exercise index". The numbers on the top of the columns indicate the percentage of the population in the corresponding activity group.

1 - 6 points: light exercise once a week or less, or moderate exercise about twice a month

7 - 9 points: light exercise about twice a week or moderate exercise about once a week or heavy exercise about twice a month

10 - 15 points: moderate exercise about twice a week or more, or heavy exercise or very heavy about once a week

16 points: heavy or very heavy exercise at least twice a week

Older subjects showed considerably greater tendency to increase physical activity in advance of a skihike than younger subjects (Fig. 3).

Of the subjects, 18.3 percent were smokers which is less than the average percentage in total Finnish population (Rimpelä, 1970). A statistically significant inverse relationship could be established between smoking and interest in physical activity.

In all age groups, most skihikers had participated in several earlier skihikes. During the winter in question the LSH subjects had participated on an average in three skihikes, the ASH subjects in two hikes. Interest in skihiking could not be explained satisfactorily by means of regression analysis consisting of 16 variables.

TABLE 1

Five most important conscious motivations for physical exercise of the skihikers. Points are the average of points (scale 1 to 5) given to the alternative items in the questionnaire.

LSH

MOTIVATION FOR PHYSICAL EXERCISE	POINTS
1. Favourable effect on general well being	4.37
2. Generally good health care	4.25
3. Favourable effect on heart and lungs	4.12
4. Recreation and relaxation	4.01
5. Favourable effect on muscular fitness	3.94

ASH

MOTIVATION FOR PHYSICAL EXERCISE	POINTS
1. Favourable effect on general well being	4.07
2. Generally good health care	4.05
3. Recreation and relaxation	3.92
4. Favourable effect on heart and lungs	3.05
5. Favourable effect on muscular fitness	3.80

TABLE 2

Motivation factors of the skihikers (n=808) for physical exercise. The factor loadings of both Promax- and Varimax- rotation of factor analysis are given. Only items with loadings higher than 0.40 are included. The six factors explained 89.4 per cent of the variance of the means of the item points.

FACTOR	PROMAX	VARIMAX
I Improvement and maintenance of health and fitness		
Protects health for the old age	0.95	0.77
Decreases the rate of deterioration of physical fitness	0.87	0.76
Good health care	0.85	0.72
Favourable effect on heart and lungs	0.85	0.74
Favourable effect on muscular fitness	0.82	0.73
Favourable effect on general well being	0.82	0.75
Prevents illnesses	0.81	0.71
Desire to increase physical performance capacity and to maintain it	0.63	0.63
Testing of physical fitness	0.59	0.62
Desire to increase the health reserves	0.58	0.62
Favourable effects on professional work capacity	0.54	0.55
Favourable effect on elasticity and flexibility	0.53	0.58
Recreation and relaxation	0.42	0.57
Decreases somatic symptoms of illness	0.42	0.46
Belongs to the life habits of our time	0.41	0.47
II Maximal improvement of physical performance capacity, desire for competition and for winning prices		
Gives possibilities to compete in sports	0.87	0.76
Development of sporting abilities and achievment of good results	0.80	0.74
Respect of good sports performances by fellow people	0.63	0.64
Possibilities to win prices and to travel	0.62	0.64
Possibilities to gain publicity	0.56	0.60
Possibilities to test performance capacity	0.52	0.54
Possibilities to meet new people	0.49	0.57
III Attempt to improve social status		
Possibilities for higher income	0.77	0.64
Possibilities to improve professional career	0.69	0.64
Recommended by the employer	0.67	0.61
Required in the job	0.56	0.54
IV Possibility to relieve stress		
Possibilities to get off from hurry	0.60	0.56
Relieves psychic symptoms and tension	0.56	0.54
Favourable effect on intellectual work capacity	0.51	0.52
V Possibility to make and maintain social contacts		
Possibility to enjoy the company of friends	0.72	0.54
Wanted and supported by family members	0.67	0.51
Possibility to be together with the family	0.62	0.49
Possibility to meet new people	0.56	0.45
Wanted and supported by friends	0.52	0.44
Favourable effect on sexual potency	0.49	0.44
VI Enjoyment of physical exercise		
Enjoyment of the tiredness caused by exercise	0.86	0.65
Enjoyment of the exertion itself	0.78	0.62
Enjoyment of the postexercise feelings	0.70	0.57

TABLE 3

Cardio-vascular and pulmonary disease and symptoms of some groups of skihikers.

DISEASE OR SYMPTOM	SKIERS (≥ 50 YEARS OF AGE) INVITED TO PARTICIPATE IN HEALTH EXAMINATION IN 1969 (REPRESENTING 95 PER CENT OF THE TOTAL POPULATION) n = 169	SKIERS (≥ 50 YEARS OF AGE) WHO PARTICIPATED VOLUNTARILY IN HEALTH EXAMINATION IN 1966 – 1970 n = 262	RESPONDERS (< 50 YEARS OF AGE) OF POSTAL QUESTIONNAIRE III n = 730
High blood pressure			
– under treatment	2	3	1
– not treated	10	4	2
Congenital heart disease	2	1	1
Acquired heart disease	2	2	3
Possible acquired heart disease	6	3	0
Cardiac insufficiency	2	0	6
Coronary heart disease			
– angina pectoris	5	2	0
– possible angina pectoris	5	2	0
– previous myocardial infarction	1	4	0
– possible previous myocardial infarction	1	1	0
Cardiac arrhythmia			
– at rest	4	1	4
– during effort	1	0	0
Chest pain at rest	12	4	14
Dizziness	4	2	16
Rheumatic fever	2	2	4
Pulmonary insufficiency	2	1	0

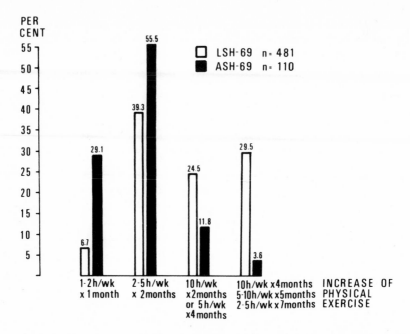

Fig. 3. Percentage distribution of increase of physical exercise prior to skihike among those skiers, who stated that the intention to participate in skihike influences their physical activity.

Major characteristics of the illnesses reported by the hikers are shown in Table 3. Five subjects were taking medicine for high blood pressure, one was treated with heart glycosides and three had medicine for cardiac sensations not, however, aside from stenocardia. Five participants had old myocardial infarctions. One deserves a more detailed description: A metal worker, born in 1914, was summoned to a health examination in 1969. He was a nonsmoker who practised physical activity regularly four times a week and had always been in good health. In his reply to the summons, he announced that he had not participated in the skihike in question due to an illness. During a skiing trip on February 9, 1969, he felt chilly and next morning he began to have severe difficulty breathing and a burning pain in his chest. In the next days, the pain was particularly severe during skiing. A sudden and violent attack of chest pain occurred on the 13th or 19th of February during exertion. During the next few days the pain was perceptible in the chest and left arm, especially on exertion. On the 23rd of February the subject took part in a 60-km-long skihike which he finished with considerable difficulty. Severe pains in the chest continued uninterrupted all through the skihike and into that evening, but began to abate during the following days. The subject consulted a doctor on March 17. Mitral regurgitation by auscultation and signs of massive anteroseptal infarction by the ECG were detected. In an examination on May 19, a paradoxal pulsation was detected signifying an aneurysm in the ventricular wall. The ECG changes had partly disappeared by the next examination on August 7, but the paradoxal pulsation was still there. This is apparently a subject who had skied a 60-km-long skihike within a fortnight after massive myocardial infarction.

About 60 percent of the subjects in the age group over 50 years of age who replied to questionnaire III and took part in the health examination reported that they had been consulting a doctor within the preceding year. Only part of these had undergone an actual health examination. One-third of the hikers had not consulted any doctor for at least three years, and one-fifth reported that at least five years had elapsed since last consultation with a doctor.

About 16 percent of the LSH subjects and 5.7 percent of the ASH subjects who replied to inquiry III had suffered from some illness during the fortnight preceding the skihike. The considerably high percentage, particularly in the LSH material, was due to an influenza epidemic at the time. Over nine percent of the LSH material, and about 5 percent of the ASH subjects experienced symptoms of illness, mostly acute respiratory infection at the moment of departure.

The most significant finding detected in physical examination was the great frequency of high blood pressure (Table 4). Cardiologic examinations for murmurs revealed patients with a previously undiagnosed luetic aortitis and a mitral valve insufficiency. No significant pathological findings were detected in laboratory tests. The predicted maximal oxygen uptake was under the average in 10.7 per cent of the

TABLE 4

Abnormal and pathological cardio-vascular and pulmonary findings in skiers 50 years of age or older, who were invited to participate in health examination in 1969. The figures give the number of cases.

FINDING	LSH n = 96	OTHER SKIHIKES n = 73
Blood pressure[+]		
- syst. and diast. >160/95mmHg	23	16
- syst. >160mmHg, diast. <95mmHg	2	4
- diast. >95mmHg, syst. <160mmHg	26	14
Cardiac auscultation		
- arrhythmias	5	7
- syst. murmurs	5	3
- diast. murmurs	1	0
Pulmonary auscultation		
- moist rales	1	0
- pulmonary friction	0	1

[+] Classification according to WHO (1962)

cases. Deviating ECG findings were frequent (Table 5, Figures 4 and 5). Among these, the most prevalent were ST-T changes during and/or after exertion. In the three years following the investigation, three myocardial infarctions are known to have occurred among the subjects, although no systematic follow-up was organized. All three cases (ages 57, 62 and 66 years at the time of the infarction) had normal blood pressure and ECGs in earlier examinations.

TABLE 5

Abnormal ECG-findings in health examination of the skiers classified according to the Scandinavian modification of the Minnesota-code (1967).[x] n indicates the number of recorded ECGs. Average heart rate was 148/min in the submaximal and 158/min in the near maximal exercise.

ECG ITEM	CODE	REST n = 169 no.	REST %	SUBMAX. LOAD n = 161 no.	SUBMAX. %	NEAR MAX. LOAD n = 160 no.	NEAR MAX. %	RECOVERY n = 168 no.	RECOVERY %
Q-wave	1.1.2.	1		1		1		1	
ST-depression, SSA	4.1.			6	3.7	6	3.8	5	3.0
	4.2	2	1.2	9	5.6	12	7.5	4	2.4
	4.3	1	0.6	9	5.6	4	2.5	12	7.1
	4.4.-5.			1	0.6			1	0.6
Total		3	1.8	25	15.5	22	13.8	22	13.1
ST-depression,H,DS	4.1.	1	0.6	7	4.4	9	5.6	6	3.6
	4.2	1	0.6			4	2.5	3	1.8
	4.3.	3	1.8	1	0.6			7	4.2
	4.4.-5.	3	1.8	1	0.6			3	1.8
Total		6	4.8	9	5.6	13	8.1	19	11.3
ST-depression,SSA,H,DS		9	6.6	34	21.1	35	21.9	41	24.4
T-wave (isolated)	5.1.-4.	10		5		6		4	
A-V conduction defect	6.2.			1					
	6.3.	1		1		1		1	
	6.4.								
	6.5.	1		1		1		1	
Ventricular conduction	7.1.	1		1		1		1	
defect	7.2.	2		2		2		2	
Ectopic beats	10.2					1			
	10.3	1							
	10.4	1		2		1		3	
	10.5	3		11		7		12	
	10.6							1	
	10.7	1		2		3		1	
	10.8	2		4		1		5	

SSA   = straight slowly ascending

H,DS = horizontal, downward sloping

x) see Appendix

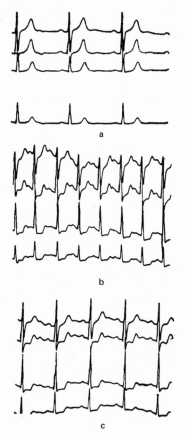

Fig. 4. ECG (Leads CH_2, CH_4, CH_5, and CH_7) of a 66 years old skier (completely symptom-
less, blood pressure 155/90 mmHg, physically very active with daily strenuous exercises)
   a)   at rest
   b)   during exercise (heart rate 149/min) and
   c)   in recovery 3 min after cessation of exercise. Note the ST-depression during exer-
      cise and in recovery

Skiing Performance

Over 90 percent of the participants reported that they had experienced at least
some perspiration and shortness of breath during the skihike, indicating a moderate
or heavy load on the cardio-respiratory system. The mean speed of the winner of the
LSH is recorded as about 15 km/h. The mean speed of all participants above 50
years of age ranged between 8.6-9.8 km/h in various years. Even during one year,
the speed has varied within a large range; for instance, in 1969 it was 6.6-14.5
km/h in skihikers above 50 years of age. About 50 percent of the hikers adjust their
speed individually. As many as 40 percent of the hikers in the ASH group tended to
adjust their speed to suit that of their fellow hiker. About 23 percent of LSH
subjects and 12 percent of ASH subjects adjusted their speed to achieve desired time
or placing.

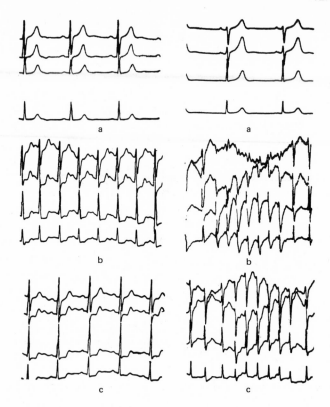

Fig. 5. ECG (leads CH_2, CH_4, CH_5, CH_7) of a 67-year-old skihiker.
a) at rest, b) 4 min, and c) 6 min after the beginning of ergometric exercise at 750 kpm/ min. Note the ventricular tachycardia (rate about 250/min). This was found repeatedly in different types of physical exercise including skiing. The subject complained of no definite symptoms of cardiovascular origin. He was daily engaged in strenuous physical exercise.

Food and Fluid Intake

The food intake of the hikers was on an average 21.9 ± 15.8 Kcal/kg (n = 59, range 1.6 ± 5.4 kcal/kg). The mean length of the hike was 65.7 km (range 30-90 km). The share of carbohydrates in food averaged 65 percent (range 34-100 percent), and on an average food intake covered about one-third of the energy consumed during skiing.

Fluid intake was 1.1 ± 0.8 1 (r = 58, range 0.2-4.8 1). If the fluids, contained in food, are added to the values above, the mean fluid intake of subjects above 50 years of age in various skihikes was on an average 1.9-2.6 1. Both food and fluid intakes were lower in older subjects (above 50 years of age) than in younger people. Losses of body weight due to skiing will be described subsequently.

Comment

All hiker groups (both ASH subjects and LSH subjects) were well represented in the participants investigated. Skihikes seem to have stimulated an interest in physical exercise with numerous participants. On the other hand, hikers appear to be physically more active than the average Finnish, and particularly American (Kenyon, 1966), population. Their active interest in sports generally lasted for years. The same persons usually take part in several skihikes during the same skiing season and tend to continue this activity for several successive years. Skihikes thus seem to attract mostly exceptionally active people; this is particularly true of middle-aged people.

Most skihikers were accustomed to physical effort. More than 50 percent of the subjects in both hiker groups (LSH and ASH) practiced physical exercise at least twice a week sufficient to cause considerable perspiration and/or shortness of breath (activity index score 10), thus providing minimum exercise to maintain sufficient physical fitness (Åstrand and Rodahl, 1970). Both populations included, however, subjects whose interest in physical exercise was not affected by their intention of participation in a skihike and who had generally little interest in sports and intended to take part in the hike untrained. Some of these subjects belonged to the age group above 50 years of age. Some disproportion may appear between these people's physical capacity and the demands of skihiking performance.

The health examinations performed on skihikers showed that the populations did not consist of merely healthy persons. Some subjects suffered from circulatory illnesses which are regarded as contraindications to heavy, uncontrolled physical exercise (Fox and Skinner, 1964). Exercise ECG showed ischemic changes in subjectively healthy persons in equal proportion to total male population of similar age (Riley et al., 1970). Lack of symptoms and good physical fitness do not, then, sufficiently guarantee the health of the circulatory system even with trained people.

Lack of symptoms of angina pectoris in this group may be due to the fact that persons suffering from these do not generally like to perform heavy physical exercise. A few subjects reported, however, that they start feeling chest pains during exertion if regular physical exercise is interrupted for several weeks. In these cases, physical exercise may have caused anginal symptoms to vanish or decrease as described for the first time by Heberden as early as 1802.

The number of LSH subjects who participated in skihikes during illness or convalescence is large enough to attract attention. Some of these hikers seem to have disobeyed all instructions concerning participation in skihikes. Many failed to undergo a health examination before the hike although the necessity for a medical examination was emphasized in the instructions given to the hikers and other people interested in physical exercise. On the other hand, it must be pointed out that without exercise ECG most pathological findings would not have been discovered in this routine medical examination.

Generally speaking, the skiers seem to adjust their performance capacity to suit the demand of the hike. A few hikers seem, however, to carry out the performance in a manner in sharp contradiction with their capacity and the instructions for skihikes. These hikers may perform the hike in a condition known as "near-accident" in occupational medicine. Since its prevalence cannot be manifested with certainty even by verifying real complications, it is also necessary to investigate the physiological and pathophysiological phenomena caused by physical loading.

II. CARDIAC LOAD DURING SKIING

An approach to this problem was made by recording some of the most important physiological factors affecting myocardial oxygen consumption, such as heart rate, systolic blood pressure, ECG, and by measuring activities of intracellular enzymes (released from the myocardium and certain other tissues) in serum and by clarifying the quantity, quality and causes of any health complications associated with skiing.

Materials and Methods

Heart Rate

During skiing, 18 hikers' heart rates were recorded by a portable tape recorder (Electrocardiocorder, Holter-Avionics Inc.). The subjects were ordinary skihikers, and the recordings were done during ordinary hikes. Heart rates during skiing were computed from recordings by playing them back on paper with an Electrocardioscanner device (Holter-Avionics Inc.) at recording speed. Heart rate was determined once per minute on the basis of the time of 30 successive R-R intervals. The changes of recording speed were corrected by calibration curves constructed at recording temperatures. After correction, the error in the recording time caused by change of recording speed ranged between 0.5-2.9 percent. The repeatability of manual determination of heart rates was better than that of computerized determinations.

Evaluation of Oxygen Consumption by Using the Mean Heart Rate

Skiing heart rate can be used in the evaluation of oxygen consumption during skiing by means of individually determined regressions of ergometric heart rate on oxygen consumption, provided that the heart rate-oxygen consumption regression equations in skiing and in ergometric load remain the same all through the skiing. The investigation was performed as follows: 10 healthy voluntary subjects performed the skiing and the ergometric tests in random order during which the submaximal and maximal heart rates were recorded (telemeter Hellige 19) and the corresponding oxygen consumptions were measured (Douglas-bag method, coefficient of variation 3.1 percent). Ergometry was performed by employing stepwise increasing loads. During skiing the measurements were made by adjusting skiing speed to cause desired heart rate levels (115-170/min) by means of telemetric recordings. The effect of prolonged exertion on the heart rate-oxygen consumption regression was studied by repeating the measurements after 20 to 30 kilometer skiing.

Blood Pressure

No successful blood pressure measurements were possible during skiing for technical reasons. The effect of skiing on blood pressure was evaluated by applying ergometry in identical manner to nine voluntary healthy subjects before and immediately after a 25-kilometer-long trip in open-air conditions, at temperatures ranging between -3 and +4 degrees C.

Serum Activities of Intracellular Enzymes

The determinations were done on voluntary skihikers who participated in Part III (see below) of the investigation. Routine laboratory methods were employed in the tests and, in several cases, ready-made kits (Boehringer Mannheim GmbH) were used. The determinations were made in each individual case within one to twelve hours so as to debar all enzyme inactivations.

Drop-outs, Attacks of Illness and Deaths

Questionnaire methods have been reported previously in this study. Detailed information of all serious complications and deaths was acquired from organizing committee, police authorities, family members, case histories and death certificates.

Results

Heart Rate

During skiing, heart rate remained rather constant from moment to moment all through the performance (Figs. 6 and 7). In all recordings, heart rate was gradually decreasing in the course of skiing as speed was reduced. The level of heart rate was comparatively high all through the performance (Table 6). The range of heart rate was 80-91 percent of individual maximal value recorded in ergometry. In three cases, maximal skiing heart rate reached or even exceeded the maximal heart rate recorded in ergometry.

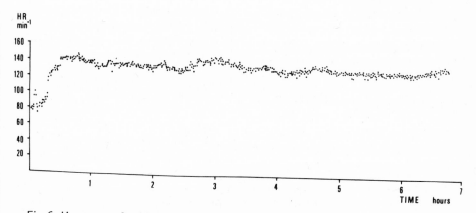

Fig. 6. Heart rate of a 64-year-old subject (no. 1) during the first 6.5 hours in a 90-km-long skihike. The subject has skied without noticeable pauses.

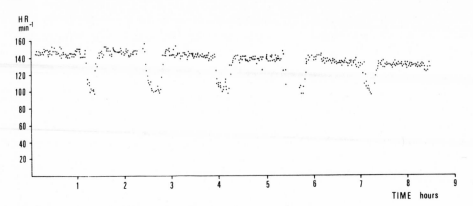

Fig. 7. Heart rate of a 63-year-old subject (no. 2) in a 66-km-long skihike. During the 8.5 hours the subject has taken five pauses.

Estimation of Oxygen Consumption in Skiing by Employing Heart Rate

During skiing, linear regressions were found to exist between oxygen consumption (x) and skiing speed (y) (at the beginning of the hike y = 0.6x + 1.02, r = 0.84, n = 79; after 25 km skiing y = 0.5x + 1.02, r = 0.79, n = 23), between heart rate (x) and skiing speed (y) (in the beginning y = 0.0249x - 0.62, r = 0.79, n = 79; after 25 km skiing y = 0.0248x - 0.090, r = 0.74, n = 23), and between oxygen consumption and heart rate (Fig. 8). Prolonged skiing transformed the oxygen consumption-heart rate regression so that heart rate for a given oxygen consumption was increased after skiing (Fig. 8). Skiing speed for given oxygen consumption was reduced, suggesting reduced mechanical efficiency of skiing. In ergometric load and at the beginning of skiing the regressions of heart rate on oxygen consumption differ only slightly (Fig. 8), which suggests roughly identical oxygen consumption for given heart rate in ergometric load and skiing (Table 7). Skihiking causes a raise in heart rate for a given oxygen consumption; thus ergometry gives, in this case, a higher oxygen consumption for a given heart rate than skiing (Fig. 9, Table 7).

The results indicate that the energy consumption in skiing can be estimated quite accurately by employing the mean heart rate during skiing, provided that the individual heart rate-oxygen consumption regression in ergometric loads is known. The energy consumption of prolonged skiing will, however, be overestimated if the calculations are not corrected for the error caused by increased heart rate during skiing.

Energy Consumption in Skihiking

The mean energy consumption during skihiking was evaluated on the basis of the mean heart rate in skiing and the regression of the heart rate on oxygen consumption measured in ergometric loads (Table 8). On an average, energy consumption was found to be 64-85 percent of the maximal aerobic power of the subject.

TABLE 6

Mean heart rates of ten skiers during 42 to 90 km skihike, the highest and lowest mean value for one hour during skiing as well as the maximum momentary values attained in skiing and in bicycle ergometer work. The Roman numerals in brackets denote the hour of skiing.

Skier no.	SKIING Length of the hike km	Duration of skiing h	min	HEART RATE min^{-1} Whole skiing	Max. for one hour	Min. for one hour	Max. heart rate In skiing	In cycling
1	90	10	54	134	138 (III)	131 (IV)	146	152
2	66	7	25	139	145 (I,II)	131 (last)	156 (III)	161
3	42	6	37	150	154 (III)	147 (I)	167 (III)	187
4	90	9	28	148	167 (I)	135 (last)	176 (I)	177
5+	90	9	25	150	154 (III)	140 (last)	168 (I)	165
6	90	9	18	147	153 (II)	138 (last)	164 (I)	171
7	66	6	20	157	164 (I)	148 (IV)	177 (I-III)	174
8	64	8	4	146	161 (I)	134 (VII)	173 (I)	177
9	64	5	19	150	153 (III)	143 (last)	172 (I)	187
10	60	6	36	165	173 (V)	160 (VI)	181 (II,III)	192

+ Recorded for 6 h 10 min.

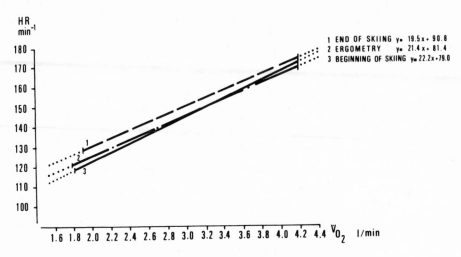

Fig. 8. Regressions of heart rate on oxygen consumption in bicycle ergometer work as well as in
in the beginning and at the end of 25 km skihike.
Correlations between heart rate and oxygen consumption:
ergometry   0.74 (n = 64)
beginning of skiing   0.90 (n = 82)
end of skiing   0.89 (n = 26)

Perceived Exertion Rate

The subjective exertion rate of ergometric load, in skiing and in running (recorded
about one month after skiing), was estimated according to Borg (1962). Perceived
exertion in skiing was lower than in ergometric load but slightly higher than in
running for given oxygen consumption. No essential effect on the regression could
be verified even after a skihike of 25 kilometers (Fig. 9).

TABLE 7

The difference (as per cent) of oxygen uptake at given heart rates between the values calculated on the basis of regression of heart rate on
oxygen uptake in bicycle ergometer work and in the beginning and at
the end of 25 km skiing.

HEART RATE	$\triangle \dot{V}_{O_2}$ % ERGOMETRY – SKIING IN THE BEGINNING OF SKIHIKE	ERGOMETRY – SKIING AT THE END OF SKIHIKE
130	−1.1	+11.5
140	−0.3	+ 7.8
150	+0.2	+ 5.3
160	+0.7	+ 3.4

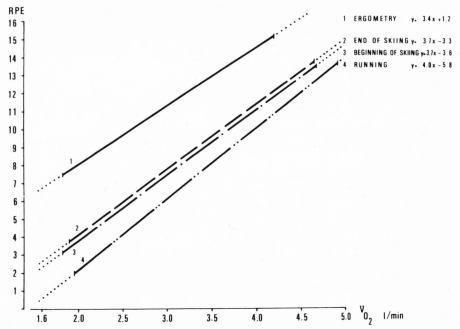

Fig. 9. Regression of rating of perceived exertion (RPE) on oxygen consumption in bicycle ergometer work, in skiing and in running.

Correlations between RPE and oxygen consumption:

ergometry	0.56 (n = 57)
beginning of skiing	0.71 (n = 82)
end of skiing	0.74 (n = 26)
running	0.74 (n = 54)

Blood Pressure

Skiing reduced systolic blood pressure in submaximal and maximal ergometric
load as compared to control measurements (Table 9). No statistically significant
changes could be demonstrated in diastolic blood pressure.

Product of Heart Rate and Systolic Blood Pressure

Heart rate in submaximal load before skiing was 154.0 ± 2.5/min, and after skiing
159.1 ± 3.5/min ($n = 8$, $p > 0.05$). In maximal load the values were respectively
176.1 ± 2.6 and 173 ± 3.2/min ($n = 8$, $p > 0.05$). Cardiac load, measured from the
product of heart rate and systolic blood pressure, decreased slightly owing to skiing,
but the differences were not statistically significant with the exception of maximal
load (Table 10).

Serum Activities of Intracellular Enzymes

The activity of the α-HBDH-enzyme which corresponds to the LDH_1-isoenzyme,
primarily located in the myocardium and red cells, was in all determinations within
normal range and no statistically significant changes could be demonstrated in the

TABLE 8

Oxygen uptake of nine skiers in maximal ergometer work (determined with Douglas-bag method) and the estimated average oxygen uptake (as absolute values and percentages of the maximal value in ergometer work) during 42 - 90 km skihike as well as the highest and lowest mean value for one hour. Oxygen uptake in skiing is estimated on the basis of the regression of heart rate on oxygen uptake in ergometer work and the mean heart rate in skiing. The results are corrected for the change of the regression caused by the skiing (see text and table 7).

$\dot{V}O_2$ l/min

SKIER no.	MAX. IN BICYCLING l/min	WHOLE SKIING l/min	%	MAX. FOR ONE HOUR l/min	%	MIN. FOR ONE HOUR l/min	%
1	3.34	2.62	79	2.76	83	2.48	74
2	3.50	2.49	71	2.76	79	2.12	61
3	3.80	2.42	64	2.59	67	2.40	63
5	3.10	2.56	83	2.66	86	2.21	71
6	3.02	2.56	85	2.65	88	2.30	76
7	4.25	3.48	82	3.84	90	3.08	73
8	4.30	3.09	72	3.78	88	2.64	61
9	4.50	3.03	67	3.22	72	2.58	57
10	3.56	2.70	76	3.00	84	2.51	71

TABLE 9

Systolic blood pressure (mean ± SEM, n = 8) at rest and in stepwise increasing ergometer work in control measurement (±23°C) as well as in cold (-3°C - +4°C) before and immediately after 25 km skiing.

| | SYSTOLIC BLOOD PRESSURE mmHg | | | |
	Control +23°C	Before skiing -3°C	After skiing +4°C	Statistical significance of difference (before—after)
Rest	125.2 ± 3.7	139.0 ± 2.8	127.1 ± 1.9	p < 0.001
Submax.load I	167.7 ± 6.8	183.8 ± 6.5	165.7 ± 7.4	p < 0.01
Submax.load II	186.1 ± 8.8	196.7 ± 8.1	179.9 ± 8.8	p < 0.01
Submax.load III	199.6 ± 10.7	207.1 ± 9.0	195.7 ± 9.7	p < 0.01
Max.load	215.7 ± 9.3	221.0 ± 9.9	211.0 ± 8.6	p < 0.05

TABLE 10

Double product (heart rate x systolic blood pressure) (mean ± SEM, n = 8) at rest and in stepwise increasing ergometer work in control measurement (+23°C) as well as in cold (-3°C - +4°C) before and immediately after 25 km skiing.

| | HEART RATE (min^{-1}) x SYSTOLIC BLOOD PRESSURE (mmHg) x 10^{-2} | | | |
	Control +23°C	Before skiing - 3°C	After skiing +4°C	Statistical significance of difference (before—after)
Rest	84.0 ± 3.8	92.0 ± 2.1	98.6 ± 6.8	p > 0.05
Submax.load I	205.9 ± 10.7	222.4 ± 9.9	219.1 ± 10.2	p > 0.05
Submax.load II	259.2 ± 14.7	270.3 ± 12.3	258.9 ± 12.6	p > 0.05
Submax.load III	294.7 ± 12.5	321.1 ± 12.2	315.0 ± 17.1	p > 0.05
Max.load	394.4 ± 24.1	394.5 ± 17.5	369.9 ± 13.2	p < 0.05

activity due to skiing (Table 11). The activity of CPK, located in the myocardium and skeletal muscles, was above control level immediately after skiing and particularly on the following day (Table 11). The highest activity, 8.5 U/1, was recorded for a 30-year-old subject on the following day after skiing. The activity increase of CPK was, relatively, the highest among all the enzymes investigated, in the subjects above 50 years of age even 10 times higher than control values.

TABLE 11

Serum activities of some enzymes (mean ± SEM, in U/1 except ICDH in umol/1 of skiers 50 years of age or older before and immediately as well as one day and 3 to 4 days after skihike. Statistical significance of difference of the results obtained in different experimental situations is also given.

		ENZYME ACTIVITY		
Enzyme	n	Before skiing	After skiing	Statistical significance of difference
HBDH	6	71.3 ± 3.9	79.3 ± 4.4	p > 0.05
CPK	11	0.43 ± 0.08	1.77 ± 0.46	p < 0.05
ALDOLASE	29	1.90 ± 0.13	2.70 ± 0.28	p < 0.05
LDH	21	111.3 ± 2.7	146.5 ± 5.4	p < 0.05
GOT	14	16.3 ± 1.7	32.9 ± 3.9	p < 0.001
MDH	17	53.6 ± 5.4	72.0 ± 4.9	p < 0.05
SDH	12	0.19 ± 0.07	0.22 ± 0.06	p > 0.05
ICDH	13	0.31 ± 0.04	0.44 ± 0.06	p < 0.05
Enzyme	n	Before skiing	1 day after skiing	Statistical significance of difference
HBDH	6	71.3 ± 3.9	68.0 ± 8.3	p > 0.05
CPK	9	0.41 ± 0.09	4.51 ± 0.76	p < 0.001
ALDOLASE	11	2.04 ± 0.27	5.41 ± 0.60	p < 0.001
LDH	6	105.6 ± 6.1	102.5 ± 13.8	p > 0.05
MDH	5	67.7 ± 6.0	58.6 ± 8.9	p > 0.05
ICDH	11	0.29 ± 0.04	0.32 ± 0.04	p > 0.05
Enzyme	n	Before skiing	3-4 days after skiing	Statistical significance of difference
HBDH	5	70.3 ± 4.6	76.3 ± 10.7	p > 0.05
CPK	10	0.45 ± 0.08	1.33 ± 0.33	p < 0.05
ALDOLASE	13	2.21 ± 0.24	2.36 ± 0.33	p > 0.05
LDH	5	101.7 ± 5.7	121.3 ± 20.8	p > 0.05
MDH	4	67.8 ± 7.7	53.6 ± 9.1	p > 0.05
ICDH	12	0.32 ± 0.04	0.49 ± 0.08	p < 0.05

The activity of aldolase, found mostly in the cytoplasm of the cells in the myocardium and skeletal muscles, was slightly above normal on the following day after skiing. The highest value, 7.9 U/1, was recorded for a subject above 50 years of age on the day following skiing.

Immediately after skiing, the activities in serum of LDH, GPT and MDH,·found in cells of the myocardium and several other tissues, were 28 percent, 99 percent and 40 percent above control values, respectively. The highest GPT-value, 67.1 U/1, was shown by a subject above 50 years of age while the highest LDH and MDH values, 202.9 U/1 and 138.0 U/1, were measured for younger participants. All the above values are slightly above normal range. The only mean activity above normal range was that of GPT.

The activity of SDH, primarily found in hepatic cells, was slightly raised, but the mean activity was not above normal range. The activity of ICDH, located in the cytoplasm as well as in the mitochondria of hepatic and several other cells, was slightly raised but remained within normal range.

The raised activities were not due to hemolysis because the activity of α-HBD located even in red cells, was barely raised. The hemoglobin concentration of the plasma was not statistically significant above control level 6.8 ± 1.5 g/1 (n = 21). Neither does hemoconcentration explain the raised enzyme activities because the hematocrit in a group of 142 skihikers before skiing was 0.44 ± 0.003, and 0.43 ± 0.003 after skiing.

ECG

One of the described ECG recordings displayed a substantial depression of ST-segment and an arrythmia for about 60 seconds with multifocal ectopic beats even in series (Fig. 10). The subject complained of no particular simultaneous symptoms.

Break-offs and Cut-downs of Skihikes

According to the information received by skihike organizers, 0.8-1.3 percent of males and 1.1-1.7 percent of females have broken off or cut down the skihike. Questionnaires sent to individual hikers gave a remarkably higher percentage for break-offs and cut-downs, *viz.* five to six percent. Older hikers broke off skiing relatively more frequently than younger hikers on short distances but not on longer trips. Weather conditions and break off rates had no distinct correlation on any distances. The results might suggest that only the healthiest old people participate in long hikes, and that in poor weather conditions generally only the most tenacious skihikers will set out. Cause of break-off in 81.6 percent of the cases was weariness or broken equipment (n = 364). Exhaustion caused 4.5 percent of break-offs and in 1.2 percent hospital care was needed after the attack of exhaustion or illness. 1.8 percent of break-offs were caused by accidents and another 0.3 percent required hospital care. 10.6 percent of break-off causes were not indicated accurately. Later personal inquiries suggested tiredness, possibly due to a low level of blood sugar, as the main cause of exhaustion or illness during skiing.

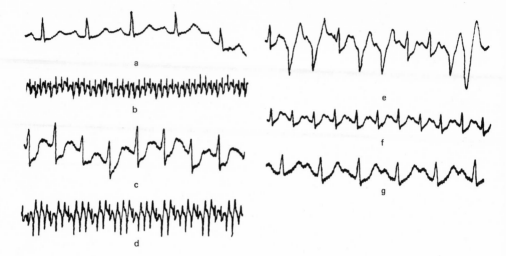

Fig. 10. ECG (lead CR_5) of a 61 years old skier recorder during a 90 km long skihike.
  a) 2 min before the start, heart rate 104/min, EKG normal.
  b) 20 min after start, heart rate 167/min, marked ST-depression.
  c) Magnification of part of recording b.
  d) 20 min 30 sec after start, heart rate 157/min, multifocal ectopic beats even in series
     (ventricular tachycardia).
  e) Magnification of part of recording d.
  f) 2 h 30 min after start, heart rate 160/min. ST-segment depressed but upward sloping.
  g) 4 h 30 min after start, heart rate 147/min. ST-depression decreased as compared to re-
     cordings c and f.

After-effects of Skihikes

About 3.5 percent of the hikers had to consult a doctor or were absent from work after skiing. The principal causes were muscular and articular troubles or symptoms of respiratory infection. There were no cardiac after-effects among the responders.

Factors Accounting for Break-offs and Certain After-effects

An attempt was made, on the ground of information obtained from questionnaire III, to explain whether certain "risk factors" might account for break-offs or some after-effects of skiing. Twenty items from the questionnaires were selected as "risk factors". All of these may be regarded as contributors to acute disturbances in the circulatory system or as contraindications to strenuous physical exercise. The prevalences of all "risk factors" were computed in the whole LSH population (n = 656) and then compared separately to the corresponding prevalences in the various groups studied (break-offs, n = 19; doctor consultations, n = 24; absences from work, n = 28). Owing to the small populations the analysis only gives general trends.

In the group of break-offs, the percentages of those who had perceived symptoms or been in bed because of acute illness prior to the hike were many times higher than in the whole population (percentages 36.9/9.4, and 15.8/3.8, respectively). The same phenomenon was noticed, though weaker, even in the groups of subjects who had to consult a doctor and in those who were absent from work. Age, excess weight and high speed during the skihike did not seem to cause drop-outs or health complications. No distinct relationship could be demonstrated between several simultaneous "risk factors" and health complications.

Deaths

Eight deaths, five serious attacks of illness and six serious accidents were reported in the several oral and written inquiries answered by the central organization of skihiking and the two questionnaires answered by organization committees of individual skihikes. These reports cover skihikes in 1955-1970 with 1,020,706 registered performances. One death in 1971 and another in 1972 have also been reported. The organization committees of the individual skihikes were not, however, asked about the last two deaths. Essential information of the cases reported is shown in Table 12.

DISCUSSION

Heart rates measured in Finnish skihikes proved slightly slower than those recorded in Sweden during the 85-km-long Vasa skihike in random tests on young subjects — 150-180/min (Hedman, 1957), 158-167/min (Åstrand et al., 1963), and 139-167/min (Fröberg and Mossfeldt, 1971). Considering the higher age and consequently lower maximal heart rates of the subjects in this study, the results are well in agreement. The maximal heart rate was reached at times which is not desirable because ECG changes, indicating myocardial ischemia and thus possibility of cardiac complications, increase with heavier loads (Doan et al., 1965).

Linear regression of heart rate on oxygen consumption, relatively slight changes in this regression during prolonged performance and comparatively small fluctuation in heart rate during skiing provide a good basis for a rather reliable estimation of energy consumption in skiing by means of the mean heart rates and individual heart rate-oxygen consumption regressions determined in ergometry. Heart rate acceleration for a given oxygen consumption in skiing must, however, be taken into account (Table 7). Oxygen consumption in skiing, as estimated on the basis of heart rate, is well in agreement with previous results (Liljestrand and Stenström, 1920; Loewy, 1923; Christensen and Högberg, 1950; Hedman, 1957). Both the absolute (2.4 - 3.51 O_2/min = 730 - 1040 kcal/h) and the relative (64-85 percent of individual maximal aerobic power, measured in bicycle ergometry) values of energy consumption are comparatively high. It proved possible to maintain this high energy consumption in skiing for a more prolonged period than in walking or in bicycle ergometer work (Michael et al., 1961; Saltin and Stenberg, 1964). This phenomenon might possibly be due to the special features of skiing performance. In skiing, a very large part of the musculature is in operation. Both the metabolic and the mechanical load on a given musculature may remain smaller than in other forms of physical

TABLE 12

Pertinent information of the deaths during or immediately after skihikes in 1959-1972 comprising about 1,300,000 performances

Year	Age years	HEALTH STATUS Previous	At the time of the hike	PHYSICAL ACTIVITY Previous	Prior to the hike	SKIHIKE Distance skied, km	Speed of skiing	Climatic conditions	Preceding symptoms	Duration of symptoms	Cause of death	Autopsy performed
1959	42	mild hypertension	resp. infection?	active athlete	regular	5	moderate	good	chest pain	30 min	myocardial infarction?	no
1960	28	(musculo skeletal?) chest pain on the left	good	active athlete	regular	40	high	good	none	0 min	subarachnoidal haemorrhage	yes
1965	54	fair.chr.bronchitis, Ca of prostate (oper.)	acute resp. infection	regular	regular	55	moderate	poor (-28°C)	not known, death during skiing	some minutes	acute cardiac failure, Co pulmonale	yes
1968	50	good, possibly occasionally chest pain in exertion	good	active athlete	regular	12	moderate	good	none	0 min	acute myocardial infarction	yes
1968	59	subjectively good, but some cardiac disease from youth	good	active athlete	regular	30	high	good	dyspnea beginning 3 to 4 hours after skiing	10-15 min	acute cardiac failure	yes
1969	53	myocardial infarction (?) 5 years previously, anginal pains	good	regular	regular	27	moderate	good	severe chest pain and dyspnea during skiing	1-3 min	acue myocardial infarction	no
1969	59	good	good	active athlete	only at work	40	high	good	nausea at the end of skiing, dyspnea, chest pain	60 min	acute myocardial infarction	no
1970	49	myocardial infarction (?) 8 years previously, anginal pains	good	regular	regular	25	moderate	poor (snow storm)	not known, death during skiing	some minutes	acute myocardial infarction	yes
1971	46	occasionally chest pain in exertion	fair	regular	rather regular	7	high	good	not known, death during skiing	some minutes	old myocardial infarction	yes
1972	49	myocardial infarction 1 1/2 years previously, good recovery	good	regular	regular	33	high	good	not known, death during skiing	some minutes	acute myocardial infarction	yes

activity in which the load is applied to a more limited muscle mass. Also, the importance of local exhaustion as a limiting factor of performance may be less significant in skiing for the same reason. The rhythmic glides in skiing generate "micropauses" (Christensen and Högberg, 1950), and thus provide a good opportunity of recovery to muscles. By means of frequent intervals (e.g., 0.03-3 seconds up to 10 seconds) of rest and exercise, the time of physical exercise can be lengthened and the total amount of work increased while the feeling of exhaustion remains small, as compared to the exhaustion caused by continuous loading during which rest and exercise intervals are of longer duration (tens of seconds) (Simonson and Sirkina, 1936; Åstrand, 1960). The gliding techniques of skiing may even account largely for the generally known observation, recorded also in the present study, that muscular and skeletal pains are relatively rare in skiing as compared to symptoms in running for the same period of time (cf. even the slight changes in the enzyme activities).

The cardiac load estimated by means of heart rate and systolic blood pressure was indirectly investigated by ergometry. The blood pressures measured supposedly reflect, however, quite well the changes caused by skiing because in combined arm and legwork (skiing) blood pressures equal those in legwork (ergometry) (Stenberg et al., 1967). Isometric phases which markedly raise blood pressure (Donald et al., 1967) do not appear in skiing. The estimated cardiac load made up of heart rate and systolic blood pressure did not seem to increase during skiing; rather, it was unchanged or even tended to decrease.

Cardiac load is apt to be at its maximum at the beginning of the hike, particularly at low temperatures. Blood pressure, peripheral resistance and left ventricular work are even at a temperature of +15 degrees C statistically significantly raised as compared to those at room temperature (Epstein et al., 1969). This may account for the pronounced anginal symptoms and ECG changes in cold weather (Blomqvist et al., 1967). Owing to adaptation phenomena (Ruosteenoja, 1954), cardiac load may even decrease during skiing. In the arrhythmia described above, the decrease of ST-segment depression during skiing may be due to this phenomenon. This observation is reminiscent of the "walk-through" phenomenon described in patients suffering from angina pectoris (MacAlpin and Kattus, 1966).

The changes in enzyme activities agree with earlier results (Donath, 1970). These enzymes were selected to represent in the best possible way cells in myocardium, skeletal muscle and hepatic parenchyma, specifically. Another criteria was the location of the enzymes in cells. Raised serum activity of mitochondrial enzymes is assumed to indicate heavier metabolic load than raised activity of cytoplasmatic enzymes.

The most pronounced increases were displayed by enzymes, located in the cytoplasm of muscle cells (i.e., CPK and aldolase). In a few cases, the values obtained were above normal range. Even other enzymes, primarily those located in the cytoplasm of various tissues (GOT, MDH and LDH, as well as SDH in hepatic cytoplasm) displayed somewhat raised activities. These values remained, however, within normal range. The smallest raise was detected in the activity of α-HBDH, located in myocardial cytoplasm and erythrocytes. The results suggest that the myocardial cells of the subjects investigated were undamaged, and that the permeability of the cellular membrance had not increased. The serum activity of ICDH, located partly in cellular mitochondria, showed little rise as compared to the activity changes of cytoplasmatic enzymes. This seems to suggest that the cells have not been totally damaged, but the permeability of the cellular membrane had possibly increased. The determined enzyme profiles suggest that raised serum activities of enzymes, located in several tissues, are due to release particularly from the cytoplasm of skeletal muscle cells. This hypothesis is supported by common subjective complaints of muscular pains in lower extremities during ergometric work after skiing. On the other hand, the activity changes were comparatively small (x 10) as compared to cases in which severe load on small musculature causes considerable pain (x 50-100) (Arnett, 1968).

The frequencies of break-offs, serious after-effects and severe complications during skihikes proved rather low. Acute illnesses were apparently the most prominent causes of break-offs, but insufficient training also seems to have been responsible in certain cases. The results show that the emphasized importance of good health and sufficient training is not merely theoretical.

There was one recorded death per 125,000 skihike performances in 1955-1970. The slight rise in the death rate in recent years may be ascribed to increased numbers of skihikers, obviously including more persons in poor health and with less training than in previous years.

The risk of sudden death during a skihike was estimated on the basis of participant numbers and deaths in 1967-1970 because these years provided the most accurate information. The age of the deceased males ranged between 49 and 59 years of age. The annual number of skiing performances for males in this age group was estimated as 2,330 (on the basis of skihike statistics). If all hikers participated in two hikes annually (*cf.* above), the number of hikers in this group is 1,165 annually. Skihikes are arranged on 12 days a year, at most. The death rate can thus be estimated as 9.0/100,000/day in the above age group. In 1968, the rate of deaths caused by cardiac or circulatory diseases in the Finnish male population in the age group 50-59 years was 2.0/100,000/day (Puska, 1972). In comparison between the sudden and unexpected deaths during skihikes and all deaths caused by cardiac and circulatory diseases in 1970. In the same age group (n = 471 = 0.58/100,000/day), the death risk during skihikes seems to be greater than that in total Finnish population. According to the control material consisting of all sudden and unexpected deaths (n = 2,606) due to any organic diseases in Finland in 1970, there were 17 deaths during skiing and two during running (Vuori et al., unpublished observations).

The estimated death risk in skiing is approximate and may involve erroneous factors. So far, however, this is the most accurate estimate of risk of serious complications in physical exercise. Skihiking thus seems to increase in some degree the risk of sudden death for middle-aged and old hikers. The amount of serious complications is bound to increase, possibly in a greater relative degree than the amount of participation, if there are continuously more middle-aged and old people taking part in strenuous physical performances.

Deaths occurred in physically active subjects under 60 years of age after relatively brief or, at most, moderate skiing. Intensive training and consequent good physical fitness did not guarantee good health (cf., the ECG findings above). No correlation between skiing length and complications could be demonstrated. All subjects who skied the longest distances did so at high speeds with one exception. Skiing speed might be even faster, however, if the trips were shorter, which is prevented as an undesirable feature in skihiking by arranging relatively long hikes.

Most deaths revealed causes which may be assumed to have contributed to the development of the complication. Three hikers had had myocardial infarction one and a half to eight years earlier, and at least one of the deceased had suffered from respiratory infection during skiing. This subject (number 3) suffered from chronic bronchitis which is often associated with reduced function of the left ventricle (Baum et al., 1971). The cause of his death was acute myocardial insufficiency. The complication may have been aggravated by cold air (-28 degrees C) which may have caused an elevated respiratory resistance (Nolte and Ulmer, 1966). In five cases the speed had been very high and in two cases the weather conditions had been unfavourable, even difficult. Only two case histories (numbers 1 and 4) were without definite risk factors, but even these subjects may have perceived symptoms of illness. None of the findings presented here or subsequently would suggest that a healthy person might succumb to the exertion caused by skiing.

III. EFFECTS OF SKIING ON CARDIAC LOAD IN ERGOMETRIC WORK

The most significant factors affecting cardiac load are presented in Fig. 11. Only a few of the primary factors can be measured on voluntary subjects. An approach to the problem was made by measuring effects of skiing on peripheral factors determining cardiac load before skiing and immediately after (15-90 min) skiing by employing identical ergometric loads. Differences between the obtained values are supposed to reflect the effects of skiing.

Material and Methods

Investigations were made on 252 voluntary participants in 10 skihikes of normal length and three especially arranged skiing trips. There were 116 subjects under 30 years of age, 14 subjects between 30-49 years and 122 subjects above 50 years of age. In separately mentioned cases, the subjects were military persons.

Field investigations were performed in temporary laboratories, mostly in school classrooms. The temperatures of these rooms ranged between +20 and +23 degrees C. Routine laboratory methods were used in the investigation. The plasma volume was determined by using J^{125} albumin (Amersham) Laurent, 1965). The measurements were made in supine position after 10 minutes' rest. The coefficient of variation of the method was ±2.2 percent. The blood volume was calculated on the basis of the plasma volume and hematocrit (Köning and Lemp, 1966). Orthostatic load was achieved by tilting the supine subject headup 70° from the horizontal position.

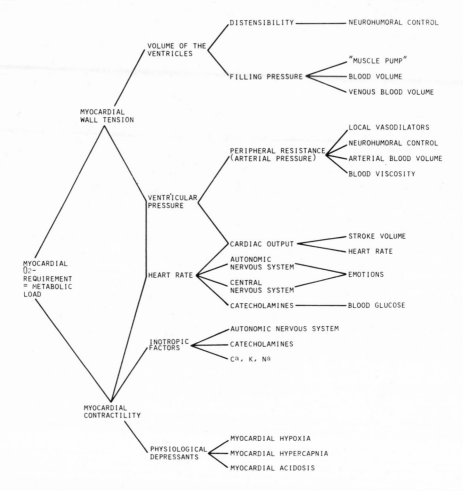

Fig. 11. Schematic presentation (modified from Rushmer, 1970) of the essential physiological determinants of myocardial oxygen consumption (Braunwald 1969, Sonnenblick and Skelton 1971).

The subjects were familiarized with the procedure during the preceding days. Skin temperatures were measured at standard points by employing a thermocouple (Ellab, Copenhagen). ECG (at least CH_2, CH_5 and CH_7, mostly all 12 standard leads) was recorded at rest, at ergometric load and in recovery for at least three minutes. The interpretation of the recordings has been described before. Ergometric tests (Monark ergometer, pedalling rate 50/min) were started with a three-minute warm-up period. The duration of the first actual load was six minutes, during which the desired heart rate was 130-150/min. The duration of the subsequent loads was generally four minutes. In maximal load, pedalling was continued, even at gradually reducing pedalling rate, until the subject felt exhausted or wished to break off. Special attention was paid to careful standardization of the ergometric tests. Oxygen consumption was measured by employing the Douglas-bag, blood pressures by using the Riva-Rocci method. Five vasovagal collapses occurred during ergometry, three before skiing and two after. The symptoms disappeared in a few minutes in supine position. No ECG changes could be observed. No other complications occurred.

Results

Heart Rate

Heart rate at rest before skiing was 68.0 ± 0.9/min for subjects above 50 years of age (n = 100). The values recorded on the next day and four days after the skihike did not differ statistically significantly from the values above.

After skiing, heart rate at all loads for subjects above 50 years of age who were not habituated to ergometry was the same or slower than before skiing (Table 13). The load was maximal according to recorded heart rate (Reeves and Sheffield, 1971) and blood lactic acid content (11.7 ± 0.8 mmol/l, n = 30) (Åstrand, 1960). Oxygen consumption at maximal load before skiing was 2.94 ± 0.17 1/min and 2.89 ± 0.19 1/min, n = 6. p < 0.05 after skiing).

Heart rate in ergometry for subjects above 50 years of age who were habituated with measurements after skiing was higher than before (Table 14). In the third ergometry, done a day or two days after skiing (n = 21), heart rate was 135 ± 2.9 1/min while the corresponding value before skiing was 145.6 ± 3.4 1/min (p < 0.001).

Blood Pressure

Systolic blood pressure decreased for all subjects, both habituated and non-habituated, but the decrease was smaller with the habituated subjects (Fig. 12). No essential changes occurred in diastolic blood pressure during or after skiing.

Product of Heart Rate and Systolic Blood Pressure

Heart rate and systolic blood pressure were measured simultaneously for nine subjects above 50 years of age. Before skiing, the product was 270.3 ± 13.2 and 257.8 ± 13.1 after skiing (unit: heart rate (min^{-1}) x syst. blood pressure (mmHg) x 10^{-2}, p > 0.05).

Orthostatic Tolerance

Measurements were done on military recruits under 30 years of age. After skiing, heart rate was higher than in control measurements throughout the tests (Table 15). Systolic blood pressure remained essentially unchanged (Table 15). Before skiing, diastolic blood pressure displayed slightly lower readings at the beginning of the tests while slightly raised diastolic blood pressures were recorded after skiing at the beginning of the tests (Table 15). Only one subject revealed vasovagal symptoms after skiing while six subjects had shown similar symptoms before skiing. Blood volume for the subjects participating in orthostatic tests was 5.57 ± 0.15 liters in control measurements and 5.08 ± 0.20 liters (p < 0.05) after skiing. Blood volume was reduced after an eight-minute orthostatic load by 3.8 and 3.9 percent, respectively, during the tests before and after skiing.

TABLE 13

Heart rate (mean ± SEM) of men (age ⩾ 50 years) not habituated in the test procedure in stepwise increasing bicycle ergometer work on identical submaximal and on maximal loads before skihike and 15 - 90 min after it.

Load	n	HEART RATE min^{-1}		Statistical significance of difference
		Before skiing	After skiing	
Submax.load I	104	141.7 ± 1.7	137.4 ± 1.5	p < 0.001
Submax.load II	45	152.2 ± 3.0	147.6 ± 2.4	p < 0.05
Submax.load III	15	150.3 ± 4.9	151.0 ± 4.3	p > 0.05
Max.load	34	160.9 ± 2.4	155.1 ± 2.0	p < 0.001

TABLE 14

Heart rate (mean ± SEM) of men (age ⩾ 50 years) habituated in the test procedure in stepwise increasing bicycle ergometer work on identical submaximal and on maximal loads before skihike and 15 - 90 min after it.

Load	n	HEAR RATE min^{-1}		Statistical significance of difference
		Before skiing	After skiing	
Submax. load I	21	127.6 ± 3.6	134.9 ± 3.3	p < 0.01
Submax. load II	15	150.3 ± 4.9	151.0 ± 4.3	p > 0.05
Max. load	17	155.6 ± 3.6	152.8 ± 3.0	p > 0.05

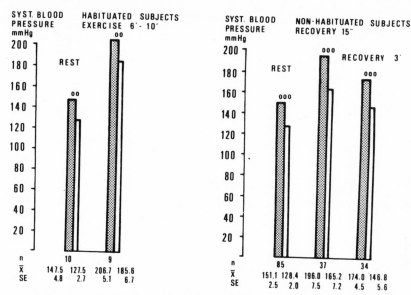

Fig. 12. Systolic blood pressure of habituated and nonhabituated subjects at rest, during exercise and in recovery (dotted bars) and within 30 min after (open bars) skihikes.
00(0.01 > p > 0.001) and 00 (p < 0.001) at the top of the bars denote the statistical significant of difference between the corresponding before and after-skiing values.

Skin Temperature

Measurements were done on 37 subjects. The only statistically significant differences were demonstrated in the age group above 50 years of age (n = 16). Here a temperature decrease in wrist skin from 32.84 ± 0.32 C to 31.53 ± 0.32 C (p < 0.01) was recorded.

Fluid and Electrolyte Balance

During skiing, hikers under 30 years of age lost on an average 1.7 percent of the body weight. Hikers above 50 years of age lost 2.3 percent. The weight change was primarily due to perspiration because food intake was insignificant and most skihikers did not urinate during skiing, however long the hikes were (even 90 km). Urination for a skiing day lasting 12 hours averaged 499 ml (range 25 - 1100 ml) in a population of 34 subjects.

Blood hemoglobin content decreased from 144.6 ± 0.9 g/l to 140.6 ± 1.0 g/l (n = 142, p < 0.001) during skiing. Hematocrit before skiing was 0.44 ± 0.003 and 0.43 ± 0.003 (p < 0.001) after skiing. No significant differences were demonstrated between the various age groups (Table 16).

Plasma volume decreased from 3.22 ± 0.07 l before skiing to 3.17 ± 0.09 l by 1.5 percent, and in blood volume the decrease was 3.5 percent after skiing (n = 20, p > 0.05). In that population, the weight loss was on an average 0.88 ± 0.63 kg = 1.3 percent of body weight. Potassium content in the plasma, in the age group

ILKKA M. VUORI

TABLE 15

Heart rate as well as systolic and diastolic blood pressure (mean ± SEM) in young (age < 30 years) healthy subjects habituated in the test procedure in orthostatic test before and 30 min after a 40 km long skihike.

HEART RATE min^{-1}

Time	n	Before skiing	After skiing	Statistical significance of difference
0'	15	62.4 ± 2.5	78.3 ± 2.7	p < 0.01
1'	15	80.1 ± 2.5	96.9 ± 4.1	p < 0.01
3'	9	85.3 ± 3.2	102.7 ± 3.8	p < 0.01
6'	10	83.8 ± 4.8	98.9 ± 3.2	p < 0.01
9'	10	82.9 ± 4.5	102.2 ± 3.4	p < 0.01
12'	9	71.6 ± 6.2	102.1 ± 4.5	p < 0.01
15'	6	74.5 ± 8.5	101.1 ± 4.6	p < 0.05

SYSTOLIC BLOOD PRESSURE mmHg

Time	n	Before skiing	After skiing	Statistical significance of difference
0'	19	126 ± 2.8	123 ± 1.9	p > 0.05
1'	10	136 ± 3.3	123 ± 2.7	p < 0.001
3'	10	132 ± 4.3	121 ± 2.9	p < 0.05
6'	10	127 ± 2.9	122 ± 2.9	p > 0.05
9'	9	124 ± 4.7	121 ± 3.4	p > 0.05
12'	5	125 ± 4.5	125 ± 4.8	p > 0.05
15'	4	127 ± 5.2	123 ± 3.0	p > 0.05

DIASTOLIC BLOOD PRESSURE mmHg

Time	n	Before skiing	After skiing	Statistical significance of difference
0'	19	85 ± 2.4	80 ± 2.1	p < 0.05
1'	10	100 ± 2.4	95 ± 2.6	p > 0.05
3'	10	99 ± 2.5	95 ± 2.6	p > 0.05
6'	10	97 ± 2.5	95 ± 2.5	p > 0.05
9'	9	88 ± 4.7	96 ± 2.0	p > 0.05
12'	5	87 ± 3.4	94 ± 2.1	p > 0.05
15'	4	90 ± 1.7	95 ± 2.1	p > 0.05

above 50 years of age, was 4.4 ± 0.11 mmol/1 at rest before skiing and 4.6 ± 0.07 mmol/1 after skiing (n = 49, p < 0.05). In maximal exercise the plasma potassium was 5.3 ± 0.11 before skiing and 5.4 ± 0.11 before skiing and 5.4 ± 0.11 mmol/1 after skiing (n = 20, p > 0.05). The plasma potassium concentration of the subjects under 30 years of age did not display any significant differences between measurements before and after skiing, neither at rest nor in exercise. The chloride content of the plasma at rest before skiing was 102.3 ± 0.6 mmol/1, and after skiing 103 ± 0.7 mmol/1 (n = 29, p > 0.05). The sodium contents in serum were respectively 136.6 ± 0.7 mmol/1 and 137 ± 0.8 mmol/1 (n = 39, p > 0.05).

TABLE 16

Plasma and blood volume, blood hemoglobin concentration, hematocrit and mean corpuscular volume (mean ± SEM, n = 20, mean body weight of the subjects 67.0 ± 1.6 kg) before and immediately after a 40 km long skihike. The time (min) indicates the time from the injection of J^{125}.

	Before skiing	After skiing	Statistical significance of difference
Plasma volume 1	3.22 ± 0.07	3.17 ± 0.09	p > 0.05
Blood volume 1	5.57 ± 0.11	5.37 ± 0.14	p > 0.05
Hb g/1 2 min	137.2 ± 2.3	132.6 ± 2.3	p > 0.05
15 min	145.6 ± 3.7	143.8 ± 3.0	p > 0.05
Hcr 2 min	0.42 ± 0.01	0.41 ± 0.01	p < 0.05
15 min	0.44 ± 0.01	0.44 ± 0.01	p > 0.05
MCV fl 2 min	103.1 ± 2.2	97.2 ± 1.6	p < 0.05
15 min	99.1 ± 2.0	104.8 ± 3.8	p > 0.05

Blood Glucose

The mean value of blood glucose concentration did not fall below normal in skiing, but in both age groups there were individual markedly subnormal blood glucose values (Table 17).

ECG

Abnormal ECG findings, recorded in control conditions mostly before skiing, are shown in Table 18. After skiing most abnormal T-waves were restored to normal. Before skiing, the two recorded atrio-ventricular conduction defects, at submaximal load, did not appear in ECG recordings after skiing at identical load. In recovery in the test after skiing, one of the cases was unchanged while the other had normalized. There was one case of WPW-syndrome whose ECG was recorded for 24 hours. The delta-wave disappeared and reappeared, varying without any significant relationship to physical load or time of the day. Skiing did not affect ventricular condition defects. Ergometric work caused ventricular tachycardia identically before and after skiing in one subject.

Ectopic beats changed as follows due to skiing: at rest they disappeared in three cases (code 10.5), remained unchanged in three cases (10.4 and 10.5), while new findings were detected in two cases (10.4 and 10.5). At submaximal load, the ectopic beats disappeared in six cases (10.4, 10.5, and 10.8), reduced slightly in frequency in two cases (10.4 and 10.8) while two new cases were detected (10.2 and 10.8). At maximal load during ergometry, ectopic beats disappeared in one case. In

TABLE 17

Blood glucose concentration (mean ± SEM) before and 5 to 90 min after 40 to 90 km long skihike at rest, in sub-maximal and maximal bicycle ergometer work and in recovery after the ergometer work. Individual minimum values in different groups before and after skiing are also given.

	Age group	BLOOD GLUCOSE mmol/1			Statistical significance of difference	MINIMUM VALUES OF BLOOD GLUCOSE mmol/1	
		n	Before skiing	After skiing		Before skiing	After skiing
Rest	< 30 years	94	5.3 ± 0.10	4.9 ± 0.09	$p < 0.001$	3.2	1.7
	≥ 50 years	76	5.7 ± 0.12	5.4 ± 0.17	$p > 0.05$	3.9	2.2
Submax.load	< 30 years	30	5.4 ± 0.21	5.0 ± 0.29	$p < 0.05$	3.0	2.9
	≥ 50 years	28	4.9 ± 0.21	4.3 ± 0.18	$p < 0.01$	3.4	2.5
Max.load	< 30 years	24	6.1 ± 0.30	4.6 ± 0.23	$p < 0.001$	4.2	2.8
	≥ 50 years	30	4.9 ± 0.19	4.5 ± 0.14	$p < 0.01$	3.3	3.2
Recovery 3 min	< 30 years	23	6.9 ± 0.35	4.9 ± 0.28	$p < 0.001$	4.6	3.3
	≥ 50 years	20	5.7 ± 0.33	4.7 ± 0.19	$p < 0.01$	3.3	3.0

TABLE 18

Abnormal ECG findings in control recordings classified according to the Scandinavian modification of the Minnesota code (1967). n indicates the number of recorded ECGs and the figures in the table the number of corresponding ECG findings. Detailed information of the material is given in the text.

ECG item	Code	Rest n = 100 no.	Submax. load n = 85 no.	Max. load n = 40 no.	Recovery n = 99 no.
Q-wave	1.1.1.-1.3.6.	3	3	0	0
ST-depression,SSA[+]	4.1			3	2
	4.2.	1	7	1	2
	4.3	3	1	1	5
ST-depression,H,DS[+]	4.1	1	8	4	6
	4.2				3
	4.3.	1			2
	4.4.-5.	1			
T-wave (isolated)	5.1.-4.	19	9	8	4
A-V conduction defect	6.2.		1		
	6.4.	1	1		1
Ventricular conduction defect	7.1.	2	2	2	2
	7.2.	1	1	1	1
Arrhythmias	8.2.		1		1
	8.3.	1	1		1
	8.8.	2			
Ectopic beats	10.4.	1	2		2
	10.5.	5	4	1	6
	10.8.		2		1

[+]SSA = ST-segment straight, slowly ascending
H,DS = ST-segment horizontal or downward sloping

recovery, ectopic beats disappeared in five cases (10.5 and 10.8), remained unchanged in two cases (10.5), and were slightly reduced in frequency in two cases (10.4), while two new cases were detected (10.5 and 10.8).

Abnormal ST-segment changes diminished or remained unchanged after skiing as compared to corresponding control recordings except in two cases at rest (Tables 19 and 20).

TABLE 19

ST-segment codes (classified according to the Scandinavian modification of the Minnesota code, 1967[x])) at rest and in recovery after submaximal or maximal ergometry in control recordings and within 15-90 min after 30-90 km skihike. Codes 4.6 and 4.7 are considered as normal. N denotes the number of recordings in both situations and no. denotes the number of codings in question.

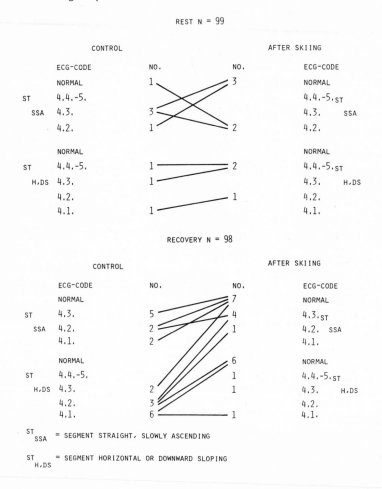

REST N = 99

CONTROL   AFTER SKIING

ST SSA = SEGMENT STRAIGHT, SLOWLY ASCENDING

ST H,DS = SEGMENT HORIZONTAL OR DOWNWARD SLOPING

Some of the subjects, from whom recordings were taken on the next day after skiing and after three to four days in addition to the pre- and post-skiing recordings (n = 21), showed abnormal ECGs. In these few cases, the ST-segment displayed the most marked abnormality in the first recording before skiing and the least abnormality in the recording done immediately after skiing (Table 21 and 22).

TABLE 20

ST - segment codes (classified according to the Scandinavian modification of the Minnesota code, 1967[x]) In submaximal and maximal bicycle ergometer work in control recordings and within 15-90 min after 30-90 km skihike. Codes 4.6 and 4.7 are considered as normal. N denotes the number of recordings in both situations and no. denotes the number of codings in question.

x) See Appendix

ST_{SSA} = segment straight, slowly ascending

$ST_{H,DS}$ = segment horizontal or downward sloping

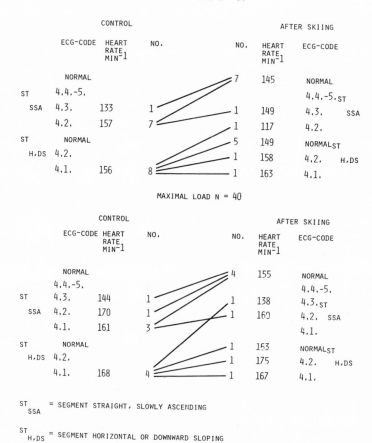

SUBMAXIMAL LOAD N = 84

MAXIMAL LOAD N = 40

ST_{SSA} = SEGMENT STRAIGHT, SLOWLY ASCENDING

$ST_{H,DS}$ = SEGMENT HORIZONTAL OR DOWNWARD SLOPING

DISCUSSION

Cardiac load was estimated primarily on the basis of heart rate and systolic blood pressure. The habituation of the subjects is known to have distinct effects on the

TABLE 21

ST -segment codes (classified according to the Scandinavian modification of the Minnesota code, 1967[x]) at rest and in recovery after submaximal or maximal ergometry before skihike and immediately (15-90 min) as well as 1 and 3-4 days after skiing. Codes 4.6 and 4.7 are considered as normal. o- and x-symbols help to follow the change of the code of the same individual in same cases. The same symbols do not necessarily denote the same subjects at rest and in recovery.

x) See Appendix

ST$_{SSA}$ = segment straight, slowly ascending

ST$_{H,DS}$ = segment horizontal or downward sloping

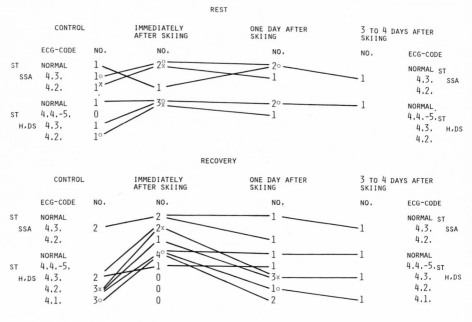

ST$_{SSA}$ = SEGMENT STRAIGHT, SLOWLY ASCENDING

ST$_{H,DS}$ = SEGMENT HORIZONTAL OR DOWNWARD SLOPING

ergometric results (Shephard et al., 1968; Davies et al., 1968). The effect of habituation is reduced with heavier loads (Shepard et al., 1968). Recordings done on even unhabituated persons at high submaximal loads are thus apt to reflect the effects of skiing quite reliabily. Nevertheless, interpretations of the effects of skiing were performed mainly on the basis of the results of habituated subjects.

Heart rate changes due to skiing were slight regarding the duration and the severity of the load (Christensen, 1931; Ekelund and Holmgren, 1964). The results well agree with previous observations of heart rate changes during physical exercise in cold weather (Kitzing et al., 1966; Ekström, 1971; MacDougall, 1972).

TABLE 22

ST-segment codes (classified according to the Scandinavian modification of the Minnesota code, 1967[x]) in submaximal and maximal bicycle ergometer work before skihike and immediately (15-90 min) as well as 1 and 3-4 days after skiing. Codes 4.6 and 4.7 are considered as normal. o- and x- symbols help to follow the change of the code of the same individual in some cases. The same symbols do not necessarily denote the same subjects at rest and in recovery.

   x) See Appendix
   ST_{SSA} = segment straight, slowly ascending
   $ST_{H,DS}$ = segment horizontal or downward sloping

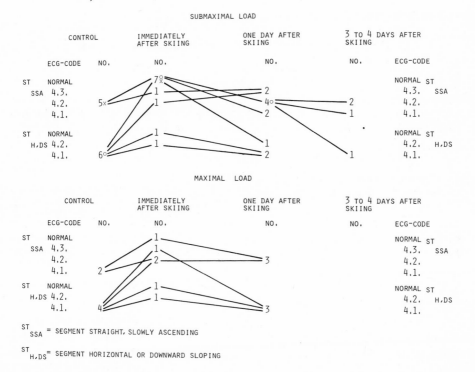

The small change of heart rate is probably due to the slight changes in blood volume and the apparently insignificant increase in cutaneous circulation. These factors, in addition to those mentioned before, apparently contribute to the skihiker's capability of maintaining high energy consumption for prolonged periods of time.

Systolic blood pressure during ergometry after skiing was 10-15 percent lower than before skiing at identical load. The result agrees with observations made previously, both in this study and in several other studies of prolonged physical exercise (Chailley-Bert, 1946; Saltin and Stenberg, 1964; Ekelund and Holmgren, 1964). The comparatively slight reduction in blood pressure may be ascribed to the same factors as for heart rate.

Cardiac load in ergometry after skiing, estimated on the basis of heart rate and systolic blood pressure, did not differ significantly from control measurements due to the slight and mutually compensating changes in the two factors. Prolonged performance does not seem to increase momentary cardiac load if other factors, such as lowered mechanical efficiency of skiing, do not have opposite effects. The exhaustion of the myocardium in healthy subjects, particularly on the basis of decreased myocardial glycogen content (Blount and Meyer, 1959), during prolonged exercise has been suggested (Rowell, 1971). The very slight share of glycogen as an energy source of myocardial work (Kaijser et al., 1972) tends, however, to exclude the shortage of this substrate as an exhaustive factor.

Changes in electrolyte content in serum were small. Owing to relatively scant perspiration and urination, it seems probable that electrolyte losses were very small as well. As a whole, changes in electrolyte balance appear too insignificant to cause any metabolic disturbances.

Decreased blood glucose concentration caused by skiing may not have essentially affected myocardial oxygen demand because the heart seems to consume glucose in equal proportion to other energy sources, largely independent of blood glucose concentration, both during prolonged exercise and at rest (Kaijser et al., 1972). Decreased blood glucose concentration may, however, have indirect effects on myocardial oxygen demand because hypoglycemia causes intense adrenalin secretion (Vendsalu, 1960) and thus increased myocardial oxygen demand. The mean adrenalin and noradrenalin contents in plasma did not, however, differ statistically significantly from corresponding values at maximal ergometric loads before and after skiing (Vuori and Pekkarinen, 1969). Although the changes of blood glucose concentration apparently had no effect on myocardial oxygen demand, the very low blood glucose concentrations measured in several hikers might have caused episodes of severe exhaustion during skiing. In the information given to skihikers, it seems essential to emphasize the importance of frequently consuming small amounts of easily digestible carbohydrates during skiing.

Skihiking did not increase the amount of ectopic beats or conduction defects at rest or in exercise. The ST-segment had in all cases either remained unchanged or slightly diminished as compared to control measurements. This phenomenon is considered to be favourable irrespective of the cause of the ST-depression. A partial explanation of the phenomenon may be found in the habituation of the subjects to the testing procedures (Furberg, 1968). This view is supported by the less abnormal ST-segment in the tests performed on the following day and three to four days after the hike, as compared to those recorded before skiing (Tables 21 and 22). The least abnormal ECG was, however, recorded immediately after skiing. At maximal loads, habituation had probably no essential effect on ECG recordings. The phenomenon of diminished ST-depression recorded immediately after skiing may partially be ascribed to circulatory and metabolic adaptation in the myocardium caused by prolonged exercise (MacAlpin and Kattus, 1966; Kattus, 1967). This opinion is supported by the increase of coronary A-V O_2 difference in prolonged exercise (Kaijser et al., 1972). Cardiac load due to skiing, as estimated from heart rate and systolic blood pressure, did not incrase in habituated subjects. They even displayed some tendency towards decreased cardiac load. No essential changes could be detected simultaneously in the other measured factors affecting myocardial oxygen demand directly or indirectly. This applies even to the release of catecholamines during ergometric work (Vuori and Pekkarinen, 1969). Carefully controlled studies seem necessary to clarify the causes of the diminished ST-segment depression. Only a few of the subjects who performed the maximal exercise test showed abnormal ECG recordings. Previously normal recordings did not show any abnormalities after skiing. Neither did any abnormalities show marked increase after skiing. Maximal ergometric load was on the average slightly lower after skiing than before. Also, the average maximal heart rate was slightly lower than in control measurements. At all maximal ergometric tests after skiing, break-off of the test was due to tiredness and stiffening or pains of the legs, but not to breathlessness or dyspnea or chest pains. In the final phase of the skihike or in any succeeding physical exercise, it may prove impossible in most cases to raise maximal cardiac load as high as it had been before the prolonged physical exercise. This is mainly due to the muscular fatigue caused by decreased glycogen content in muscles (Karlsson and Saltin, 1971). Long duration as such does not seem to increase the risk of cardiac complications in this type of physical performance.

CONCLUSION

1. Skihiking seems to achieve, at least partially, the objectives of motivating interest in physical exercise because 35-40 percent of the ASH group and 65-86 percent of the LSH group in all age groups indicated that they were going to intensify physical activity when intending to participate in a skihike. On the other hand, middle-aged and old skihikers were almost exclusively previously active in physical exercise.

2. Skihikers seem to be mostly persons whose physical fitness can be regarded as sufficient for participation in a skihike. A few hikers suffer, however, from latent or symptomatic illnesses regarded as contraindications to strenuous uncontrolled physical activity. Acute illnesses seem to be associated with drop-outs and subsequent health complications. The necessity of sufficient training and health examinations of middle-aged and old people should be emphasized in skihike information.

3. Cardiac load during skiing must be regarded as severe. It remains, however, relatively stable if too high speeds are avoided, particularly in the beginning and when skiing uphill. The highest cardiac load may frequently occur at the beginning of the skihike, but it does not seem to increase. On the contrary, the load may even decrease in later phases. This is suggested by the constant or slightly decreasing product of heart rate and systolic blood pressure, and the diminished abnormal ST-segment changes during skiing. At the end of the skihike, maximal performance capacity is generally reduced owing to limiting peripheral factors. This phenomenon is apt to decrease the risk of cardiac complications.

4. Cardiac overload may occur with subjects suffering from latent or symptomatic circulatory illnesses. In these cases, the risk of sudden death during skiing seems to be pronounced as compared to the corresponding risk in total Finnish male population of the same age. The risk seems to be primarily associated with high speeds and poor weather conditions. No essential differences in physiological responses were found between subjects under 30 years of age and subjects above 50 years of age but competition and other factors which would possibly increase speed of skiing should be avoided.

5. The capability of maintaining great relative energy consumption in skiing may be ascribed particularly to micropauses during skiing, distribution of load on large musculature, well-retained fluid and electrolyte balances due to cold climate, and to the probably favourable distribution of blood circulation. Skihiking seems to cause few complications in musculoskeletal structures, and the risk of accidents is relatively small. These factors accentuate skiing as recommendable form of physical exercise for various population groups. The results of this study cannot, however, be generalized or applied as such to other types of physical activities or to activities performed in other climatic conditions.

SUMMARY

Some physiological and pathophysiological effects, particularly on the heart, of a strenuous form of mass-sport, skihiking, have been presented. Most hikers were healthy, physically active persons. The investigated populations included, however, subjects (6 to 16 percent of total) who participated in a skihike during illness or convalescence. Six subjects had had myocardial infarction and about 10 percent of the subjects above 50 years of age displayed ischemic changes in exercise ECG. Circulatory load in skiing proved heavy because the mean heart rates during a five to 11-hour skihike were 134-165/min and V_{O_2} was estimated as 2.4-3.5 1/min (86-91 percent and 64-85 percent of individual maximal values, respectively, (n = 10, mean age 50.7 years, range 32-64 years). The serum activities of myocardial enzymes did not show any considerable changes. Even the activities of enzymes released from skeletal muscles changed only moderately. Break-offs were recorded for 0.8 — 1.3 percent of participants (n = 55,676) but only 7.8 percent of the break-offs were due to health complications. Skiing during illness or convalescence seems to be frequently associated with break-offs. At least 10 deaths occurred between 1955-1972 during skihikes (n = 1,300,000). Participation in skihikes seems to increase the risk of sudden death for male skihikers above 50 years of age, as compared to total male population of the same age. The risk can, however, be largely detected by medical examination including exercise ECG. Product of heart rate and systolic blood pressure in ergometry did not increase due to skiing. Changes of fluid and electrolyte balance due to skiing were small. The ST-T changes recorded in the electrocardiogram were less pronounced after skiing than before skiing, both at rest and at identical ergometric loads. Thus momentary cardiac load did not seem to increase due to skiing.

The results of this study suggest that skihiking involves comparatively small health risks. The risk is, however, increased by skiing during illness, neglecting health examinations and skiing at high speeds and in poor weather conditions. Age in itself does not seem to be a contraindication to participation in skihikes. The results cannot be generalized or applied, as such, to other physical performances.

The study has been supported financially by grants from the Finnish Research Council for Physical Education and Sports (Ministry of Education) and from the Finnish Heart Foundation.

APPENDIX: PART OF THE SCANDINAVIAN MODIFICATION OF THE MINNESOTA CODE (1967)

ST-depression (leads CR_{2-7} or CH_{2-7})

4.1 ST-J depression of 1.5 mm or more and ST segment straight and slowly ascending, horizontal or downward sloping

4.2 ST-J depression of 1.0-1.4 mm and ST segment straight and slowly ascending, horizontal or downward sloping

4.3 ST-J depression 0.5-0.9 mm and ST segment straight and slowly ascending, horizontal or downward sloping

4.4 No ST-J depression as much as 0.5 mm but ST segment downward sloping and reaching 0.5 min or more below P-R baseline

4.5 No ST-J depression as much as 0.5 mm but ST segment horizontal or downward sloping but reaching less than 0.5 min below P-R baseline

4.6 Isolated ST-J depression of 1.5 mm or more, ST segment upward sloping

4.7 Isolated ST-J depression of 0.5-1.4 mm or more, ST segment upward sloping

A-V conduction defect

6.2 Partial (second degree) A-V block in any lead

6.4 Wolff-Parkinson-White

Ventricular conduction defect

7.1 Complete left bundle branch block

7.2 Complete right bundle branch block

Arrhythmias

8.2 Ventricular tachycardia (over 100/min)

8.3 Atrial fibrillation or flutter

8.8 Sinus bradycardia (under 50/min)

Ectopic beats

10.2 Frequent (more than 5 out of 20) unifocal ventricular premature beats

10.4 Unifocal (2 to 4 out of 20) ventricular premature beats

10.5 Occasional ventricular premature beats

10.8 Occasional supraventricular (including nodal) premature beats

REFERENCES

Arnett, J.H. (1968) *Penn Med* 71, 74.

Åstrand, I. (1960) *Acta Physiol Scand* 49 (suppl. 169) 11.

Åstrand, P.-O., Hallbäck, I., Hedman, R., and Saltin, B. (1963) *J Appl Physiol* 18, 619.

Åstrand, P.-O., and Rodahl, K. (1970) *Textbook of Work Physiology*, McGraw-Hill Book Company, New York.

Åstrand, P.-O. and Ryhming, I. (1974) *J Appl Physiol* 7, 218.

Baum, G.L., Schwartz, A., Llamas, R., and Castillo, C. (1971) *N Engl J Med* 285, 361.

Blomqvist, G., Astrand, I., Ekblom, B., and Hall, P. (1967) in *Physical Activity and the Heart* (M.J. Karvonen and A.J. Barry, eds.), Charles C Thomas, Springfield.

Blount, D.H., and Meyer, D.K. (1959) *Am J Physiol* 197, 1013.

Borg, G. (1962) *Physical Performance and Perceived Exertion*, Thesis, Lund.

Chailley-Bert, P. (1946) *Sporte, education physique, leurs reactions sur l'appareil circulatoire* Bailliere, Paris.

Christensen, E. H. (1931) *Arbeitsphysiologie* 4, 453.

Christensen, E.H., and Högberg, P. (1950) *Arbeitsphysiologie* 14, 292.

Davies, C.T.M., Tuxworth, W.T., and Young, J.M. (1968) *J Physiol* (Lond) 197, 26.

Doan, A.E., Petersen, D.R., Blackmon, J.R., and Bruce, R.A. (1965) *Am Heart J* 69, 11.

Donald, K.W., Lind, A.R., McNicol, G.W., Humphreys, P.W., Taylor, S.H., and Stauton, H.P. (1967) *Cir Res*, suppl. I, 15.

Donath, R. (1970) *Med Sport* 10, 2.

Ekelund, L.G., and Holmgren, A. (1964) *Acta Physiol Scand* 62, 240.

Ekström, N.Å. (1971) in *Second Intern Symp on Circumpolar Health*, Oulu.

Epstein, S.E., Stampfer, M., Beiser, G.D., Goldstein, R.E., and Braunwald, E. (1969) *N Engl J Med* 280, 7.

Fox, S.M. III, and Skinner, J.S. (1964) *Am J Cardiol* 14, 731.

Fröberg, S.O., and Mossfeldt, F. (1971) *Acta Physiol Scand* 82, 167.

Furberg, C. (1968) *Acta Med Scand* 183, 153.

Heberden, W. (1961) in *Classics in Cardiology*, vol 1. (F.A. Willius, and T.W. Keys, eds.), Dover, New York.

Hedman, R. (1957) *Acta Physiol Scand* 40, 305.

Kaijser, L., Lassers, B.W., Wahlqvist, M.L., and Carlson, L.A. (1972) *J Appl Physiol* 32, 847.

Karlsson, J., and Saltin, B. (1971) *J Appl Physiol* 31, 203.

Kattus, A.A. (1967) in *Int. Symp. on the Coronary Circulation and Energetics of the Myocardium, Milan 1966*. Karger, Basel.

Kenyon, G.S. (1966) in *International Review of Sport Sociology*, vol. 1, Polish Scientific Publishers, Warsaw.

Kitzing, J., Kutta, D., and Bleichert, A. (1966) *Int Z Angew Physiol* 23, 159.

Koning, E., and Lemp, A. (1966) *Klin Wschr* 44, 862.

Laurnet, B. (1965) in *Kliinisen Kemian laboratorio-opas* (in Finnish) (A. Hyvärinen, J. Jannes, E. Nikkila, and N.E. Saris), WSOY, Porvoo.

Liljestrand, G., and Stenstrom, N. (1920) *Scand Arch Physiol*. 39, 167.

Loewy, A. (1923) *Schweiz Med Wochenschr*.. 53, 657.

MacAlpin, R.N., and Kattus, A.A. (1966) *Circulation* 33, 183.

MacDougall, D. (1972) in *Scientific Congress*, München.

Michael, E.D., Hutton, K.E., and Horwath, S.M. (1961) *J Appl Physiol* 16, 997.

Nolte, D. and Ulmer, W.T. (1966) *Beitr Klin Tuberk* 134, 54.

Punsar, S., Pyörälä, K., and Siltanen, P. (1968) *Ann Med Intern Fenn* 57, 53.

Puska, P. (1972) *Suom. Lääk. -L.* (in Finnish) 27, 3071.

Reeves, T.J., and Sheffield, L.T. (1971) in *Coronary Heart Disease and Physical Fitness* (O. Andree Larsen and R.O. Malmberg, eds.), Munksgaard, Copenhagen.

Riley, C.P., Oberman, A., Lampton, T.D., and Hurst, D.C. (1970) *Circulation* 42, 43.

Rimpelä. M. (1970) Stencil (in Finnish), Turku.

Rose, G.A. (1962) *Bull W H O* 27, 645.

Rowell, L.B. (1971) in *Physiology of Work Capacity and Fatigue* (E. Simonson, ed.), Charles C Thomas, Springfield, Ill.

Ruosteenoja, R. (1954) *Acta Physiol Scand* 31, 248.

Saltin, B., and Grimby, G. (1968) *Circulation* 38, 1104.

Saltin, B., and Stenberg, J. (1964) *J Appl Physiol* 19, 833.

The Scandinavian Committee on ECG Classification (1967), *Acta Med Scand*, suppl. 481.

Shephard, R.J., Allen, C., Benade, A.J.S., Davies, C.T.M., di Prampero, P.E., Hedman, R., Merriman, J.E., Myhre, K., and Simmons, R. (1968) *Bull W H O* 38, 765.

Simonson, E., and Sirkina, G. (1936). *Arbeitsphysiologie* 9, 267.

Stenberg, J., Astrand, P.O., Ekblom, B., Royce, J., and Saltin, B. (1967) *J Appl Physiol* 22, 61.

Vendsalu, A. (1960) *Acta Physiol Scand* suppl. 173.

Vuori, I., and Pekkarinen, A. (1969) *Scand J Clin Lab Invest* 23, (suppl. 108) 42.

Physical Exercise and Cardiovascular Fitness

Daniel Brunner, M.D.

INTRODUCTION

With advancing age, significant structural and functional changes occur in the cardiovascular system (Åstrand, 1960; Åstrand, 1956; Brimby and Bengt, 1966; Strandell, 1964). However, it is difficult to distinguish between the process of aging *sensu strictori* and environmental influences such as lack of exercise and overeating.

The present study was undertaken to assess physical fitness of healthy middle-aged and elderly male city dwellers, who participated for many years in a regular exercise program of calisthenics and sports.

MATERIAL

Forty-five men, 55-71 years old, were examined. All were members of a health club. Thirteen were 55-59 years old, 15 were 60-64 and 17 were 65-71. In the youngest group, seven were engaged in sedentary work, two in vocational pursuits which required much walking and four were manual workers. In age group 60-64 years, five had sedentary occupations, four were in jobs involving moderate physical activity and six were manual workers. Ten in the oldest age group were engaged in sedentary work, two were in jobs involving moderate physical activity and five were engaged in manual work. No special diets or eating habits were observed. However, all subjects reported that they carefully watched their body weight. Eight subjects were vegetarians and five were naturalists. All subjects were non-smokers, in accordance with the regulations of their club.

PROCEDURE AND METHODS

All subjects underwent clinical examinations and were interviewed on their medical and vocational history, and their sport activities. No signs or symptoms of clinical disease were detected. A 12-lead electrocardiogram was taken at rest. Arterial blood pressure was measured, and each subject performed a multistaged, sub-maximal workload test on a bicycle ergometer.

The test was performed in sitting position on an electrodynamically braked ergo-meter bicycle. The electrocardiographic response, employing lead V_s, was con-tinuously monitored on a nearby oscilloscopic screen. In addition, a trace of lead V_s was obtained every two minutes on a direct writing electrocardiographic unit until 10 minutes after the exercise, or until the electrocardiogram returned to the pretest pattern. Blood pressure was recorded every two minutes on a standard sphyg-momanometer.

The fitness test started with a workload of 150 kpm/min for 6 minutes. In subse-quent stages the workload was increased to 300, 450, 600 and 750 kmp/min. Each stage lasted six minutes. Between each stage, a rest period of four minutes was interposed. No attempt was made to increase the workload to a higher level than 600 kpm/min. If a subject could not sustain a certain workload for more than three minutes, the next lower workload stage was considered to be his maximal tolerable workload.

Reasons for the discontinuation of the test short of 600 kpm/min were: (1) ST-depression of more than two mm; (2) positive T-waves becoming flat or negative; (3) negative T-waves becoming positive; (4) appearance of intraventricular conduc-tion disturbances; (5) appearance of a pulse rate of 90 percent of the age-specific maximal heart rate, or systolic blood pressure of 250 mm Hg or more and/or diastolic blood pressure of 120 mm Hg or more; (6) development of severe anginal pains; (7) development of marked dyspnea; and (8) appearance of marked ex-haustion.

RESULTS

Table 1 presents anthropometric and physiological findings. The subjects were grouped into three classes according to their physical fitness. Twenty-one subjects who were able to complete a workload of 600 kpm/min for six minutes comprised class A. Seventeen subjects who were not able to exercise for more than four minutes at a workload of 600 kpm/min were in class B. Class C consisted of seven subjects whose maximal tolerable workload was only 450 kpm/min for six minutes (Table 2).

Of the youngest age group (55-59 years), nine were in class A, three in class B and one in class C.

Of fifteen subjects of age group 60-64 years, eight were in class A, six in class B 3, and one in class C.

Of the oldest age group (65-71 years), four were in class A, eight in class B and five in class C (Table 2). The average age of the subjects in class A was 61.6 years, 64.7 years in class B and 66.1 years in class C (Table 3).

Heart Rate: The average pulse rate of class A subjects at rest was 69 per minute and 119 at the end of the fitness test. In class B, the average rest pulse rate was 66, and effort rate 131. The corresponding figures for class C subjects were 83 and 145.

TABLE 1
Determinations Taken at Rest
Means, Standard Deviation and Range

No.	Age group 55-59 13	Age group 60-64 15	Age group 65-71 17
Heart rate	73.7	67.1	69.8
	*15.0	12.2	8.8
	**53-98	48-93	51-78
Weight (kg)	71.8	66.5	63.1
	11.0	6.7	7.4
	57-91	57-78	49-72
Height (cm)	166.7	165.4	163.6
	6.9	6.7	7.1
	159-180	158-177	151-178
Systolic blood pressure (mm Hg)	126.9	134.7	143.2
	18.8	26.1	22.0
	105-180	90-205	100-190
Diastolic blood pressure (mm Hg)	84.6	85.7	90.0
	6.9	11.6	10.0
	75-90	70-120	60-100

*Second line: standard deviation.
**Third line: range.

TABLE 2.
Trained Elderly People — Fitness Test

Age	No.	Sedentary Workers	Light Physical Workers	Physical Workers	600 kpm/min for 6 minutes Class A	600 kpm/min for 4 minutes Class B	450 kpm/min for 6 minutes Class C
55-59	13	7	2	4	9	3	1
60-64	15	5	4	6	8	6	1
65-71	17	10	2	5	4	8	5
Total	45	22	8	15	21	17	7

After a rest period of four minutes, the pulse rate of class A and class B subjects decreased to 84, of class C to 101. Class C subjects displayed higher pulse rates and slower return of the recovery pulse to the pretest level than class A subjects. Class B was between the other two.

TABLE 3
Response of Pulse Rate and Blood Pressure
To Workload

	Class A	Class B	Class C
No.	21	17	7
Average age	61.6	64.7	66.0
Non physical work	9	9	5
Light physical work	7	———	1
Heavy physical work	5	8	1
Pulse rate			
At rest	69	66	83
At effort	119	131	145
Recovery 2 minutes	86	83	104
Recovery 4 minutes	84	84	101
Blood Pressure Systolic/diastolic mm Hg			
At rest	132/87	119/72	165/98
At effort	186/104	185/102	194/103
Recovery 2 minutes	134/85	135/81	137/92
Recovery 4 minutes	125/87	132/81	137/92

Blood Pressure (Table 3): The average systolic blood pressure at rest in subjects of class A was 132 mm Hg. The average diastolic blood pressure was 87 mm Hg. At the end of the exercise test, average blood pressure values were 186 mm Hg, and 104 mm Hg. The blood pressure returned rapidly to pre-effort levels. After a rest of four minutes, it amounted to 125/87 mm Hg.

Average blood pressure values at rest of class B was 119/72 mm Hg. At the end of the exercise test, average blood pressure was 185/102 and after a rest of four minutes, 132/81 mm Hg.

Average blood pressure values of class C subjects at rest were in the "moderate" hypertensive range (165/98 mm Hg). Peak values at the end of the fitness test were 194/103 mm Hg and after a four-minute rest, 137/92 mm Hg. Thus, the smallest blood pressure increase was found in class A with complete return to rest level, or even lower, in the four-minute recovery period. Class C subjects not only had the greatest effort-induced increase of blood pressure, but also their rest level of systolic blood pressure was higher than in the other two groups.

Maximal oxygen consumption per minute and maximal oxygen consumption per kg body weight per minute were determined by extrapolation according to Åstrand's nomogram (Åstrand and Rodahl, 1970). Average maximal oxygen consumption in class A subjects was 2.4 liters per minute, or 35 ml per kg body weight per minute, which are high values for elderly people. Fifty percent of the veteran athletes reached these high values. Class B subjects showed maximal oxygen consumption of 2.5

TABLE 4
ECG Findings

	Class A 600 kpm/min for 6 minutes		Class B 600 kpm/min for 4 minutes		Class C 450 kpm/min for 6 minutes	
	At Rest	After Effort	At Rest	After Effort	At Rest	After Effort
Normal	17	16	14	13	7	5
Incomplete Left Bundle Branch Block	1	1	1	1		
Incomplete Right Bundle Branch Block	2	2				
T-wave Changes	1	1	1	1		2
ST Depression 2 mm		1		1		
Left Vent. Hypertrophy			1	1		

liters per minute, and 29.5 ml/kg body weight. The corresponding figures for class C were 1.4 and 21 ml/kg of body weight.

Tension-Time Index, the product of heart beat per minute and systolic blood pressure, was used to measure myocardial oxygen consumption (Katz and Feinberg, 1955; Sarnoff et al, 1958). The Tension-Time Index in class A was 220, in class B, 239, and 278 in class C.

Electrocardiograms (Table 4): Thirty-seven subjects had a normal electrocardiogram at rest. Two subjects had an incomplete left bundle branch block; two had an incomplete right bundle branch block. Two subjects had negative T-waves—in one, the tracings were consistent with the diagnosis of left ventricular hypertrophy. In two subjects of class C, positive T-waves became negative at the effort test. ST-depression of more than 2 mm appeared in one subject of class A and in one of class B ST-depression which was already present in the rest ECG and increased in the effort ECG. These changes disappeared in less than four minutes after the effort. No extrasystoles or disturbances of rhythm were detected during or after work.

Body Weight: The average body weight was similar to the standard average relative body weight (average weights as reported in "Build and Blood Pressure Study", Society of Actuaries, Chicago, 1959). In the youngest age group, 55-59 years, the average body weight was 4.5 percent higher. In the oldest group, 65-71 years, it was 6.5 percent lower than the average relative body weight for subjects of their height and age; in class B subjects, 60-64 years old, average body weight was 4 percent lower.

Lipoproteins: Lipoprotein values are presented in Table 5. Serum cholesterol and serum beta-cholesterol percentage of the veteran sportsmen in the age ranges 55-59 years and 60-64 years are compared with lipoprotein values found in population studies in Israel (Brunner et al., 1974). (No comparable data for subjects 65-71 years old from Israeli population studies are at our disposal.) The average serum cholesterol level of 13 veteran sportsmen 55-59 years old was 205.6 ± 27.6 mg%, and that of 15 subjects aged 60-64 was 203.3 ± 39.9 mg%, which is significantly lower than

TABLE 5
Lipoprotein Patterns

	No.	Total Cholesterol, mean standard deviation	Significance	Beta-cholesterol percentage mean standard deviation	Significance
Age 55-59 years					
Veteran sportsmen	13	205 ± 27.6		77.6 ± 5.1	
			p < 0.001		N.S.*
Population study	496	232 ± 40.7		79.6 ± 6.0	
Age 60-64 years					
Veteran sportsmen	15	203 ± 39.9		78.4 ± 6.3	
			p < 0.01		N.S.*
Population study	310	223 ± 37.1		79.5 ± 5.7	

* N.S. — Not significant.

those found in the general male population of this age (232.1 mg%). No significant difference was found with regard to beta-cholesterol percentage.

DISCUSSION

The aim of this study was to assess the fitness of elderly men who are habituated to physical exercise. Although the subjects under study had a very high grade of physical fitness considering their age, a gradient with age is evident. The youngest age group did best. Nine of 13 subjects of age group 55-59 were in class A. Of the oldest age group, only four out of 17 subjects could perform the mean workload of class A; eight were in class B and five in class C. The achievement of 15 60 to 64 year old subjects was half way between the two groups. Eight of the latter group were in class A, six in class B and one in class C.

There was no difference in the pulse rate at rest between class A and class B. However, the pulse rate at rest of class C subjects was significantly higher. The relatively small increase of pulse rate during exercise in class A subjects who completed a workload of 600 kpm/min for six minutes with an average pulse rate of 119 beats indicates high fitness similar to that of young athletes. The highest exercise heart rate in this group was 140. Two subjects in this group had an incomplete right bundle branch block, one had an incomplete left bundle branch block, one had negative T waves and, in another, ST-depression was recorded at the end of the six-minute effort. However, these ECG abnormalities did not influence or limit their performances.

Four subjects of class B responded to exercise by a pulse rate of 150 beats per minute. The tests were therefore discontinued. In one subject of class B and in two of class C, T-wave changes or ischemic ST-displacement appeared during exercise. Their tests were discontinued. Exhaustion and severe fatigue were the reasons for discontinuation in two subjects with incomplete left bundle branch block, two with incomplete right bundle branch block, one with evident damage in the posterior wall and one with left ventricular hypertrophy.

Four subjects of class C could not proceed to a workload of 600 kpm/min because of exercise tachycardia of above 150 beats per minute at the end of the six-minute exercise at a workload of 450 kpm/min. The average pulse rate of class C subjects at the end of the test was 145 beats. In two subjects of class C, T-wave changes appeared, accompanied by severe fatigue but no pains.

All class A and class B subjects had normal blood pressure at rest. On the other hand, all seven class C subjects had diastolic blood pressure at rest over 90 mm Hg, and systolic blood pressure of 165 mm Hg.

It seems remarkable that the Tension-Time Index is lowest in class A, indicating that these subjects performed their relatively high workload with a relatively small myocardial consumption. This may serve as an additional suggestion that physically active subjects profit from a more economic use of oxygen in their heart muscle at effort.

Since increased serum cholesterol is considered to contribute to the development of coronary heart disease, the conspicuously low serum cholesterol values of the veteran sportsmen might suggest a beneficial effect of regular physical training on cholesterol metabolism in elderly people. However, such assumptions must be made with reservation because of the small number of subjects under investigation in this study.

No difference in beta-cholesterol percentages was found between trained and untrained males of comparable age. In earlier studies, we reported that the high beta-cholesterol percentages, irrespective of total cholesterol levels, are an indicator of increased coronary proneness.

No influence of occupational work or fitness was noted. In each age group 30-40 percent of the subjects were engaged in manual work. In class A, there were nine sedentary and seven manual workers, while seven had occupations involving moderate effort such as a good deal of walking. The corresponding figures in class C were five sedentary, one manual worker and one who walked much. In class B, there were nine sedentary and eight manual workers.

All veteran sportsmen were middle-class people with a wide spectrum of occupations. The only common denominator of their group was their adherence to a regular exercise regime. Twenty-eight of them indulged in sports and calisthenics for half an hour per day, or for about 60-90 minutes twice weekly. Only 17 spent more time with physical training. It seems that regular training of about 30 minutes per day is sufficient to keep elderly people in a state of high fitness and to engender a feeling of well-being.

CONCLUSION

Forty-five males, 55-71 years old, who participated in a regimen of regular calisthenics and sport activities, were examined to evaluate their physical fitness. Multistaged ergometric maximal workload tests with electrocardiographic monitoring and blood pressure measurements were performed.

Twenty-one subjects were able to perform workloads of 600 kpm/min for six minutes (class A), 17 completed workloads of 600 kpm/min for at least four minutes (class B) and seven performed workloads of 450 kpm/min for six minutes (class C). Thirty-eight subjects had normal ECG tracings at rest. Three subjects had ST-depression or negative T-waves at rest. No correlation was found between ECG abnormalities and work tolerance. The mean pulse rate at the end of the exercise was 119 in class A, 131 in class B and 145 in class C. Blood pressure increased in all subjects in response to the effort, but returned to the pre-effort level in less than four minutes. The maximal oxygen consumption per kg body weight/min was 35 ml in class A, 29.5 ml in class B and 21.0 ml in class C subjects. The veteran sportsmen had lower serum cholesterol values than untrained males of comparable age. There was a slight but distinct decline of exercise tolerance with age. Nevertheless, even in the age group 65-71 years, 12 out of 17 subjects could perform a workload of 600 kpm/min for at least four minutes.

It seems that regular physical exercise of about 30 minutes per day or two to three hours per week is sufficient to keep elderly people in a state of high fitness.

REFERENCES

Åstrand, I. (1960) *Acta Physiol Scand suppl* 169.
Åstrand, P.-O. (1956) *Physiol Rev* 36, 307.
Åstrand, P.-O., and Rodahl, K. (1970) *Textbook of Work Physiology*, McGraw-Hill Book Company, New York.
Brimby, G., and Bengt, S. (1966) *Acta Med Scand* 179, 513.
Brunner, D., Altman, S., and Loebl, K. (1974) unpublished data.
Katz, L.D., and Feinberg, H. (1958) *Circ Res* 6, 656.
Sarnoff, S.J., Braunwald, E., Welde, G.H., et al. (1958) *Am J Physiol* 192, 148.
Strandell, T. (1964) *Acta Med Scand suppl* 175, 414.

Multi-Stage Cardiovascular Testing

Edward Terry Davison, M.D.

INTRODUCTION

Over the past five years multi-stage exercise stress testing has become an integral part of cardiologic evaluation in most major medical centers in this country. Such testing provides a noninvasive technique for:

1. Detection or confirmation of overt or latent coronary heart disease.
2. Evaluation of cardiovascular functional capacity, particularly as a means of clearing individuals for strenuous work or exercise programs.
3. Detection or confirmation of arrhythmias.
4. Increase of individual motivation for entering and adhering to exercise programs.

Increased longevity and development of successful exercise programs in the elderly, as well as reduced mortality for the elderly undergoing aortocoronary artery bypass, suggests the need for a more aggressive approach toward the determination of cardiovascular function in the elderly (Hamby et al., 1973).

Types of Test

In principle, there are only two basic types of exercise stress tests. One is submaximal; the subject usually does not attain his top performance or functional aerobic capacity, but stops at some arbitrary end point such as a predetermined heart rate based on his age and activity adjustment. Sheffield (1965) employs increasing work loads on a treadmill either until the subject is stopped by the onset of symptoms or until his heart rate reaches 90 percent of the expected maximal heart rate predicted according to his age (Table 1). Hellerstein (1969) uses a bicycle ergometer to measure the amount of work that must be done by middle-aged persons to achieve a heart rate of 150 beats per minute.

The other type is maximal exertion in which the subject is presumed to have reached the limit of his oxygen uptake (V_{O_2} max). The Bruce test consists of six

EDWARD T. DAVISON

TABLE 1

Predicted Maximal Heart Rates By Age, And
Recommended Target Heart Rates For Submaximal Exercise Testing

Maximal and Submaximal Heart Rates Predicted by Age														
Ages (yrs)	20	25	30	35	40	45	50	55	60	65	70	75	80	85
Maximal heart rate (untrained)	197	195	193	191	189	187	184	182	180	178	176	174	172	170
90% of maximal heart rate	177	175	173	172	170	168	166	164	162	160	158	157	155	153

Data from Sheffield, L.T., Holt, J.H. and Reeves, T.J. (1965) *Circulation* 32, 622.

stages of treadmill walking, with each stage lasting three minutes (Bruce et al., 1969). There is a stepwise progression of workload from stage to stage (Table 2). It begins at a low level that can be accomplished by almost any patient and ends with a high demand load that can be completed only by a well-conditioned athlete.

Maximal and submaximal exercise tests generally employ the treadmill, the bicycle ergometer or steps. Each method has its own characteristics but the ability to attain predictable work loads with the least variance is accomplished with a treadmill which controls the rate of expenditure of energy involuntarily.

TABLE 2

Energy Expenditure for Men and Women
at Various Treadmill Grades and Speeds

	Speed		Grade		Mean O_2 Cost (ml/kg x min*)	
Stage	(mph)	(Kmph)	(%)	(degrees)	Men	Women
I	1.7	2.74	10	5°43'	17.4	16.9
II	2.5	4.02	12	6°51'	24.8	23.2
III	3.4	5.47	14	7°58'	34.3	32.2
IV	4.2	6.76	16	9°06'	43.8**	49.1***

    * For healthy persons who have not attained maximal exertion at stage specified.
   ** Disproportionate increment in O_2 uptake is attributable to decreased mechanical efficiency when individuals begin to jog or run upgrade.
 *** Unusually well-trained, athletic young women.
    Data from Bruce, R.A. and McDonough, J.R. (1969) *Bull N Y Acad Med* 45, 1288.

Certain requirements must be met in planning a multi-stage exercise test. First, the workload should start at a low level and progress to higher levels in regular sequence, with load increments that demand increases in O_2 uptake no greater than 10ml/kg/min at each stage. Each stage should be at least three minutes in duration; this is the time required to insure a near steady state of aerobic demand. There is little to be gained by using stages of longer duration. Four to six stages are reasonable; more than that unduly prolongs the procedure. It is preferable not to halt the subject abruptly at the end of a session, but to let him continue exercising at a low level for a minute or two. The subject should be monitored for the first five to 10 minutes of the recovery period or until the heart rate falls to within 10-15 beats of the pre-exercise period. The most well-defined and practical parameters of exercise response are those recorded by electrocardiogram, blood pressure, heart rate, duration of exercise and measurement of oxygen uptake.

The physical workload during a treadmill test or a step test will define oxygen uptake in terms of "ml/kg x min" while the bicycle ergometer load determines oxygen uptake in absolute units or as liters per minute.

Lead Systems

Three different classes of ECG lead systems are being used: (1) simple bipolar chest leads, (2) conventional or modified 12-lead system and (3) orthogonal or vector three-lead system. Each lead system has specific advantages and disadvantages with respect to ease of application, sensitivity, specificity and relative freedom from noise during exercise. S-T depressions of the type generally recognized as ischemic tend to be oriented spatially in a direction opposite to that of the mean QRS vector (Blomquist, 1965). Electrode positions corresponding to precordial leads V_5 and V_6 offer the best compromise between sensitivity and specificity if a single lead is to be used.

The location of the negative electrode is variable. A high anterior chest or high back position (right subscapular, manubrium or right inferior scapular border) includes a vertical component and performs better than a strictly horizontal lead. Available data suggest that the use of a multiple rather than single lead is associated with a small but significant increase in sensitivity probably of the order of magnitude of 10 percent (Blackburn, 1969).

EXERCISE END POINTS

Peak work load and the point at which the test is discontinued are always determined by criteria referring to the patient's response. The target load for asymptomatic patients may be either maximal oxygen uptake or heart rate during exercise corresponding to 85 percent of the mean age-specific maximal heart rate. Most physicians discontinue the test at lower work levels if any of the following events is encountered:

1. Angina
2. Claudication
3. Dizziness

4. Symptoms or signs suggesting cerebral ischemia
5. Fall in blood pressure or heart rate with increasing work load
6. ECG consistent with ventricular tachycardia
7. Significant electrocardiographic abnormalities if not present at rest
   a. Progressive horizontal S-T depression of 5mm or S-T elevation of more than 1mm, multifocal PVCs, any sustained atrial tachyarrhythmia, and atrioventricular block

Risks and Safety Procedures

Mortality and morbidity attributable to exercise testing have recently been examined by Rochmis and Blackburn (1971). Data obtained from 73 physicians and physiologists, representing the experience of 170,000 tests with a predominance of multi-stage progressive tests (73 percent), gave a total of 16 deaths (1/10,000) attributable to the test. Absolute contraindications include fresh myocardial infarction, uncontrolled cardiac arrhythmia and acute general illness (See Table 3).

TABLE 3

I. Absolute Contraindications
   1. Acute myocardial infarction
   2. Acute pulmonary embolism
   3. Ventricular tachycardia and other dangerous dysrhythmias (multifocal ventricular activity)
   4. Uncontrolled congestive heart failure
   5. Active myocarditis
   6. Digitalis or quinidine toxicity
II. Relative Contraindications
   1. Rapidly increasing or unstable angina pectoris
   2. Complete A-V block
   3. Severe aortic stenosis
   4. Cerebral vascular insufficiency
   5. Untreated severe pulmonary or systemic hypertension
III. No Contraindications
   1. Stable angina pectoris
   2. Healed myocardial infarction (more than two weeks)
   3. Most chronic valvular cardiac disease
   4. Most patients with a past history of supraventricular or ventricular dysrhythmia

Stress Testing in The Diagnosis of Ischemic Heart Disease

Exercise testing, whether submaximal or maximal, is one of the clinician's most useful tools in diagnosing coronary artery disease with non-invasive techniques. S-T segment changes on the ECG represent actual functional changes at the myocardial cell membrane (Bruce et al., 1969). S-T depression, which is upsloping (Fig. 1), is associated with a significant efflux of potassium (Case et al., 1966). This may be a normal response to exercise or may reflect a deficient enzymatic $Na^+ - K^+$ exchange at the myocardial cell membrane. The more advanced ischemic response of hori-

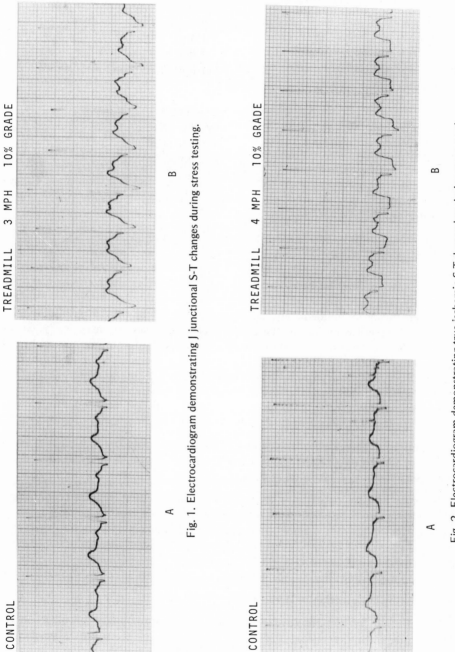

Fig. 1. Electrocardiogram demonstrating J junctional S-T changes during stress testing.

Fig. 2. Electrocardiogram demonstrating true ischemic S-T depression during stress testing.

zontal and downsloping S-T segments occurs in the presence of lactate excretion and a fall in pH, reflecting probably intracellular acidosis (Fig. 2).

S-T segment depression is thought to represent subendocardial ischemia. This is the region most sensitive to alterations in coronary flow due to the peculiar architecture of the intramural arteries (Estes et al., 1966). For submaximal or maximal multistage testing, S-T segment depression of 2.0 mm or more (.10mv) after exertion at 60 milliseconds beyond the J point, whether upsloping, horizontal or downsloping, is abnormal.

The frequency and depth of postexercise ischemic S-T depression are closely related to hemodynamic factors (particularly the pressure-time index) which influence myocardial oxygen requirements (Detry et al., 1970). Since patients with significant coronary atherosclerosis have limited ability to increase myocardial flow (and oxygen supply) during stress, it is not surprising to find that these patients have a greater frequency of positive exercise tests than do symptomatic patients with either normal coronary arteriograms or nonobstructive coronary atherosclerosis.

In a recent study by McHenry et al. (1972), graded treadmill exercise testing and coronary cinearteriographic studies were carried out on 86 patients with angina pectoris. All patients revealed at least 75 percent stenosis in one or more major coronary arteries, and 83 of 86 exhibited 90 percent or greater stenosis in at least one artery. In 70 of the 86 (82 percent) patients, a positive S-T segment response developed during or immediately after exercise. In 12 of the 16 with a negative response, disease was limited to the right or left circumflex coronary artery. Of the 12 patients with an isolated stenosis of the left anterior descending artery, 11 (92 percent) had a positive S-T segment response. Of 55 patients with two or three vessel diseases 51 (93 percent) demonstrated a positive S-T response. The results of the above study are in agreement with other reports demonstrating increasing frequency of positive stress tests with more severe coronary disease angiographically (McConahay et al., 1971; Bartel et al., 1974).

In addition, the presence of deeper S-T segment depression (2.0 mm) and predominant S-T elevation were associated with more severe coronary disease and less "false positives" (McHenry et al., 1972).

The rate of false positives is approximately five to eight percent (Estes et al., 1966). False positives occur more frequently in females and, as expected, in the presence of "minor S-T segment abnormalities". Potassium-43 exercise myocardial scanning appears to be an accurate non-invasive method of assessing patients with suspected false-positive exercise tests and provides a means of increasing the specificity of exercise testing (Zaret et al., 1973).

Stress Testing in Detection of Arrhythmias

Unexplained palpitations, dizziness and syncope are common problems in the elderly. Although the resting 12-lead electrocardiogram often provides a limited sample of transient rhythm changes, exercise testing utilizing the treadmill is a more satisfactory method for unmasking an underlying arrhythmia (Fig. 3) or conduction disturbance (Fig. 4) as the cause of these symptoms. Early recognition and treat-

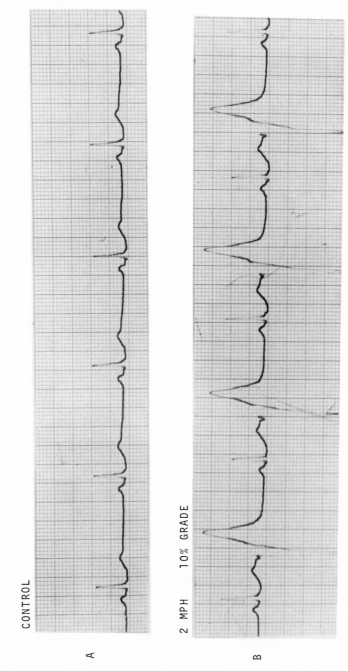

Fig. 3. Bigeminal PVCs occurring during treadmill testing in cardiac patient complaining of palpitations during exertion. Resting electrocardiogram was normal.

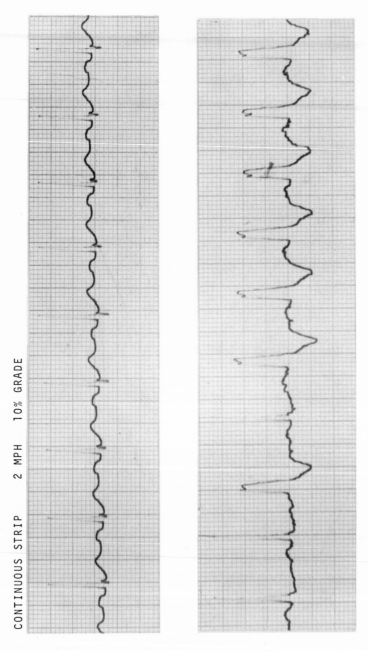

CONTINUOUS STRIP   2 MPH   10% GRADE

A

B

Fig. 4. Left bundle branch block during exercise testing in 60-year-old male, four months post anterior wall myocardial infarction.

CONTROL

A

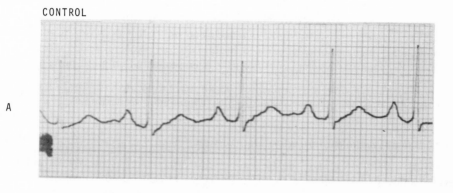

TREADMILL   3 MPH   10% GRADE

B

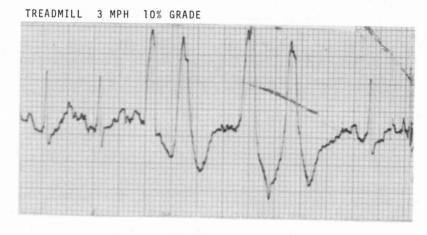

Fig. 5. Ventricular tachycardia during treadmill testing in 54-year-old male with postmyocardial infarction who complained of palpitations and syncope. Holter monitoring failed to reveal any arrhythmia.

ment of ventricular tachyarrhythmias (Fig. 5) in ambulatory patients with coronary artery disease is a major problem. Ventricular premature beats in the presence of coronary artery disease may be the prelude to sudden death (Chiang et al., 1963).

Both treadmill exercise testing and prolonged ambulatory electrocardiographic monitoring, compared by Kosowsky et al. (1971) for their ability to reveal ventricular ectopic activity in 81 patients, proved more effective than a three-minute standard electrocardiogram in displaying ventricular arrhythmias. Of 66 patients in whom the resting ECG was normal, prolonged monitoring was positive for arrhythmias in 18, or 27 percent, whereas exercise was positive in 26, or 39 percent. In 12 cases, ventricular arrhythmia was recorded only with exercise. In addition to displaying an increased incidence of arrhythmia, exercise also revealed more serious rhythm abnormalities, which could not have been suspected on monitoring alone.

Serial exercise testing is a simple method for evaluating the effect or lack of effect of antiarrhythmic drugs or potential life threatening arrhythmias (Gettes and Surawicz, 1961; Gooch and McConnell, 1970).

Detection of Preclinical Coronary Heart Disease

Brody (1959) presented the first systematic study of 756 unselected asymptomatic subjects. Twenty-three of these subjects had ischemic S-T depression of 0.5 mm or more at the initial examination, and 16 of the 23 men (70 percent) developed classical angina or had a myocardial infarction during a three-year follow-up period. Corresponding figures for the 733 with a negative exercise test were 55 (0.75 percent). The predictive power of the exercise ECG thus appears to be very high. However, the incidence of positive tests in an asymptomatic middle-aged population is fairly low, or about four percent in both Brody's series and in the population studied by Doyle and Kinch (1970).

Treadmill Exercise Assessment of the Functional Capacity of Patients with Cardiac Disease

Estimation of the impairment imposed by cardiac disease as outlined by the New York Heart Association functional classification is an integral part of a complete cardiac evaluation (The Criteria Committee of the New York Heart Association, 1953). Because the history is subjective, a more objective evaluation is desired in many circumstances. Exercise testing is an acceptable objective means of evaluating cardiac symptoms. It is possible to classify cardiac impairment into four groups, physiologically as well as clinically, and in general, the clinical evaluation corresponds to that of the exercise test. When a discrepancy exists between measured performance capacity and clinically related functional class, hemodynamic data obtained during cardiac catheterization usually indicates that graded exercise more accurately reflects the degree of cardiac impairment.

Patients with cardiac disease who have a work capacity of 22ml O_2/Kg per min or greater have sufficient reserve to perform routine physical activity and are usually symptom-free. Patients with a working capacity of 16ml O_2/Kg per min or less have decreased myocardial reserve both clinically and at cardiac catheterization. As long as a patient's level of fitness or cardiovascular reserve exceeds 16ml O_2/Kg per min, he will be relatively symptom-free (Patterson et al., 1972).

CONCLUSION

Multistage stress testing has been reviewed in terms of clinical uses, contraindications, hazards and advantages and methods. Such testing provides valuable information in the diagnosis of ischemic heart disease and for the methodology of cardiovascular epidemiology. Additional applications of testing include evaluation of medical and surgical therapy in cardiac disease, preclinical myocardial ischemia, assessment of cardiovascular fitness in the context of physical exercise reconditioning programs, detection of life-threatening arrhythmias and effectiveness of drug therapy in the treatment of arrhythmias.

REFERENCES

Bartel, A.G., Behar, V.S., Peter, R.H., Orgain, E.S. and Kong, K. (1974) *Circulation* 59, 348.

Blackburn, H. (ed.) (1969) *The Ernst Simonson Conference: Measurement in Exercise Electrocardiography* Charles C Thomas, Springfield, Ill.

Blomquist, G. (1965) *Acta Med Scand* 178 (suppl 440), 1.

Bruce, R.A. and McDonough, J.R. (1969) *Bull NY Acad Med* 45, 1288.

Bruce, R.A. and Hornstein T.R. (1969) *Prog Cardiovas Dis* 11, 371.

Brody, A.J. (1959) *JAMA* 171, 1195.

Case, R.A., Roselli, H.A. and Crampton, R.A. (1966) *Cardiologia* 48, 33.

Chiang, B.N., Perlman, L.V., Ostrander, L.D., et al (1963) *Ann Internal Med* 70, 1159.

Detry, J.R., Prette, F. and Brasseur, L.A. (1970) *Circulation* 42, 593.

Doyle, J.T. and Kinch, S.H. (1970) *Circulation* 41, 545.

Estes, E.H., Entman, M.L., Dixon, H.B. et al. (1966) *Amer Heart J* 71, 58.

Gettes, L.S., and Surawicz, B. (1961) *Amer J Med Sci* 254, 257.

Gooch, A.S., and McConnell, D. (1970) *Prog Cardiovas Dis* 13, 293.

Hamby, R.I., Wisoff, G.B., Kolker P. and Hartstein, M. (1973) *Chest* 50, 46.

Hellerstein, H.K. (1969) *J SC Med Assoc* 65 (Suppl 1 to No. 12), 46.

Kattus, A.A., Jorgensen, C.R., Worden, R.E. and Alvaro, A.B. (1971) *Circulation* 44, 585.

Kosowsky, B.D., Lown, B., Whiting, R. and Guiney I. (1971) *Circulation* 44, 826.

McConahay, D.R., McCallister, B.D. and Smith, R.E. (1971) *Amer J Cardiology* 28, 1.

McHenry, P.L., Phillips, J.F., and Kniebel, S.B. (1972) *Amer J Cardiol* 30, 47.

Patterson, J.A., Naughton, J., Pretroe, R.J. and Gunnar R.A. (1972) *Amer J Cardiol* 30, 757.

Robb, G.P., Marks, H.H., and Mattingly, T.W. (1956) *Trans Assoc Life Insur Med Dir Amer* 40, 52.

Rochmis, P. and Blackburn, H. (1971) *JAMA* 217, 1061.

Sheffield, L.T., Holt, J.H., and Reeves, T.J. (1965) *Circulation* 32, 622.

Zaret, B.L., Strauss, H.W., Martin, N.D. et al. (1973) *N Engl J Med* 288, 809.

The author thanks Mrs. Arlene Butterman for help in reviewing the literature and Mrs. Emma Hertlein for secretarial assistance in preparing the manuscript.

The Soft Signs of Neurological Problems of Mobility

David Green, M.B., B.S. (Melb.)

INTRODUCTION

"Soft signs" is clinical shorthand for early and subtle signs of disease. The term is often used as contrast with the phrase "hard signs" which implies unequivocal and pathognomonic signs of disease. It also implies debatable or at times rather indefinite clinical signs which often merge imperceptibly into the usual normal physical findings of a particular age group. Thus, before commenting on specific "soft signs" of neurological disease in patients above the age of 50 years, it would seem worthwhile to list the findings in the physical examination and fragments of the clinical history in the late middle-aged and the elderly which are not uncommon nor critical indicators of disease. These relatively common and normal variants are often mistaken as clinical signals of serious ongoing intracranial disease and are the subject of unnecessary consultations, laboratory work and admissions to hospital. Were they recognized for what they are, that is, the normal changes in the central and peripheral nervous systems occurring with age, a great deal of anxiety and fear in patients could be allayed and considerable money saved when unnecessary and often dangerous laboratory work is eliminated. The following list contains a number of these normal and common variants found in the examination of the late middle-aged and elderly:

1. Talkativeness and vagaries of speech.
2. Indistinct pronunciation to a modest degree.
3. A hesitant, staccato type of speech.
4. Some inattention and restlessness.
5. Poor vision and cataracts.
6. Moderate deafness, either unilateral or bilateral.
7. Unequal pupils, poorly reactive to light.
8. An absence of the convergence reflex.
9. Incomplete upward gaze.
10. Inadequate lateral gaze.

11. Tinnitus: whistles, hissing steam, resident bees, bells, chimes and dripping water. This symptom is rarely of diagnostic significance.
12. Neck stiffness, usually reflecting cervical osteoarthritis.
13. A brief aortic systolic murmur radiating into both common carotid arteries. This murmur is probably the most common incidental cardiac bruit heard during the examination of the elderly and may be pathognomonic of atherosclerotic aortic stenosis. It usually is not a signal of serious functional cardiac disease or a cause of Stokes-Adams attacks, although it can certainly play this role at times.
14. Deep tendon reflexes may be hyperactive, normal or absent.
15. Vibration sense, often said to be absent at the ankles at seventy years, but present in many patients well into their eighties.
16. Absence of ankle jerk, always remarked on in the examination of the aged. However, the ankle reflex as well as the triceps reflex are the weak sisters among reflexes and one often absent or difficult to elicit in the young while in the usual recumbent position. The ankle reflex can often be detected after being thought absent by having the patient kneel in a chair. It must be searched for in a patient with sciatica. In a routine examination it is best to remain simple and do routine tests gently and gracefully.
17. Alternate motion rate test in either of the upper and lower extremities not done as vigorously as in the younger patient. One must train oneself for these nuances in the physical examination much as the neurologist who examines infants and young children. There, too, the examination must be tailored and not kept in a rigid mold.
18. Snout reflex, often found in normal elderly patients.
19. Asymmetry of strength. This is an important finding and indicative of disease. Minimal generalized weakness is frequently encountered. An older patient has limited strength, and the examiner must over the years become accustomed to this. One must test strength slowly and carefully explain what is wanted; be prepared to mimic or act out some of the extremity movements to help the patient understand what is wanted before making a final judgment.
20. Often thin and generally wasted. This is not as important in neurology as is local wasting. The intrinsic hand muscles are conspicuous in their wasting during old age. The interosseous spaces are often somewhat hollowed out. If this is not asymmetrical and unassociated with a complaint of recent hand weakness, sensory loss or fasiculations, it is probably benign and part of the price of aging.
21. Hesitant, shuffling and short-paced gait which must be distinguished from the gait of Parkinson's disease or a minimal hemiparesis. The important thing to watch for is associated movements of the upper extremities because, if these are absent or diminished and asymmetrical, it is a fine clue toward the diagnosis of either corticospinal-tract or extrapyramidal-tract disease on that side.
22. Mild intention tremor, a modest but almost invariable price we pay for longevity.

23. A certain languor and deliberativeness in the movements of an older person's extremities. This must again be distinguished from the slow-motion, stuck-in-molasses movements of a patient with Parkinson's disease. Although an elderly person's joints are stiff and somewhat slow to move, there is not any cogwheel rigidity present which is so characteristic of Parkinson's disease (Green, 1974).

MAJOR NEUROLOGIC DISORDERS

These early and subtle signs and symptoms of neurological disease in the middle-aged and elderly which affect a patient's capacity to move about easily and gracefully are most important and informative clinically in patients with

(1) Parkinson's disease
(2) Hemiparesis secondary to cerebrovascular atherosclerosis
(3) Toxic effects of tranquilizing drugs
(4) Foot drop gait associated with either metabolic disease such as diabetes mellitus or mechanical causes such as excessive leg crossing.

Parkinson's Disease

James Parkinson's "An Essay on the Shaking Palsy" published in 1817 still contains the best description in English of the "soft signs" of that disease. Parkinson's own words on the early stages of the illness are as follows:

> So slight and nearly imperceptible are the first inroads of this malady, and so extremely slow is its progress, that it rarely happens, that the patient can form any recollection of the precise period of its commencement. The first symptoms perceived are, a slight sense of weakness, with a proneness to trembling in some particular part; sometimes in the head, but most commonly in one of the hands and arms. These symptoms gradually increase in the part first affected; and at an uncertain period, but seldom in less than twelve months or more, the morbid influence is felt in some other part. Thus assuming one of the hands and arms to be first attacked, the other, at this period becomes similarly affected. After a few more months the patient is found to be less strict than usual in preserving an upright posture: this being most observable whilst walking, but sometimes whilst sitting or standing. Sometime after the appearance of this symptom, and during its slow increase, one of the legs is discovered slightly to tremble, and is also found to suffer fatigue sooner than the leg of the other side: and in a few months this limb becomes agitated by similar tremblings, and suffers a similar loss of power.

> Hitherto the patient will have experienced but little inconvenience; and befriended by the strong influence of habitual endurance, would perhaps seldom think of his being the subject of disease, except when reminded of it by the unsteadiness of his hand, whilst writing or employing himself in any nicer kind of manipulation. But as the disease proceeds, similar employments are accomplished with considerable difficulty, the hand failing to answer with exactness to the dictates of the will. Walking becomes a task which cannot be performed without considerable attention. The legs are not raised to that height, or with that promptitude which the will directs, so that the utmost care is necessary to prevent frequent falls.

In 1819, a former medical student at Guy's Hospital and Diplomate of the Apothecaries Society of London, John Keats, distilled the definition of aging, lack of mobility and perhaps the Shaking Palsy in the "Ode to a Nightingale"

The Weariness, the fever, and the fret
  Here, where men sit and hear each other groan;
Where palsy shakes a few, sad, last gray hairs,
  Where youth grows pale, and specter-thin, and dies.

Parkinson's disease is the Myxoedema of Neurology. This means that just as the physician has great trouble recognizing early hypothyroidism, so does the neurologist have similar difficulty with the diagnosis of early Parkinson's disease. The elderly patient with a slow deliberate manner, rather deep voice, sallow complexion, puffy facial features and annoyingly slow capacity to think, has myxoedema. When described in these words, the diagnosis is obvious. But if the physician accepts the patient in the first few minutes of the clinical interview as being just elderly, obese, slow-witted and a bit cantankerous, he can easily miss the diagnosis entirely and fall back on the remark that he or she is just another old, slow-moving and slow-witted person with no particular disease.

All who practice medicine have had this experience and sadly a remediable illness goes on untreated at times for years. Early Parkinson's disease has a similar destiny. If one accepts the diminished capacity to move gracefully, the lowered and sometimes monotonic speech, the lack of eyeblink and thus the somewhat hostile stare, the ironed out facial features and infrequent change of expression as belonging to a phlegmatic, somewhat depressed, laconic and annoyingly hostile person, then the diagnosis of Parkinson's disease is lost and buried in a sea of wrong clinical thinking. Parkinson's disease should be diagnosed on the basis of clinical impression and not on the late signs of rigidity and tremor. Correct and early diagnosis is helpful now that reasonably good therapy is available and should be offered to the patient.

Hemiparesis Secondary to Cerebrovascular Atherosclerosis

It is easy enough to recognize a patient with a severe hemiplegic gait by the spastic, clumsy, shuffling, circumducting leg and the partially flexed upper extremity. However, it is the subtle, mild hemiparetic patient who presents a challenge in diagnosis. His illness can be identified by watching him walk, not for the gross features described above, but for the subtle loss of associated movement of the upper extremity or the natural swing of the arm. This single physical sign is often more important than much of the rest of the physical examination and all the laboratory work that can be done. When hesitancy of gait is combined with the loss of associated movement of the upper extremity, hemiparesis or Parkinson's disease is very likely to be present. Parkinson's disease has other distinguishing features as outlined in the preceding section. Hemiparesis secondary to cerebrovascular atherosclerosis and thrombosis is distinguished by the presence of diminished alternate motion rate or swing of the extremity, drift of the forearm and hand when held in front of the patient and hyperreflexia or at least asymmetric deep tendon reflexes.

Toxic Effects of Tranquilizing Drugs

All too often patients who seem stunned, benumbed, bemused, who walk in an agonizingly slow, clumsy, hesitant or unsteady fashion, whose speech is slowed or slurred, whose thinking is limited and hesitant and who have the features of Parkinson's disease minus tremor are patients who are toxic because of phenothiazines. Tranquilizing drugs generally not only tranquilize but also benumb the intellect. Such drugs are frequently overprescribed or overused and their expense is a national scandal. In truth, the demand and appetite for these drugs is a reflection of clever advertising by the pharmaceutical companies and a mindless demand for the medication by patients. Osler very rightly observed "the desire to take medicine is perhaps the greatest feature which distinguishes man from animals" (Seldes, 1966).

Physicians share the blame in the overuse of these drugs. It is true that the drugs blunt anxiety and restlessness, but they also cause dullness and ataxia. It is almost heretical at this time to say the anxieties of life are more preferable and tolerable than this perpetual, drugged, toxic, somnolent and often ataxic state. If the Parkinsonian patient seems to have his feet stuck to the floor in molasses, the toxic patient seems to have molasses in his brain and his thinking is slowed down accordingly.

Foot Drop Gait

The foot drop gait can often be seen and occasionally heard as the patient approaches the office door because of the slapping sound the foot makes as it strikes the floor. However, many times the foot drop or weakness of the anterior tibial compartment may be missed in the patient complaining vaguely of weakness in the extremity until the patient is asked to try to walk on his heels. It is then that the foot drop becomes evident. Diabetes mellitus is a common cause and at least ten percent of diabetics at some time in their lives have a peripheral neuropathy; a fair percentage have significant motor involvement and either a foot drop or diffuse weakness of the leg muscles. A special variety of diabetic mononeuropathy is involvement of the femoral nerve and, thus, weakness of the quadriceps muscles. Diabetic neuropathy is frequently asymmetric.

Another unfortunate cause of gait dysfunction occurs in the elderly who tend to sit a lot more than they should. While sitting, daydreaming or watching television endlessly, they cross their legs for hours and compress the lateral peroneal nerve against the neck of the fibula. These patients can never date the onset of the foot drop and their complaint is weakness of the leg rather than the foot. Their fear, often expressed early, is that they may have had a stroke. The history of leg crossing, the restriction of the deficit to the foot drop, the sensory loss on the lateral aspect of the leg and dorsum of the foot and the improvement when leg crossing is discontinued – all tend to support the diagnosis. In this instance, a nerve conduction time study of the peroneal nerve gives convincing evidence of peripheral nerve disease and helps reassure the patient.

There is, of course, a type of difficulty with gait so common and so subtle in its onset that it is hardly ever given a paragraph in a medical text. It is the slow, stooped, hesitant gait of the elderly. What was once an elastic, bouncing gait is now measured and it seems as if each step requires thought. Often this gait and the presence of senile tremor excites the thought of definable disease, but a firm diagnosis cannot be offered.

Keats described this final state of man well in his poem, "The Eve of St. Agnes," when describing the Beadsman who does "harsh penance on St. Agnes Eve":

His prayer he saith, this patient, holy man;
Then takes his lamp, and riseth from his knees,
And back returneth, meager, barefoot, wan,
Along the chapel aisle by slow degrees.

CONCLUSION

Hopefully, the precepts and principles of exercise and activity discussed in the other chapters of this book, if applied, may delay or at least hold at bay for some the common destiny of the elderly to gradually lose their capacity to get about easily.

REFERENCES

Green, D. (1974) *N Y State J Med* 74, 6.
Seldes, G. (ed.) (1966) *The Great Quotations*, Lyle Stuart, New York.

Section III

Motivation and Planning

Motivation for Fitness

Frederick A. Whitehouse, Ed.D., F.A.P.A.

INTRODUCTION

The concepts of "motivation" and "fitness" present the same problems as the concepts of "beauty," "goodness" and "sin" since such words may mean different things depending upon the viewpoint. Here, motivation is considered as "efforts made to encourage the patient to act for his benefit."

"Fitness" carries the same problem of specification. Here, it implies a psychophysical combine and the necessity to consider both interdependent aspects to produce a state of physical and mental well-being with the adaptive capacity to remain so. The content of the paper will further clarify the meaning.

Preachers try to motivate their parishioners, teachers their students, parents their children and physicians their patients, and frequently they fail. All, in one way or another, profess to make this effort for the individual's own good and buttress their words by claiming special knowledge about the subject or problem. But, all of them seldom look at the issue from the consumer's side because they are so filled with their own convictions: Who can be wrong or do wrong when one is on the side of God, logic, reason, science and good intentions?

Why do they fail? Often because too broad, too noble and too generalized reasons are given. Furthermore, their views are usually an imposition, a demand, a know-it-all or even a threat to the individual's own sovereignity of spirit and personal propensities and needs. The imposition of another's will is, at best, only a short-term gain. The recipient of persuasive efforts must not only make up his own mind, be convinced of the message, feel it satisfies what he sees as his needs, but also wish to exert some freedom of choice about it. It isn't easy to persuade people to behave as we believe, especially since our message is but one of the many competing for their attention. In fact, in self-defense, we all have had to practice resistance to the bombardment of many causes thrust upon us in a complex society.

Our culture, generally speaking, tends to interpret fitness as either beauty or muscle. We are more concerned with appearances than health, with show rather than substance. Usually a higher price in effort is paid for what is considered attractiveness than for physical well being.

However, fitness programs need to tell the truth and not 'ape' the superficial pitch of the huckster. We should not wish to entice people for the wrong reasons to satisfy our sense of noble purpose. Yet, as products of the American culture, we can be trapped by overselling because it is so common and acceptable.

Those espousing the value of fitness have been physicians, physical educators, athletic coaches and other people who naturally stress and talk about the physical benefits and are less skilled and insightful in interpreting the psychological values. Since the mental, emotional and the physical are so bound together, greater emphasis should be placed on the psychological and emotional benefits of achieving physical fitness. The release of aggressions, the lessening of mental tensions, the greater feeling of confidence, a sharper alertness, the joy of movement, the feeling of pride in self-discipline and other things can be said that are modest promises. Furthermore, mentally fit individuals appear to have fewer physical problems and those physically fit, fewer emotional problems. Studies in industrial populations (Hinkle et al., 1960) support this view.

Mental practice in self-discipline, in the surmounting of problems, in resistance to the tough cost of physical achievement, becomes beneficial not only in terms of the accomplishments of the goals of fitness but in the practice of the qualities of remaining fit.

This is why in striving for fitness we need to involve and engage the whole person in our efforts to motivate.

THE ISSUES OF NEEDS

One method of approaching the problem of motivation is to study human needs. From such an examination, one could then attempt to use the results in planning an execution of programs. An investigator could easily fill a book by merely listing the various needs cited by prominent authors who range from the less expansive who would hardly go beyond the instinctual (such as hunger, thirst and sex), holding that all other needs stemmed from these, to the views of Gardner Murphy who believes that in motivation ". . .there is an almost infinite number of needs and tensions." In between are such well-known writers as Fromm with five categories, Maslow with six, Horney with nine and Murray with 20 (Hall and Lindzey, 1957). Horney later reduced her list of nine to three: "Moving towards people, moving away from people and moving against people."

In an effort to summarize the many points of view, the following three major categories are offered:

1. *Physical needs:* the instinctual classes of hunger, thirst and sex and the broader sensory and physiological needs. Our muscles demand usage, crave movement and action. We feel deprived and upset if we cannot see, hear, smell, touch and experience our senses. Even in sleep, we toss and turn and use our muscles related to both

bed pressure and our dreams. Prolonged physical immobilization causes mental and physical deterioration.

Sensory deprivation experiments show how, when we cannot obtain sensory stimulation, we rebel and may insist upon leaving the setting. If we stay, we manufacture our own sensory usage by hearing, seeing and smelling things that aren't there. We may see ghostly images and hear music in our effort to satisfy the craving (Ruff and Levy, 1959: Ruff et al., 1959; Levy et al., 1958; Zubek, 1964; Jackson et al., 1962).

2. *Psychological needs*: the desire for information, knowledge of the world about us, novelty, aesthetic satisfactions, sense of worth, self-identification, achievement, security power, mastery, transcendence, etc.

3. *Social needs*: friendship, membership, love, admiration, prestige, submission to social conformities, etc.

It is important to consider such classifications in planning and carrying out fitness programs so that as many as these needs may be touched upon and each individual's special needs may be understood.

INDIVIDUALIZING MOTIVATION

The medical and psychological literature is replete with advice that the patient should be treated as an "individual." While individualization is a matter of degree, the more this can be achieved increases the chances for successful results. If we are to deal with and attempt to help and influence a person toward better fitness, it is valuable to know his background, life style, interests, concerns, habits, present physical condition, stated expectations and personal goals for the enterprise. This gives the opportunity for clarification and the correction of false hopes as well as the offer for real benefits.

Fitness programs are therapeutic programs, in whatever form they take, and should be as individualized as can be reasonably done, psychologically as well as physically. A mass approach may entice a group that finds the incentive attractive, yet the group won't continue participation unless the program gives evidence which satisfies mental and emotional needs.

Motivating the individual won't take place unless he believes what one says. But before that, he must first understand the information presented. Information and advice that is too broad or general leaves such a vague impression that an individual doesn't quite know what to think about on his own or how to relate it to his own interests. If we say, "This program will make you healthier and gives you a greater chance for a longer life," it sounds impressive to the giver but the receiver often is reminded of the preaching of parent or clergyman upon the rewards of being good and holy. He may feel a bit guilty about his nonacceptance but relieves his conscience and his vague feelings of confusion by an underlying resentment against the would-be persuader's expectation of acceptance. Such levels of advice are really careless, unconcerned retreats from greater responsibility and only serve to get oneself off the hook. For example, consider a judge who may feel he has done his duty by asserting to the delinquent that "he should behave himself, go to school, get a job or attend church regularly." Talking to an individual privately doesn't mean we are individualizing motivation, especially when we give each one the same general advice.

While we surely espouse the principle that patients require individual treatment and would deplore the "Madison Ave." mass motivational technique, we may be trapped by generalities. A physician who obviously doesn't prescribe the same medicine in the same dosage for all his patients may give rather global advice about physical fitness. Some patients do not take medicine or follow recommendations at least in part because the reasons have not been made clear to them. Consequently, advice which takes the form of "getting an outdoor hobby" or "joining the Y" may not be effective unless additional information is given as to need and purpose.

Another mistake made in the name of good, well-intentioned advice is the use of such sentimental homilies as "You owe it to those you love," "Nature meant our bodies to be fit," "Your wife and children depend on you," which are often received with more irritation than inspiration. Guilty feelings have limited staying powers for motivation. The same can be said for appealing to a noble principle. True, the society holds up to us the model of those who sacrificed all for principle. Most of us verbally agree with the altruism but would not act if too much personal sacrifice is required unless the return for self-enhancement is apparent and fairly certain.

Related to the "noble principle" motivation is a highly respected social folklore. We say that a mark of maturity is the ability to delay immediate gratification for long-term benefit. Quite so, but this approach has limited appeal. Even mature individuals are highly selective about what they choose to delay. Usually there is a need for some gratification along the way in terms of evidence that signals progress. These small rewards tend to continue stimulation towards the more important goal.

It is wise for physicians to detail a patient's improvements and to tell him how gains may be estimated before he begins (Whitehouse, 1970a, 1970b). A pat on the back and the message that one is coming along fine is not as motivating as telling the patient that his heart rate or respiration rate has declined, his blood pressure has dropped or other possible physiological parameters have improved even if the gain has been slight. Not only will the patient feel better, he will be reinforced in the conviction that his efforts make a difference in a tangible way.

With few exceptions, none of us like to be told what to do, have no voice in the planning nor any opportunity to express ourselves creatively. As much latitude, choice, novelty, options or alternatives as possible ought to be integrated into such programs. True, some time will be wasted but, in the long run, an individual will put more of himself into actions about which he feels some sense of mastery and personal choice.

Fear and threats, whether implicit or explicit, have never proven to be good motivating forces. They sometimes seem to work but they have poor lasting power and eventually create a resentment barrier. A good example is the man who recently had a coronary occlusion. He never could stop smoking, overeating or underexercising before but now reforms immediately. Sometimes the reality of the threat which he experienced is strong enough to maintain the change, but even those fears lessen and he doesn't stay reformed unless other supporting incentives come into being. Now a coronary occlusion is, in a sense, a supreme threat; yet it may not work on some or remain for others. Those who seem not to have been influenced at all are the ones who subconsciously are the most fearful, too fearful even to make any change lest it certify reality. So they seemingly ignore it because they cannot endure the dreadful truth of threatened existence.

SOCIAL SUPPORT

A major support to the individual seeking and participating in any improvement routine is the encouragement of family and friends. It's nice to be admired and sustained by kind strangers but it is vital that one feels that effort is appreciated by those who mean the most and who will share happily in any triumph. Therefore, efforts to use such individuals, especially in some assisting capacity, is usually profitable.

If a diet is to be altered or exercise to be done, one's spouse, for instance, ought to know about it and the possible ways of helping. An individual may find it easy to quit on himself, but because he values the high estimation of those he loves, he perseveres.

One major problem of motivating individuals after 50 years of age is that, in many, their personal reaction to aging, their decline in physical powers, the usually increasing isolation from children as they leave home and friends as they die, the frequent loss of ambitions once cherished and the incidence of actual or beginning illnesses all serve to depress their image of self-worth. The challenge is seen as too large to even try, and the tide of events may defeat them to the point of not fighting back. Such people need to cope first with what they conceive to be bigger questions than "fitness." They need "mental fitness" even more than physical fitness as a force!

An incident illustrating this need happened some years ago when I was director of rehabilitation for the American Heart Association which sponsors programs for women with heart disease, especially for those whose physicians recommend less physical expenditure as homemakers. The typical homemaker often uses more physical energy than her husband who works in industry. Studies of energy cost equivalents show this (Hellerstein and Hornsten, 1966). The Homemaker's Course was to show them how to do their tasks with less energy stress on their cardiovascular systems. The instructor was showing how it was important to sit and peel potatoes on a paper towel. During this demonstration several women asked completely irrelevant questions that had nothing to do with the instruction. It was immediately apparent that there were other things on their minds and that their questions, while not actually saying so, were leading to their more basic feelings of "am I going to be able to be a wife and mother" and "what is the real significance of my condition?" Clearly they needed their physicians to be sympathetic enough to sit down with them and discuss the issues. In addition, perhaps some counseling or group therapy was indicated before they were ready to cope with some of the lesser issues represented in homemaking.

Some older individuals, in a sense, accept the challenge and resist, but instead of altering their self-image in reasonable conformance to the reality of aging, they react irrationally by trying to maintain an earlier youthful ego. They may begin to "live it up," take to increased drinking, neglect their responsibilities and marriages, and alienate or abandon old friends because they represent the past. The inevitable result is often tragic psychologically and physically.

One cannot sell such people on the logic and the benefits of fitness. They need personal counseling first to get themselves together. And this may not help either!

COUNSELING FOR FITNESS

It would be wise to evaluate the need for counseling. A few of those over 50 may need nothing more than a personal talk with a knowledgeable individual; a small number may need some combined help from their physician and fitness experts; a fair number may need more structured and continuing counseling for some period; and some will need rather intensive psychotherapy if they are to alter their present outlooks on life.

One cannot say what the proportions are or give concrete evidence since there will be much variation. This suggestion is made on the basis of the aging complex and upon the known difficulty of changing possible life-long habits and life styles. If merely presenting the logic of fitness for such a group was sufficiently good persuasion, it would be simple but humans are polymorphic and live simultaneously at several levels of consciousness, with cognitive control of the internal consultants along with deep-seated influences.

Probably no program can help everyone to a desirable degree. Consequently, one screens to permit certain efficiencies and economies, with consideration for his resources. However, the message is this: incorporate as much counseling as is feasible and there will be a greater likelihood of a more effective program.

Finally, counseling is no panacea and this way of reaching the individual is not always successful. Yet, it is the best way to remove or decrease psychic barriers and to open up individuals to their potentials for self-decision and self-direction.

SOME CONSIDERATIONS IN PLANNING A FITNESS PROGRAM

Earlier it was mentioned that a fitness program was one kind of a therapeutic endeavor. As such, it may be useful to review the basic issue of a therapeutic enterprise. In an article on the concept of therapy (Whitehouse, 1967), I listed a variety of therapeutic systems, methods and techniques which numbered around 350, with such categories as psychotherapeutic, psychophysical, psychosocial and somatic. This outlay in no way encompassed all therapies since there are about 600 kinds, chiefly in the psychotherapeutic area.

What does this cornucopia imply? Obviously, there isn't a single standard method for everyone, and the medical dictum that "no one medicine cures all" is apt. Clearly, it also implies that many methods have been devised presumably to meet particular kinds of individual problems and that therapists alter methods and use systems compatible with their own personal interests. In my opinion, this is the basic reason for such variation although the originator usually claims to have created the approach because of the patient's particular problems. Such patients are apparently only a stimulus to the therapist's desire to practice and gain satisfaction through the means of a method he devises and projects in the exchange with the patient. This point does not rule out the somatic therapies in which somewhat the same process takes place by choice of specialty and procedures used.

Another reason for the diffuse number is the need for the patient and the therapist to locate a compatible system of mutual accommodation. This is very important in the psychotherapeutic realm and usually quite necessary in the somatic areas. In the latter case, the placebo literature strongly supports a concordant relationship.

The final reason for the wealth of therapies is that they are a reflection of the American culture; enterprise, impulse for change, affluence and less rigidity than older cultures create a broader therapeutic market.

With these observations in mind, one would surmise that a parallel takes place in fitness programs and there are many kinds with different emphases, a variety of philosophies and a multitude of ways of execution in keeping with leadership personalities.

THE QUESTIONNAIRE AS A DEVICE

Perhaps as a step to planning a viable fitness program, one may ask the participants why they entered. If this is done, a variety of answers will be found — plausible ones, lengthy ones, pithy ones, etc. But, unfortunately, few people know what really persuaded them to do such a thing. They may give an answer which was given to them as a good reason before they began or parrot the words of the physician who referred them. Some may regurgitate the current social message about fitness. One may get back what the leader put into the program as a claimed value. Furthermore, answers will be made which tend to present the responder as intelligent, thoughtful and constructive or reflect what the individual considers appropriate to justify his actions. Finally, one may also receive an answer which pleases the questioner. The participants don't wish to be though ungrateful and unappreciative of the efforts made on their behalf.

To be sure, these reasons are given with reasonable sincerity, but an individual really doesn't know what the impulse was. He knows what he tells himself and this is his honest reply, or he feels it's honest enough. Those who have been personally engaged in psychotherapy appreciate that what we may have been telling others and ourselves for years may not be necessarily true of ourselves. What's more, sometimes we knew it but felt we had to suppress it.

Furthermore, a number of other variables may influence an answer. Replies depend upon who asks the questions, what the apparent purpose was as seen by the responder, when the question is asked (for example, at what point in time of his feeling of success or failure) and what the surrounding circumstances were. For example, was it answered in the gym, in a group of others or alone in his own living room?

While many illustrations could be cited to support these statements, let me confine myself to a simple story. Consider Mrs. Jones. Some time ago, she felt rather angry with the attention her husband showed to that slender Mrs. Smith down the block. She looked in her mirror more critically and decided "fitness is healthier" and that's the answer she may give if questioned. Mrs. Jones then completes a fitness program and, upon being asked again (with Mrs. Smith still getting too much attention), may say, "I lost ten pounds and I don't lose my breath going up the stairs, but I think the program is deficient." If, however, Mrs. Jones is now getting the attention she desires, she may say, "It did wonders for me, I feel better, it gave me more poise and confidence, I'm a happier, more alert person, etc."

THE ISSUE OF INFORMATION

Frequently, the professional assumes too much about how well-informed and understanding of procedure the patient may be. In fitness programs, a few good slogans, some specialized advice by a physician and some general statements about a program are often enough for some patients but not for others. Many individuals beginning a new endeavor are lucky to retain half of what is put before them. They, as many medical patients are at particular times, are not ready to listen as they are preoccupied with acquiring some accommodation to the setting and program. In addition, probably most individuals entering these enterprises have only sketchy information about the human body and its functioning so that comments about certain benefits don't register.

Written material for reinforcement that one may take home and read and show to spouse and friends should supplement verbal interpretation. The patient may "hear" it wrong, miss the point when the chap beside him coughed or misunderstand the technical word used. Therefore, such review material may encourage his motivation. Spouting information when patients are busily engaged in physical activity will not reach those concentrating upon the effort.

Of course, a good demonstration and a helpful, interested, cheerful attitude by the program leader will ensure better group communication and participation. Every means that will put the message across — cognitively, physically and emotionally — should be employed.

THE PROGRAM LEADER

Perhaps, the appropriate way to begin this section is with a key quote from Emerson: "The only gift is a portion of thyself." In an age when we use printed greeting cards for all occasions, which someone else has thought up what we ought to say and which may even have our names printed on them, it is not unusual to find that much human interaction is lost and evidently felt to be unnecessary. We, who work with human beings, must not succumb to the debasement of values around us. The more sensitive we become, the happier we will be in our work, thus improving our performance with consequent greater benefits to our patients. So the first consideration is: "What kind of person is the leader?"

The people we help must believe in us and our credibility as concerned helpers. For example, such belief is what makes a pharmaceutical more effective – not only because of its ingredients, but because of the placebo element. Some patients do not obtain good results from the medicine prescribed by their physicians while in others, even a placebo works as well or better than the same medicine (Wolf, 1959). At the basis of this response lies the nature and personality of the giver, among other components.

What factors encourage high credibility in the leader, and, therefore, are influential? I enumerate them:

Belief in Self

You must believe in your own worth as a leader. You must be personally convinced that what you do will be beneficial, that you have the knowledge and qualities to assist in your patient's accomplishments. Personal ambiguity tends to be projected, leading to uncertainty on the part of the patient.

Belief in Subject or Field

It is important that you believe the means and techniques you use are useful and appropriate. You must have faith in the therapeutic principles which guide you.

Belief in the Patient

Perhaps the most important asset is your belief in the patient's ability to profit. This is something that you really cannot hide because it will be apparent to your participants. If you are saying to yourself "I wonder if I am wasting my time with this group of fat, old ladies," or, "this gang I got is 'for the birds;' I wish I had a more eager, gung-ho group," it will get across. Your language, tone, body movements, facial changes and everything about you will be read or sensed. There is no escape from projective disclosure. This is true of physicians, college professors, sales clerks and everyone in a human interpersonal relationship (Whitehouse, 1970c, 1968).

Sincerity of Interest

Concern needs to be shown by your interest in your means and procedures, and in the attention you manifest in the individuals with whom you deal. Ann Morrow Lindbergh said, "There is nothing more exhausting than insincerity." Genuiness or phoniness is soon spotted. When you fake it, so will your participants and relieve themselves of this false game by quitting."

Enthusiasm for Subject

You have all experienced the value of enthusiasm and how impelling it can be. Most of you know the home team advantages in sports and the stimulus of the fans behind the individual or group. Let me cite two dramatic examples from the medical literature.

Surgeons, operating for ulcers, who were skeptics of the surgical procedure, obtained only half as many five-year cures as the enthusiasts, and the skeptics had 20 times the incidence of recurrent marginal ulcers as the enthusiasts (Beecher, 1961).

An even more remarkable story is the history of the rise and denouement of the internal, mammary-artery ligation operation which was intended to improve coronary blood flow for patients with angina. First performed in Italy, it was taken up in this country and reported with enthusiasm by eminent surgeons. After some time, when suspicion arose as to its efficacy, an investigation was done in which half of the patients received the true operation and the other half a sham procedure which merely left a real chest scar without the actual operation. The results were that both groups benefited with little essential difference between them. Pain was lessened in both groups and one patient in the false group even went back to the work he couldn't perform prior to the episode because of chest pain (Cobb et al., 1959).

To be a good motivator, you must obtain personal enjoyment and satisfaction in your work. And, I would warn you that this aspect should not be delayed until you complete a program and assess it. It must take place along the way, every day if possible, and not depend solely upon the final benefit to your clients.

One aspect that tends to rob a ministrator of needed satisfaction for personal motivation is to be obsessed with perfection only upon complete final success. There is a trap particularly for the most dedicated and sincere, especially when we see others who "don't really care." However, we must realize that we must be concerned with ourselves as well if we are to provide the best service. Proper balance means acknowledging the fact that, for reasons often beyond our control, failure will result.

Recognition of the Patient's Problems and Fears

Patients are encouraged to continue their struggles if they believe the person helping them is aware of their doubts, problems and fears. If patients have someone who understands, who is treating them as individuals even though they may be operating in a group program, it is supportive. Furthermore, getting a few things "off one's chest" opens the door to greater mobilization of effort which may have been blocked. Consequently, whenever opportunity is available or definitely made available to talk to patients individually, it will be beneficial to the patient.

Clarity of Verbal Presentation

It has been found that people are more influenced by an opinion if the conclusions are explicitly stated rather than merely left to the receivers to draw their own inferences as to what one really means (Karlins and Abelson, 1970). Not only is it a good practice to explain what is going to be done and what the purpose is, but to clearly state what the benefits are purported to be and why. The more one leaves a group in the dark, the less cooperative they are and the more resentful they become. When possible, each individual should know how it will benefit him personally and not that which is just generally useful to the group.

Avoid False Claims or Exaggerated Promises of Benefit

This is rather obvious but sometimes in a would-be effort to motivate, examples of extraordinary benefit of a few or even one individual are held up as models. It's as if everyone could do it with exceptional effort. Famous athletes' extraordinary efforts overcoming physical adversity to perform successfully are not exactly models for the over-50, since people would tend to be more influenced by the achievements of others who they think are more like themselves. So examples when given should be those with which a patient can identify comfortably.

Creative Effort

Creativeness on the part of the leader or motivator is not only a source of personal satisfaction but it tends to spark those who are the recipients. Departures from routine, a new order in the business, or a spontaneous, different way of performing creates excitement, perhaps laughter, and less tension and, somehow, a greater sense of oneness in a group.

Human Relations

So much of motivation lies in good human relations which incorporates respect for the individual, an avoidance of pretense, an absence of false jollity and abstinence from artificial praise. We recognize that blacks don't wish to be patronized or called "boy" but frequently younger therapists believe it is encouraging to greet clients over 50 with: "How's the boy today?" or "All together boys." Those over 50 come from an era when politeness was valued so they probably won't say, "Cut it out." They may even smile, or a group of women may giggle when called "girls." It is supposed to be a light touch but it really is a put-down and, while most may not think twice about it if said once, it is a nonpayoff in the long run and tends to build resentment and resistance. Patients are equals and not sheep to be herded. Blacks may accept being called "boy" by another black; those over 50 may enjoy it greatly if somebody in his 70's calls them "boy," but not by therapists younger than their children.

People over 50 are sometimes slower to respond and it isn't because they are getting senile. Age brings more reflection. One has a greater reservoir of reference points and one has seen the error of jumping or deciding too soon. The younger person with more animal spirits and energy to burn feels he can afford to waste effort. Consequently, patience should be a factor, and the current social trend to instant everything or short-cutting ought to be avoided. Of course, the younger leader will find more rigidity in his older patients and must take this into account.

A psychiatrist I know is so open, friendly and unpretentious that people are inclined to say with delight as well as relief in their tone, "Is he really a psychiatrist?" Many of us might well ask ourselves whether we come across as human and not as setting ourselves apart behind a professional facade.

Clergymen and physicians, traditionally awesome figures, have been getting this message. The stiff, formal posture and the fond, gold-headed cane attitude is out and no longer viable. Respect doesn't come from awe but from humanness. Respect comes from giving respect.

The following investigation on the home life of a group of children provides a supportive parallel. It found a number of factors about which psychologists might well be appalled. Some children came from homes in which the father was rather tyrannical. He dominated the home and his word was law. In other families, the mother played the dominant part and the husband was passive. Some children were never allowed to go to the movies during the week; others went frequently. Some had too little, if any, spending money; others had too much. Some children were physically spanked; others were never censured. These things and similar situations found are usually felt to be harmful influences. Yet, this was actually a study of the home life of well-adjusted children. How come? The authors concluded that it really didn't much matter how children were treated on the surface as long as they felt loved and accepted by their parents (Stout and Langdon, 1950).

So, many of the things we are frequently concerned about are not important as they may be superficial. What is vital is that we look for the basic qualities in our programs which make individuals feel secure, concerned about, accepted and treated with respect. The quantity of the equipment, the beauty of the surroundings and the credentials of the leaders may be helpful and contributory but don't rate as high and will not in themselves provide effectiveness unless the human qualities are attended to first.

Decision Making

We who may be the motivators or persuaders often fail to take into account the need for the patient or client to have made his own decision. We are often in positions in which people are dependent upon us for services. Frequently, they solicit our advice, or we give it to them without such request because of the nature of the relationship. However, many errors are made both in everyday life and in therapeutic realms because we didn't permit the individual a choice. We made the decision for "his own good" and for our own good also, as we obtain the feeling of satisfactory service.

Sometimes, we let ourselves be trapped into this. Many people do not wish to take personal responsibility for a decision because they wish an out which will not injure their own self-esteem or a possible exit from something displeasing. They would then have someone to blame if magic results are not achieved, and it makes it easier to quit when things get tough because they are not quitters on themselves but on you, the persuader. Furthermore, this nonresponsibility makes it legitimate to beat the game in any way they choose. They circumvent the persuader or punish whoever is in charge by performing routinely and casually, absenting themselves and not living up to what has been set out for them. Then, when the inevitable poor result comes about, it isn't their defeat but yours. The minor guilt they feel may be absolved by hostility and ridiculing the process or by expressing some pity for the fools who haven't escaped.

Another way the motivator fails is that he doesn't recognize that many people, after hearing the well-meaning persuader give all kinds of good reasons indicating at least his own firm convictions about it, may be reluctant to say no. They haven't had time to think about it and are too polite or too much in awe, or feel it isn't cricket to discourage someone who believes, especially when he says it is for their own good. So they say yes and don't show up or follow through and if they do, it is only a polite try once or twice. They not only never were convinced but, in addition, now reject the persuader and are annoyed with themselves for complying.

Subtle Transference

The following classical story illustrates a lot of what I have been saying about your proper role as leader. A patient had long suffered from chronic asthma. His physician was sent a sample of a new "drug" which was then tried on the patient with a dramatic alleviation of his complaints. However, when a "placebo" was substituted by the physician without the patient's knowledge, his asthma returned as before. Several trials were made back and forth, all without the patient's knowledge, and each time the "drug" was effective and the "placebo" was not. Eventually, the physician needed a new supply of the drug which he now believed to be meritorious. At this point the pharmaceutical company revealed that since they were not sure of the efficacy of the new product, even though they had received favorable responses from others, they had originally sent him a placebo (Boshes, 1960). In other words, as long as the physician believed that a true drug was given, and perhaps had confidence in it, the patient also believed. As long as the physician knew it was a placebo, somehow the patient got the message.

This story is in no way unique. The fields of medicine, psychotherapy, pharmacology and others are replete with marvelous examples of the importance of who the ministrator is, what he believes, how confident he is, the trust and expectations of the patient, the circumstances of the occasion and even the atmosphere of the setting, among other factors. It is such factors that affect all therapy and all interpersonal engagements.

PROGRAM MANAGEMENT

The management of a "fitness" program is something best left to those who are more skilled than I. Nevertheless, as a psychologist I have a few suggestions. One ought to state to the group one's personal expectations, what standards one believes ought to be maintained and, if possible, set certain dates for general accomplishments. Patients usually do not mind the imposition of some rules of the game as long as they know what they are and why. You have a right, as do your patients, to have prospective hopes; it is expected of you. Such delineation actually makes people more comfortable.

Efforts should be made for feedback of views by participants. Before each new session, a few minutes' time for discussion, asking for advice and offering of some alternatives, will usually give feedback. If you don't get it, the chances are that you are to blame. And so feedback can be technically important and a measure of the relationship as well.

The size of your group is important and this is true with the physical educator in a gym or the teacher in a classroom. Optimal size would usually range from an economic minimum to a size which still permits a good interpersonal relationship. Too small is harmful to the social aspects between individuals and doesn't enable some to profit from compatible associates. Too large a group changes many things. It is discouraging to the leader who cannot get to know each patient as a person, and in effect makes individuals feel lost in the mob with the implication in a symbolic sense that they are not important.

If the most is to be made of the social factors and a group or team spirit, such groups should be socially compatible and probably roughly in the same age bracket. This composition should be with such people as they may associate with in everyday life. It's difficult enough to cope with the self-discipline of personal reform without needing to accommodate to companions with a totally different life style. Whether there ought to be a mix of the sexes obviously depends upon so many factors, and particularly the nature of the program, that it is difficult to make general statements. Certain programs at certain stages would probably benefit by the association. One might ask, "Why all this stuff about mixture?" We have an exercise program and muscles have no distinctions. That's true, but one is dealing with human beings first and their eccentricities of status, background and variance in experience. However, it is obvious that in a practical way, neat compatibilities usually are not feasible and in some cases, even a degree of incompatibility can lead to worthwhile competition. Such factors ought to be borne in mind.

Finally, attention should be given to the embellishment of the routine. Some colors are found to create more optimistic and happier moods than others. This has been shown in hospital wards. Generally, it is the lighter, cheerier pastels rather than the institutionalized dark greens and muddy browns that are more conducive to optimism and cheerfulness. Poor lighting, extraneous sounds and echoes and general clutter are certainly not supportive of such a feeling. An environment gives people messages, be it a hospital, house of worship, a library or a night club. People respond in kind with an attitude.

Some Considerations on Means and Methods

It would be wise to consider that many participants can profit by certain physical activities from a psychological standpoint even though such are not in the prescribed physical routine. For example, a quiet, shy bookkeeper, who remembers going bowling once 10 years ago as his major physical activity, may walk past a punching bag, for example, as if it weren't there. But, if encouraged to give it a punch or two, he does so with a rather demonic light in his eyes. He hasn't ever had much chance to express his aggressions and the thirst has been building for a long while. I would suggest that initially patients be given a choice of equipment use and, after a while, encouraged to try each one so that some personal spark may be generated.

Equipment should as much as possible have dials and measuring means. Our inhibited bookkeeper, after he has beaten up his boss enough through the punching bag, may now be ready for more modest aggression against the dials and friction. Performance on the bicycle ergometer in which one has tangible read-outs of performance and improvement is very motivating for most people. Individual charts of progress may take time but they tend to arouse interest.

The mirrors used in ballet classes should be used in other realms, including gymnasiums, to get visual pictures of oneself that one can carry away and retain. They show quite patently that we are exercising, although, of course, our muscles know it.

You may begin to know more about your clients by the way in which they use and respond to equipment. Such responses may give you clues as to how to help them plan. In everyday life, most of us express our aggressive, or what is often called animal impulses, through some form of sublimation. The businessman may do this by contending with his competitors; the medical man by becoming a surgeon which is a noble form of sublimation, except when too many operations are performed. Physical activity tends to balance and moderate this aggressive tension. The businessman may not make as many errors as his anger subsides. The surgeon may enjoy banging that golf ball, perhaps hard if not accurately, and not make that questionable decision to operate. The homemaker may have more patience with her children. It may make the truck driver more cautious in traffic for, as you know, far too many of us become aggressive drivers. And so, it's nice to take out hostility on equipment in a socially approved and sanctioned way.

I have often thought that one of the things that holds a marriage together is that each partner will permit a certain amount of aggression against himself or herself which each cannot otherwise express in their daily routine.

Of course, your work in fitness programs is a nice sublimated form of aggression. In one sense you have a captured group and you put them through a routine of some discomfort if they are to improve, but you have the balance of a noble constructive purpose.

So your work must blend the psychological, emotional and physical sides of human effort. The Japanese have a form of therapy called Morita Therapy, part of which is heavy manual labor, part of which are games and part of which is intellectual, using Zen techniques (Kora and Ohara, 1973). Consider how narrow much of psychotherapy is in this country, in which often the therapist is not concerned at all with the physical, nor at what job one works, nor how one may spend his life, but only in the "dials" of the mind. It goes along with our cultural denial of somatic realities. The body is animal and tends to interfere with the intellectual and spiritual. Prejudices against the handicapped who show physical atypicality may obviate our consideration of their minds or aspirations.

We all have a mental impression of our body image. If we are ashamed of our physical status, it tends to depress our confidence and mental outlook. Individuals who suffer loss of body members are often quite upset not only because of the public attitude and the physical limitations, but because it does things to them psychically.

Much of our living and our jobs get to be routine. While some are so conditioned to habituation that they can take more of it, most of us resist mere repetitiveness. While some prescribed exercise is necessary, as far as possible games even of a simple nature ought to be used, as they make for more total pleasurable involvement.

From the beginning, it would be motivating if some measure of improvement could be certified even in a minor way. This is why factual measurements are important.

Occasion should be made for social reinforcement of gain — a chart showing everyone the evidence of progress, congratulations made to each other, personal approval by the leader and the social interaction that goes into a team effort. It is also beneficial if the group is encouraged to express themselves on what they personally see as the mental and emotional benefits of the program. Sometimes people think about such feelings but they don't speak out because of embarrassment. For example, one may be reluctant to say, "I feel more self confident," as if he had been weak. But if the brave one does say so, others are motivated to express this opinion or similar ones. As the leader becomes experienced, he learns the ways in which improvement may be voiced and encourages such comment by leading questions if necessary.

It is important, as referred to earlier, for the engagement to become more personalized — one in which the leader can talk individually to each participant about their interests and goals and plans made which will be of particular benefit. Not only do individuals then feel some sense of alliance, purpose and belonging which tend to support affinity and to develop personal investure in an enterprise, but also it encourages a social interplay between members of the group which helps them reinforce each other. Under such circumstances, the group begins to reinforce each other and to believe that others are concerned about them. Such a situation achieves some of the beneficial effects of group therapy.

There are programs which recognize the physical and psychological coin of fitness. A report of a hospital-based program cited in the *N.Y. Times* says this: "Once a week the group meets at the hospital. They lie on the floor and learn exercises to improve their strength and circulation. They discuss diet and the general effect of nutrition on health. They talk about their fears — not of dying, but of becoming infirm. . .they visit each other's homes between meetings. . .more importantly, the number of physical complaints has been reduced" (1973).

Continuance In A Program

There is no doubt that retention of participants in a fitness program is one of the biggest barriers to success. This is certainly clear from our knowledge of diet, smoking, drug and alcoholic programs. People start out with an apparent good purpose but for one reason or another, quit.

While no one can say that they have the solution as such courses of disaffection are apt to vary with the individual, perhaps some of the suggestions offered may be contributory to an answer. The following assessment may also be of use:

1. It is important to remember that the stimulus which prompted the individual to get involved in a fitness program may not at all be the incentive which causes him to continue. If the individual entered the engagement on the basis of some felt fear or threat which, as said earlier, usually doesn't persist, it tends to dissipate in a short time.

The early behaviorists found that if a child was afraid of dogs, a gradual acquaintanceship by moving the dog closer a bit at a time usually removed the fear. In this sense, the individual's fear of whatever consequences he is concerned about may be removed by his having done something about it, by joining and saying, "At least I tried." The fear or threat recedes as it is not reinforced, or they get used to tolerating the fear. If the bad coughing spell comes back or they experience overweight button popping in public, perhaps another attempt will be made to reinstitute the smoking or food deprivation.

Consequently, if one enters a routine without sufficiently good motivation, it doesn't last. The only thing to do is to intrude with stronger constructive motivations as substitutes.

2. There are the "rainbow seekers"; a fitness program will solve all their problems and without much effort. The lady will find a husband, the man will recover from his impotence, the individual will become the admired person he wishes to be. These people have tried and will try anything to ease their discouragement with their lot in life and tend to go through the motions of compliance. Short of psychotherapy, I don't have any suggestions. The more you present the reality about the actual benefits and the cost in effort it will take, their fantasy evaporates as a motive.

3. The leadership of the program is a big factor in continuance and this is true in professional, academic, sports and business efforts. Individuals become fascinated by good leaders, identify with them, give them loyalty, try to remain associated and place faith in their ministrations even when they lack such faith in themselves.

4. One good measure for retention of people in a physical fitness program is to encourage opportunity for individual creativity, and to devise a number of options for personal choice. These opportunities, if available, lend more a sense of self-investment, of self-management, than if one is forced into a prescribed routine. Of course, there are limits to this, but as much leeway as feasible ought to be accepted. Through such procedures, an individual often finds an incentive he didn't know he had, and what's good about it is that he arrived at it himself without imposition. Naturally, this approach is not foolproof. Some who are more dependent prefer placing the responsibility in the lap of the expert. Yet this is shakier ground and such individuals have a greater tendency to quit when the going gets tough.

5. I have written earlier about the importance of social motivation. By being involved with others and suffering through a shared experience, we obligate ourselves to each other. We become ashamed to be the goof-off, the quitter, the one who would arouse discouragement in others by our departure.

6. Finally, when we are treated with respect for individual propensity, it enhances our sense of identity. Such regard implies in turn a faith in us by the leader. This reinforces our self-worth and provides the psychic nourishment to sustain the discipline required by the physical stress which is part of the price for achieving physical fitness and good health.

CONCLUSION

Attention to the following psychological factors will promote mental and emotional benefits and assist in the incorporation of motivational elements in physical fitness programs:

1. Recognition that the approach requires both mental, emotional and physical engagement.

2. Individualization of the program to the group and to the person.

3. Satisfaction of some of the participant's basic psychic needs.

4. Provision of choice elements and alternatives.

5. Social support and reinforcement.

6. Continuous productive measurement certifications from the beginning by assessment devices.

7. Incorporation of creative opportunties such as novelty, change of pace, improvisations.

8. Engagement of recreational elements; play and game qualities.

9. Personal projections of the leader as a concerned, interested, competent and helpful person.

10. Attention to the aesthetics of the environment and the propitious atmosphere.

11. Counseling to some degree as an adjunct.

Those whom we would serve as leaders in fitness programs for individuals over 50 are faced with the products of a cultural mistake which neglected to provide them with an early infusion of health and body knowledge which should begin with elementary school instruction in the first grade. Our present emphasis upon the mind and its education tends to push aside the fact that we are psychophysical entities and healthy minds and healthy bodies depend upon each other. Neglect in either takes its toll of both.

When individuals arrive at mature ages, so many poor habits and so much misuse and disuse have been suffered that many of our restorative efforts reap only feeble results. In fact, we are dealing with the survivors, as many others have been eliminated by tragic health and neglected opportunities. Nevertheless, we must salvage and do what we can. With our insight we also owe some effort toward prevention. Most of the patients served in the therapeutic fields are not as much injured by fate and poor constitutional factors as by the general unconcern of society about cultivating and preserving health and health habits at an early age. Our rectification effort by fitness programs may be late but it is worthy, for no one lies beyond our interest and everyone is due our concern. The interdisciplinary fields involved with this effort have an important quality in common: a mutual respect and consideration for human well-being and a dedication to this responsibility.

REFERENCES

Beecher, H. K. (1961) *JAMA* 176, 1102.

Boshes, B. (1960) *Ann Int Med* 52, 182.

Cobb, L. A., Thomas, G. I., Dillard, D. H., Merendino, K. A. and Bruce, R. A. (1959) *N Eng J Med* 260, 1115.

Hall, C. S., and Lindzey, G. (1957) *Theories of Personality*, John Wiley & Sons, Inc. New York.

Hellerstein, H. K., and Hornsten, T. R. (1966) *J Rehabil* 32, 48.

Hinkle, L. E., Jr., Redmont, R., Plummer, N., and Wolff, H. G. (1960) *Am J Public Health* 50, 1327.

Jackson, C. W., Jr., Pollard, J. C., and Kansky, E. W. (1962) *Am J Med Sci* 243, 558.

Karlins, M., and Abelson, H. I. (1970) *Persuasion*, Springer, New York.

Kora, T., and Ohara, K. (1973) *Psychol Today* 6, 63.

Levy, E. Z., Ruff, G. E., and Thaler, V. H. (1958) Military Medicine Section, Am. Med. Assoc.

New York Times (1973) June 10.

Ruff, G. E., and Levy, E. Z. (1959) *Am J Psychiatry* 115, 793.

Ruff, G. E., Levy, E. Z., and Thaler, V. H. (1959) *Aerospace Med* 30, 599.

Stout, I. W., and Langdon, G. (1950) *J Educ Sociol* 23, 442.

Whitehouse, F. A. (1967) *Rehabil Lit* 28, 238.

Whitehouse, F. A. (1968) *Hofstra Rev* 3, 28.

Whitehouse, F. A. (1970a) *N Y State J Med* 70, 522.

Whitehouse, F. A. (1970b) Metrop. Washington Reg. Med. Conf. on Coronary Risk Factors, Arlington, Va. Sept. 26.

Whitehouse, F. A. (1970c) *Proc Am Psychol Assoc* 775.

Wolf, S. (1959) *Pharmacol Rev* 11, 689.

Zubek, J. P. (1964) *Brit Med Bull* 20, 38.

Gerontological Aspects of Physical Activity—Motivation of Older People in Physical Training

Eino Heikkinen, M.D. and Birgit Käyhty, M.Sc.

INTRODUCTION

Aging influences physiological, psychic and social properties of man. Of these, changes of the physiological properties are best known. Most of these physiological changes are characterized by a gradual, even decline from the age of 25-30 years (Skinner, 1973). Maximum performance capacity decreases with age about 20-45 percent, depending on the function (Table 1). The metabolic alterations which precede the decline of the physiological functions and the mechanisms which regulate the processes of aging are poorly understood.

TABLE I

Comparison of the average physical fitness of 20 - 25 and 70-year-old men

Variable	Age (years)		Percent decline	Reference
	20-25	70		
Max. ventilation volume ($1/min/m^2$)	80	55	31	Grimby & Söderholm, 1963
Max. heart rate/min	195	155	21	Åstrand & Åstrand, 1955; Hollmann, 1963
Max. oxygen uptake (ml/kg x min)	45	25	44	Åstrand, 1960; Shephard, 1966
Manual cranking ability (kg M/min)	1900	1350	29	Shock & Norris, 1970

Recently, some attempts have been made to measure the biological age of man (Bourlière, 1970; Dirken, 1972; Heikkinen et al, 1974). Table 2 presents some tests

TABLE 2

Tests used in or suggested for the measurement of biological age in man

Test	Correlation to chronological age	References
Osteoporosis index of metacarpal bones	-.79	Comfort, 1969
Audiometry (6000 Hz)	.76	Morgan & Stevens, 1972
Graying of hair	.72	Hollingsworth, 1965
Skin elasticity	.60	"
Audiometry (4000 Hz)	.60	"
Vibration sense	.54	"
Systolic blood pressure	.52	"
Light adaptation	.49	"
Reaction time	-.48	Comfort, 1969
Vital capacity	-.40	Hollingsworth, 1965
Grip strength	-.32	"
Heart size	.29	"
Serum cholesterol	.23	"

which have been used in or suggested for the measurement of biological aging. An index of a biological (physiologic) age can be constructed by combining several tests. Correlations of the indexes to chronological age are rather high (.80-.90) showing that they can be used in epidemiological field studies. But variation between individuals is so high that the specificity and sensitivity of the tests must be increased before they are used for comparison between single subjects.

Variation in the rate of aging in man is determined by heredity, living habits and environmental factors. Leisure time physical activity as a component of living habits has become increasingly important during the development of our technological culture, in which the number of physically inactive people seems to be increasing. Physical activity decreases with advancing age (Cunningham et al., 1968), but only few epidemiological studies have been carried out on exercise habits in different age, social and occupational groups.

Decreased physical activity is supposed to contribute to the exponential growth of the incidence of many diseases after the age of 30 (Mellerowicz and Meller, 1972). The rate of aging (Shock, 1967) cannot presumably be retarded by habitual physical training, but it can prevent premature appearance of symptoms and diseases and, in this way, improve the quality of life of old people. The trainability of old people is better than it was supposed earlier (deVries, 1970; Hollmann, 1973; Adams and deVries, 1973). The maximal oxygen uptake is improved 10-15 percent among 65 to 70-year-old sedentary men with two months' physical training, and the activity of metabolic enzymes in skeletal muscles is also increased (Liesen et al., 1975). The activities of muscle and connective tissue of m.vastus lateralis were higher in habitually training 33 to 70-year-old men when compared to sedentary controls (Suominen and Heikkinen, 1975). These findings provide sufficient reasons to recommend physical exercise for old people as a good tool in the prevention and treatment of degenerative conditions (Mellerowicz and Meller, 1972; Biener, 1972).

With the increasing interest in the physical activity of old people, it has become apparent that information about the exercise behavior of old people and the physiological, psychological and social factors which influence their physical activity is insufficient.

Therefore the studies reported in this chapter were planned to find out:

a) Biological aging, physical fitness and physical activity of men living in the western and eastern parts of Finland
b) Health and living habits of 66-year-old persons of Jyväskylä
c) Physical fitness of 68-year-old persons of Jyväskylä
d) Motivation of 66-year-old persons of Jyväskylä and factors preventing it. Such information should be useful to arrange and develop more appropriate exercise and health education programs for older people.

MATERIAL AND METHODS

The biological age of 460 unselected men, ages 25 to 57, was estimated from the results of the tests for vital capacity, digit-symbol, thresholds for vibratory and auditory stimuli, simple reaction time and cortical thickness of metacarpal bone. An index of biological age was constructed from the results of vital capacity and thresholds for auditory (at 4000 Hz) and vibratory stimuli. The methodological part of the study has been described elsewhere (Heikkinen et al., 1974).

The physical activity and physical fitness of unselected men, ages 25 to 59, were evaluated by a questionnaire in connection with the North Karelia Project in the eastern part of Finland (Puska, 1974).

Investigations on the living habits, health, physical fitness and factors affecting physical activity were performed in the city of Jyväskylä where all the 66-year-old persons were interviewed in 1972 and, about two years later, examined by fitness and health tests (Fig. 1).

The parameters evaluated in the fitness and health examinations of the 68-year-old persons are presented in Table 3.

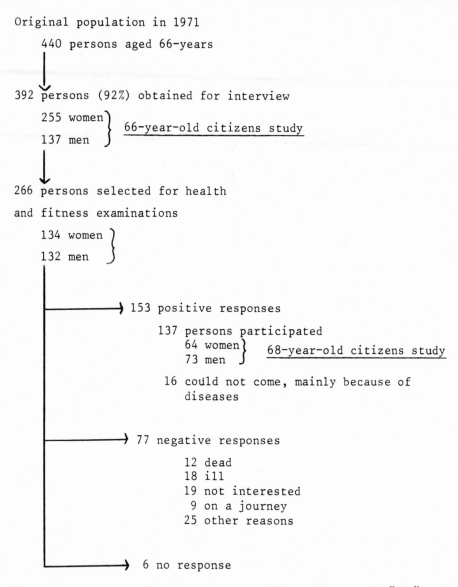

Original population in 1971

    440 persons aged 66-years

392 persons (92%) obtained for interview

    255 women ⎱
            ⎰ 66-year-old citizens study
    137 men ⎰

266 persons selected for health
and fitness examinations

    134 women ⎱
    132 men ⎰

        ⟶ 153 positive responses

            137 persons participated
              64 women ⎱
                    ⎰ 68-year-old citizens study
              73 men ⎰

           16 could not come, mainly because of
           diseases

        ⟶ 77 negative responses

              12 dead
              18 ill
              19 not interested
               9 on a journey
              25 other reasons

        ⟶ 6 no response

Fig. 1.   Selection of subjects for the studies of 66-year-old persons of Jyväskylä.

RESULTS AND DISCUSSION

Biological Aging

The results of various parameters of biological aging changed almost linearly between the age groups 25-27 and 67-68, except those of vital capacity which

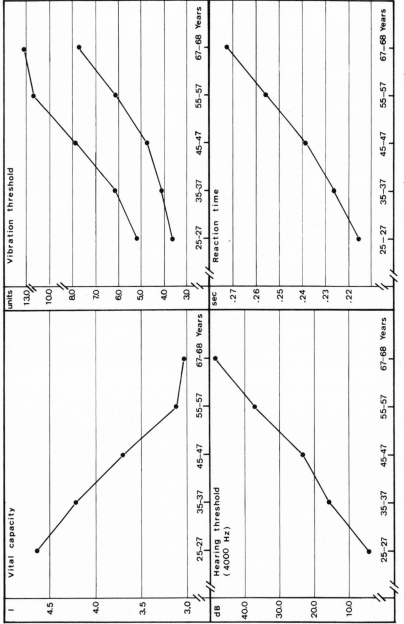

Fig. 2. Results of some tests used in the measurement of biological aging (Heikkinen et al. 1974). The age group "67-68 years" refers to the study of 68-year-old persons (see Material and Methods). The upper curve of the vibration threshold represents the results of measurement at the wrist and the lower curve, at the ankle.

TABLE 3

Parameters measured or evaluated in the study of 68-year-old citizens of Jyväskylä

Object	Parameter
1. Social situation	Interview: Living habits, life satisfaction, opinions about health and social services
2. Fitness	Ergometer test Sit-up test Handgrip test
3. Biological age	Vital capacity Thresholds for vibratory and auditory stimuli Reaction time Digit-symbol test
4. Health	Physician's examination, physiotherapist's examination (in particular findings which might influence physical activity)

declined very little between the two oldest age groups (Fig. 2). An index of biological age (IBA, which was formed from the weighed means of the results of vital capacity and thresholds for auditory and vibratory stimuli) changed about one percent a year from 43 to 61 units in 30 years (between 25-27 and 55-57 years).

Equal decrease in physiological functions with aging has been observed by Dirken (1972) with industrial workers in Holland. The correlation coefficient of IBA to chronological age was .786 in our study. The results show that biological aging can be estimated with reasonable accuracy in an epidemiological field study. The measurements could be used to investigate the effects of various environmental (e.g., work conditions) and individual (e.g., habitual physical activity) factors on biological aging.

Functional Capacity and Health

Increasing age is associated with decreasing functional capacity and degenerating health. About 50 percent of the population over 65 felt that they were in good health (Koskinen, 1971) but, in objective investigations, about two thirds of them had at least one chronic disease (Sievers, 1970). According to self-evaluation, the fitness of men in North Karelia decreases considerably with age (Fig. 3). The figure of low fitness increases from 8.7 percent to 31.2 percent between the youngest (25-34 years) and the oldest (45-59 years) groups. The figure for good fitness decreases, respectively, from 43.6 percent to 12.3 percent.

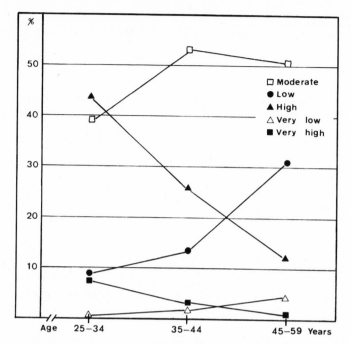

Fig. 3.   Percent distribution of 25 to 59-year-old North Karelian men in various categories of physical fitness according to self-evaluation.

Forty-seven percent of the 66-year-old persons of Jyväskylä felt their health was good and significant negative correlation was found to incomes. Forty percent of the people of low income and 54 percent of the people with higher income felt their health good. About 80 percent of the subjects were able to move outside without difficulty and about six percent needed a walking stick. The rest of the subjects needed more help for outdoor living and 1.3 percent of the subjects were confined to indoor living.

The health examination of the 68-year-old persons of Jyväskylä showed that about two thirds of them could be exposed to the stress of a submaximal ergometer test without a noticeable risk of cardiovascular symptoms or complications (Table 4). About one third of the subjects were evaluated sufficiently fit to participate in the physical rehabilitation program without considerable health risks. About one half of the subjects would need careful individual instructions and medical supervision, at least in the beginning of the training program. On the other hand, about 20 percent of the subjects had diseases which restricted strenuous physical exercise. The figure of the healthy people may be higher than in the original population of the 66-year-old persons because selection removed some sick people from the sample.

The symptoms of effort in relation to the level of physical activity among 68-year-old subjects are presented in Table 5. One to eight percent felt symptoms already in everyday duties. Uphill climbing and hurrying caused dyspnea in one third

TABLE IV

Fitness of 68-year-old citizens of Jyväskylä for performance tests and for physical rehabilitation programs according to physician's evaluation

Variable	Evaluation	Men % (N=73)	Women % (N=64)
Fitness for ergometer test[1]	+	67.1	73.4
	-	32.9	25.0
	later	-	1.6
Fitness for sit-up test[2]	+	57.5	67.2
	-	42.5	32.8
Fitness for physical rehabilitation program[3]	+	39.7	40.6
	-	60.3	59.4

1. Subjects who had manifest coronary heart disease or other diseases which would evoke symptoms during the test were excluded

2. Subjects who had back diseases or other diseases which would limit performance were excluded

3. Only apparently healthy subjects were evaluated as fit for later physical rehabilitation program (The purpose of the program is to find out the trainability of healthy 70-year-old persons)

TABLE V

Symptoms of effort provoked by various degrees of physical activity among 68-year-old citizens of Jyväskylä

Symptom	Rest or very low physical activity Men %	Women %	Efforts of normal every day duties Men %	Women %	Uphill walking stair climbing Men %	Women %
Dyspnea	-	1.6	5.5	9.4	32.9	28.1
Chest pain	1.4	1.6	8.2	1.6	20.5	20.3
Back troubles	-	-	4.1	3.4	12.3	9.4
Claudication intermittens	-	-	1.4	1.6	9.6	9.4
Troubles in the joints of lower extremities	-	-	2.7	1.6	8.2	9.4

of the subjects, angina pectoris in one fifth, back troubles and claudicatio inter- mittens in one tenth of the subjects. Many symptoms, however, were such that physical exercise in appropriate doses could diminish them or prevent their be- coming worse.

Exercise Behavior

The effects of aging on the physical activity of human populations are not well known. According to Cunningham et al. (1968), both the amount of physical ac- tivity and its intensity decrease with advancing age. The leisure time physical activity in the unselected adult population in eastern Finland decreased in intensity with aging (Fig. 4). Among the 66-year-old persons of Jyväskylä (Table 6), slow walking

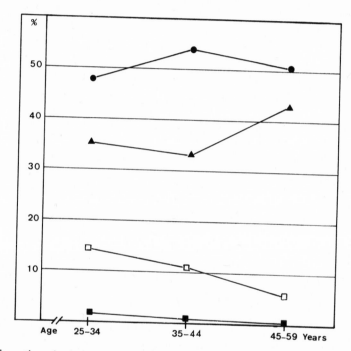

Fig. 4. Leisure time physical activity of 25 to 59-year-old men in North Karelia.
● = Low physical activity, ▲ = Moderate physical activity (walking, cycling, etc., at least 4 hours/week), □ = High physical activity (jogging, skiing, swimming, ball games etc. at least 3 hours/week), ■ = Very high physical activity (participation in competitive sports).

is the most usual form of physical activity. The exercise of men was more intensive than that of women. Men also walked longer distances (Fig. 5). The time devoted weekly to physical activity is shown in Table 7. About one fifth of men walked more than 21 hours a week, according to their own evaluation. Besides walking, the most popular forms of physical activity were swimming, gymnastics, cycling and skiing (Fig. 6).

TABLE VI

Intensity of walking among 66-year-old citizens of Jyväskylä. Percent distribution to three different categories of physical activity are presented for groups standardized by sex and health

Group	Intensity of walking			Statistical significance of the difference
	I	II	III	
Men	63 %	30 %	7 %	p < .001
Women	81 %	17 %	2 %	
Healthy	68 %	24 %	8 %	p < .001
Unhealthy	85 %	11 %	4 %	

I   = Is accustomed to walk slowly without sweating and becoming breathless

II = Is accustomed to walk briskly, sweating a little and becoming somewhat breathless

III = Is accustomed to walk vigorously, sweating amply and becoming breathless

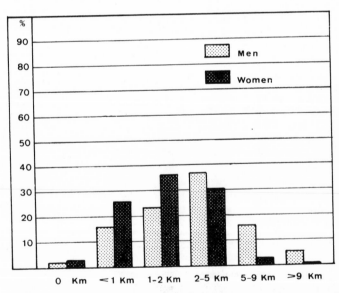

Fig. 5.   Amount of habitual daily walking among 66-year-old persons of Jyväskylä.

TABLE VII

Time used for physical activity in a week among 66-year-old citizens of Jyväskylä (N-392)

Time hrs/week	Men %	Women %	All %
0	5.8	5.8	5.8
1 - 4	17.3	34.2	28.7
5 - 14	40.8	44.7	43.3
14 +	35.1	15.3	22.2

Physical activity among 66-year-old people is common but only about 10-30 percent of men and five to 15 percent of women exercised in a way which produced a training effect on the heart and circulation by attaining a pulse rate of more than 170 minus their age in years (Cureton, 1956; Karvonen et al., 1957; deVries, 1971).

Factors Affecting Physical Activity

Exercise habits are regulated by various individual and social factors like motivation, attitudes, earlier habits, possibilities for physical activity (e.g., health and fitness, economic situation, availability of suitable places), and the values and norms of

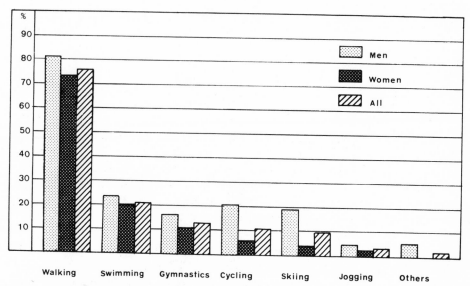

Fig. 6. Preference of various kinds of sport among 66-year-old persons of Jyväskylä. The bars show the percent number of subjects engaged in the indicated kind of sport at least once a week.

environment. Because contacts with health care personnel are common among old people, instructions by doctors and nurses could constitute an important method to promote exercise habits of aged people. For instance, people over 65 in Finland make, on an average, three visits to doctors per year (Purola et al., 1971). Instructions for physical activity are, however, relatively uncommon. About 60 percent of 68-year-old men and 70 percent of 68-year-old women in Jyväskylä had not received any advice for physical training (Table 8). Detailed instructions were given only to 14 percent of men and three percent of women.

TABLE VIII

Quality of instructions for physical activity by health care personnel	Percent distribution of 68-year-old citizens in various categories of instruction for physical activity	
	Men N=73 %	Women N=64 %
No instructions	58.9	71.1
Strenuous physical activity forbidden	15.1	4.7
Some specific forms of physical activity forbidden	–	3.1
General encouragement for physical activity	6.9	7.8
Detailed instructions for physical activity	13.7	3.1
Physical training arranged under medical supervision	5.5	3.1

The 66-year-old subjects were asked to evaluate the importance of various factors for their physical activity (Fig. 7). In this group good physical fitness, pleasure and recreation, moving in nature, preservation of youthfulness and weight regulation were the five most important factors. When a similar question was presented to university students, the main difference was that social contact (possibility to be in good company) was considered more important than among old people (Heikkinen et al., 1969).

Although physical training had a positive value among old people and most would like to participate in it, several factors caused obstacles to participation (Fig. 8). The

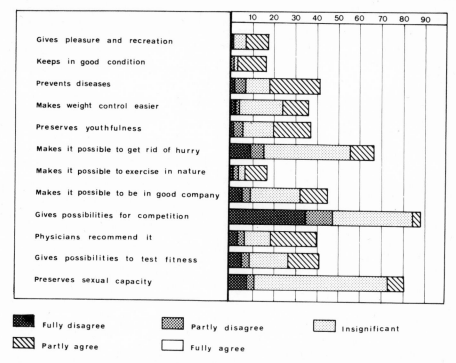

Fig. 7. Reasons to practise sports among 66-year-old persons of Jyväskylä. The subjects were asked to evaluate the validity of the given statements for their physical activity.

most important were disease (56 percent), invalidity (33 percent), lack of supervised training (27 percent) and lack of company (22 percent). Lack of knowledge (19 percent) and lack of suitable places for exercise (18 percent) were also felt to be important limiting factors. About one third of the subjects were not interested in physical activity. Most of the 68-year-old persons (68 percent) thought they would increase their physical activity if training were possible under appropriate guidance and supervision.

In practice, the drop-out frequency from the training program depends largely on the composition of the program and the ability of the trainer and/or leader. If training consisted only of jogging, the drop-out percent was usually high. On the other hand, if the program consisted of several forms of exercise, the results were better. In a study of 55 to 70-year-old men living in Cologne, the drop-out was only 10 percent during two months' training which consisted of walking, jogging, ball games, gymnastics and swimming for three to five hours a week (Liesen et al., 1975). In another investigation (Heikkinen et al., 1975), all of the 26 subjects, age 69 (14 men and 12 women), were able to complete an eight to 10-week physical rehabilitation program which was constructed according to the experiences gained in Cologne study. However, the trained groups consisted of selected people, mostly men, and it is not possible to generalize the results to the whole population of old people.

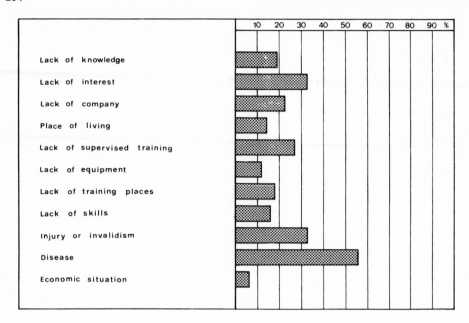

Fig. 8.   Factors inhibiting physical activity among 66-year-old persons of Jyväskylä according to
their self-evaluation. No factor excludes another.

CONCLUSION

Human aging is characterized by a constant and gradual decline of physiological
functions in which the average rate of decline is about one percent per year after
20-30. Variation between functions and individuals is large.

The biological age of men can be assessed with satisfactory accuracy in an epidemiological field study by using an index constructed from relatively simple measurements (e.g. vital capacity, thresholds of auditory and vibratory perceptions). To
evaluate the biological age of an individual in a valid way, it is necessary to increase
the accuracy and the sensitivity of the tests.

Physical performance capacity and health decrease with advancing age. Two thirds
of the people over 65 have at least one chronic disease. About half of them, however, feel their health good. Of the 66-year-old persons, about 80 percent, according
to our study, are capable of taking care of the normal daily tasks without considerable difficulties. The number of people who feel their physical fitness is good decreases from 44 percent to 12 percent between the age groups of 25-34 and 45-59.
Of the 68-year-old persons of Jyväskylä about two thirds were in such good condition that they could be exposed to the stress of a submaximal ergometer test
without an apparent risk of heart and circulatory complications. About 30 percent
of the subjects were regarded fit for physical training programs without strict medical supervision.

Old people are interested in physical activity but only about 20 percent of 68-year-old persons, for instance, exercise with such intensity that improvement of cardiovascular function can be expected. The exercise behavior of old people is not sufficiently known. Also, factors which cause obstacles to the appropriate training have not been investigated.

Good physical fitness, pleasure and recreation, moving in nature, preservation of youthfulness and weight control were the most important aims for physical activity among 66-year-old persons. Physical activity is inhibited by several factors of which disease and disability, and the lack of supervised training, company, knowledge and suitable places were considered as most important.

Physicians and nurses could provide an important source of information about health living habits. Only a minority of 66-year-old persons had received instructions for physical exercise and less than 10 percent of them had received detailed instructions.

The results also indicated that people with higher income were healthier and physically more active than people with low income.

REFERENCES

Adams, G.M., and deVries, H.A. (1973) *J Gerontol* 28, 50.

Åstrand, I. (1960) *Acta Physiol Scand* 49. suppl. 169.

Åstrand, P.-O. and Christensen, E.H. (1964) *Oxygen in the Animal Organism*, (F. Dickens. E. Neil, and W.F. Widdas, eds.), Pergamon Press, New York.

Biener, K. (1972) *Sporthygiene and Präventive Sportmedizin*, Verlag Hans Huber, Bern.

Bourliére, F. (1970) *Public Health Papers* 37. WHO, Geneva.

Comfort, A. (1969) *Lancet* 1411.

Cunningham, D., Montoye, H., Metzner, H., and Keller, J. (1968) *J Gerontol* 23, 551.

Cureton, T.K. (1956) *JAMA* 1139, 162.

deVries, H.A. (1970) *J Gerontol* 325, 25.

deVries, H.A. (1971) *Geriatrics* 94, 26.

Dirken, J. U. (1972) *Functional Age of Industrial Workers*, Wolters-Noordhoff, Groningen.

Grimby, G., Söderholm, B. (1963) *Acta Med Scand* 173, 199.

Heikkinen, E., Vuori, I., Ojala, A., and Seppälä, P. (1969) *Sos Lääket Aikak* 59, 7.

Heikkinen, E., Kiiskinen, A., Käyhty, B., Rimpelä, M., Vuori, I. (1974) *Gerontologia* 33, 20.

Heikkinen, E., Suominen, H., Parkatti, T., Forsberg, S., Pohjolainen, P. and Rahkila, P. (1975) *Nordisk Gerontologi* (Eds. B. Steen and A. Svanborg), Astra Läkemedel AB, Lund.

Hollingsworth, J.V., Hashizume, A., and Jablon, S. (1965) *Yale J Biol Med* 38, 11.

Hollman, W. (1963) *Höchst-und Dauerleistungsfähigkeit des Sportlers,* Barth-Verlag, München.

Hollman, W. (1973) *Sport in the Modern World – Changes and Problem*, Springer-Verlag, Berlin, Heidelberg, New York.

Karvonen, M.J., Kantola, E., and Murtola, O. (1957) *Ann Med Exp Biol Fenn* 307, 35.

Koshkinen, S. (1971) *University of Tampere. Institute of Social Policy. Research Reports* 21.

Liesen, H., Heikkinen, E. Suominen, H., Michel, D. (1975) *Sportarzt and Sportmedizin* 26, 26.

Mellerowicz, H., and Meller, W. (1972) *Training*, Heidelberger Taschenbücher, Berlin.

Morgan, F.R., and Stevens, S.T. (1972) *Percept Mot Skills* 415, 34.

Purola, T., Nyman, K., Kalimo, E., and Sievers, K. (1971) *Publications of the Social Insurance – Series A*, Helsinki.

Puska, P. (1974) *Publications of the University of Kuopio. Community Health – Series A 1.*

Shephard, R.J. (1966) *Arch Environ Health* 664, 13.

Shock, N.W. (1967) *Can Med Assoc J* 96, 836.

Shock, N.W., and Norris, A.H. (1970) in *Medicine and Sport*, (Brunner, D. and Jokl, E. eds.), Vol. 4, S.Karger, Basel.

Sievers, K. (1970) *Suomen Lääkärilehti 3364, 35.*

Skinner, J.S. (1973) *Limiting Factors of Physical Performance* (J. Keul, ed.), George Thieme Publishers, Stuttgart.

Suominen, H., Heikkinen, E. (1975) *Eur J Appl Physiol* 249, 34.

Across the Nation—Habilitation

The Mission is Possible

Lawrence J. Frankel

INTRODUCTION

More than 20 million Americans are 65 and older. In the United States, yielding to old age has become a socially accepted behavior pattern, as demonstrated by proliferating numbers of nursing homes, spiraling numbers of patients in hospitals and extended care facilities, and the vast number of old people supported by welfare. Inquiry into the causes of cardovascular disease, the number one killer in the United States, engages the interest of the medical profession and appears related somewhat to aging. In 1969, of the 1,002,111 people who died from heart and blood vessel diseases, almost 75 percent were 65 and older. In 1968, Jean Mayer, Ph.D., Professor of Nutrition at Harvard University School of Public Health, declared, "There never has been a group on earth less physically active than the modern American" and tied the rising heart attack rate to our lack of vigorous exercise.

PROJECT PREVENTICARE

Delayed Echoes

Sixty-two years ago, rompered, buster-brown haircut and reluctant, I accompanied my mother to a home for the aging in lower Manhattan to see a kinswoman who had emigrated to America from the same village in Lithuania where my mother was born. While they visited animatedly, my eyes wandered around a large dormitory-type room, filled with dozens of white iron bedsteads, each one occupied by a tiny, wrinkled, little old lady grasping a brown paper bag from which were withdrawn scraps of bread, then eagerly pushed into toothless mouths. Appalled, even at that tender age, I later inquired, "Mama, what are all these old ladies doing in that great big room?"

Wistfully smiling down at me and tightly grasping my hand as we walked homeward, Mama said, "They are there because they are old and their children do not want them any more."

Bravely, I looked up and said, "Mama, I would never, never, let anything like that happen to you."

In the last dozen years the recollection of that visit has returned time and again, like a delayed echo.

Changing patterns of life and a changing world mold our philosophies and our sense of values. I have experienced incomparable reward and spiritual enrichment by devoting many years of my life toward the physical problems of the lame, the halt and the blind. Now full circle, six decades after my childhood experience, the challenge of helping by "Project Preventicare" to break the worldwide conspiracy of silence, as Simone de Beauvoir calls it, towards its largest growing segment, the aged, has moved us to attempt perhaps a revolutionary concept in motivating the multimillions of aging people to improve their old age by engaging in sports and exercise. These are the people whose socio-economic, cultural and educational backgrounds precluded involvement in any sport, recreation or program for physical enhancement for most of their lifetimes.

History

Late in 1970, helped by a grant-in-aid from the West Virginia State Commission on Aging, we were charged with developing a physical fitness program for the elderly, relevant to their years, state of detraining and physician recommendation. With the advice of our own foundation medical advisory committee and the blessing of the local medical society, we initiated a pilot study with 15 subjects ranging in age from 60 to 80 years. In April of 1972, our foundation, impressed with the initial results, broadened its horizons to develop its current demonstration project in order to reach older people in outlying communities, residents of federally built housing complexes and a group within a home for the elderly.

METHOD

For those in our less ambulatory groups, exercises were designed that could be performed in chairs, couches, wheelchairs or on carpeted floors. Performing the exercises slowly to music, and as rhythmically as possible, enhanced both mood and tolerance. For the exercises used, see Chapter 24.

All participants in this program have their heart rate and blood pressure recorded every two weeks and, with exception of those in the home for elderly, are ergometrically evaluated on the Monarch Bicycle every three months. Åstrand's submaximal test is used with subjects performing at loads of 50 to 75 watts.

RESULTS

Questioning doctors like Dr. J. D. frequently ask me, "What data are you collecting? You will undoubtedly need to substantiate many of your contentions." And yet, Dr. J. D., who had often queried me about data, one day after his annual physical apparently was concerned about himself and requested that we plan an exercise program for him particularly to augment cardio-respiratory fitness. At his beginning program, his resting pulse was 80 or 82 and his blood pressure in the hypertensive range Nothing much more was said for several months while he pursued a devoted daily regimen.

During a casual conversation one day, Dr. D. said, "Larry, I am quite impressed; my resting pulse is 52, blood pressure in normal range. There must be something to all this!" Guardedly, I replied, "Many of our friends would say, 'This is but one case, and not statistically significant'," His answer was, "It is significant as hell to me!"

A personal communication from the late Dr. Paul Dudley White noted, "There are large numbers of the elderly who might never consent to enter into formalized programs, but who nonetheless need to be convinced that they must use their muscles and their minds." Therefore, we should assemble those who would adopt a missionary approach toward reaching those large numbers who are rapidly declining toward total immobility.

We are not certain at this stage that the collection of hard data within the age group with which we are concerned will match in relevance, the incomparable clinical experiences we noted in almost all our subjects — in their mental attitudes, the reduction in their subjective symptoms, reduced visits to physicians, lessened medication and an almost infectious joie de vivre.

Can we feed into a computer for statistical analysis the following examples from our delightful subjects?

C.B., age 81, two years prior to our program was totally incapacitated after a spinal tumor — subsequently after months in a wheel chair seldom was without a cane. Only weeks later, the cane was discarded, his ambulation greatly improved and he learned to walk with reasonable grace on our two-inch balance beam. His zest for life was reflected in the final words of a poem he composed concerning his program here, "My life has just begun — for I am only 81"

A year later this gentleman entered the hospital for an exploratory operation. When a saddened physician told him he had a carcinoma of liver, pancreas and intestine and a prognosis of only a few days, C.B. looked up with a smile and said, "Doc, you can't win 'em all." During his last days, he requested that his gym clothes be brought to the hospital so he might perform for his roommates in his hospital room. C.B. passed away shortly thereafter in his sleep. I was asked to be one of his pallbearers. Imagine my feelings as I noted in the center of his casket a small trophy we had awarded to him for his earlier rapid progress among his peers in our classes. Dr. W.R., chairman of our medical committee, who often observed our classes remarked to me: "There is no question that because of his involvement in our program, C.B. faced death with poise, grace and equanimity."

While we were interviewing prospective subjects at a nearby federal housing development, a twinkly "young" lady of 82 remarked to me: "Mr. Frankel, don't you think at my age it is rather late in life to start exercising?" In a feeble attempt to be facetious I replied, "You know that Sarah, it was told in the Bible, conceived and bore a son when she was past 80." Her retort, which left me with mouth agape, "Well, Mr. Frankel, get me a good man and I'll try to emulate Sarah."

About three months later, I was called by one of our board members who reported that a client of his, G.A.C., residing at Carroll Terrace, a high-rise residence for the elderly where each week we conduct classes, was bedfast and required neighbors to bring her bedpan, prepare her food and bathe her. She would, therefore, be required to transfer to a hospital or extended care facility. He asked, "Would we look in and see if there was any hope?" The subject was desperately fearful of going to a hospital. First requiring the subject's physician to initiate an exercise program, we started G.A.C. on exercise a week before Christmas. Three months later she was completely ambulatory, cooking all her meals and among the group performing on stage for visitors who come to see "Project Preventicare." With some humility, we must ascribe her result to 3M — motivation, movement, miracle.

These are a few of many, many experiences we have encountered, but they are sufficient to convince us that planned fitness regimes in such population groups may decelerate the aging process. enhance the joy of living for the multimillions often living alone in darkness and despair outside the pale of less than desirable institutionalization.

DISCUSSION AND PRIORITIES

The vast majority of elderly people in the United States live within the community. Only one in 25 lives in an institution, such as a rest home, nursing home or medical facility. And yet, there has been a vast proliferation of nursing homes throughout the United States, representing billions of dollars in investment, much of it with federal aid. It is also known that in the transition from family situation to that of nursing home, the mortality rate increases by 25 percent among similar age groups. Inactivity, boredom and a sense of uselessness play a major part in such mortality. We do not suggest that all nursing homes contribute to rapid human obsolescence, but three recent communications in our own experience are most provocative:

1. From a large university medical center, "We are thinking about embarking on a program similar to yours, perhaps on a more extensive basis, since we have a number of physiotherapists and many surrounding nursing homes which I think could benefit from a program such as yours. Here are some questions I would like to ask, etc." Two years later, nothing was started yet.

2. We received an inquiry from a large home, sponsored by one of America's richest churches, about "Project Preventicare" and sent instructions and advice. The following reply was mailed to us a year later: "I wish I could report all kinds of good things going on here. We are in the talking stage of a program designed for our members who are ambulatory and physically able to profit from preventative exercise. I have given your report to our physician, and hopefully he will give his permission for this. I wish it were possible to visit you to see your program at work."

3. From a home sponsored by a prominent fraternal order with 850 guests, many in their 80s, we received a request for information and a year later got the following letter: "I unfortunately do not have a great deal to report at this time. Sheets were distributed to guests to perform and continue exercises in their own rooms. There is no follow-up system in existence at this time. I wish I could report concrete success to you. Perhaps in near future it will be the case . . ."

After a story concerning our program had national distribution via a wire service, this sample letter was received along with many similar ones:

"I am very irritated by the fact that many White House Conferences are called to study problems of health but few efforts made to pursue programs prove worthwhile. I believe a real effort should be made (somehow) to inaugurate your exact program for elderly in every Golden Age and Senior Citizen group in the United States. I am showing your article to my N.Y. State Congressman."

We have three very beautiful high-rise residence complexes for the elderly in our city. We have paid more than one visit to observe in each lobby area large numbers of somnolent guests dozing or watching television, later returning sleepily to their apartments. There is almost total disregard on part of the greatest majority to become interested even vaguely in any physical enhancement. Yet, the bingo syndrome is rampant.

Continued inactivity by this segment of our elderly must soon lead to immobility and a further exacerbation of the problems of the taxpayer to support still larger numbers who must be ultimately moved to extended care facilities or nursing homes.

There is a constantly rising cost for proper care for which social security and health insurance are inadequate. Hence, millions of elderly citizens will be swept out of sight in substandard nursing homes; and when these multitudes can expect their final years to be spent in pain, solitude and squalor, our nation cannot boast about the quality of life it has achieved.

"FITNESS IS AGELESS – FOREVER YOUNG AT HEART"

I find a good bit of relevance in Dr. Alexander Leaf's *National Geographic* (1973) sponsored study of the "Mysteries of Human Longevity", and our own firm contention that fitness yields a high degree of agelessness and a spirit eternally young. Provocative is Dr. Leaf's awe, more of the fitness of the subjects he studied than of their advanced years, often considerably over 100 years. The photographs he collected among natives of the Ecuadoran village of Vilcabamba, and of the Abkhazians living in the Caucasus Mountains in southern U.S.S.R. are most intriguing and revealing.

His observation that aged Georgians consume around 1800 calories a day, which are 600 less than that recommended by the U.S. National Academy of Science for males over 55, might be worthy of emulation in our overfed, underexercised society with the highest coronary death rate in the world. The weight of current medical opinion concurs that the sparse diets described by Dr. Leaf would delay development of atherosclerosis in our nation. I note a more than average range of obesity among residents of the high-rise complexes we visit. They shuffle, not walk, slowly pushing grocery carts loaded with empty calorie foods, sugared soft drinks, sweet rolls, ad nauseam.

Dr. David Kakiashvilli, a Georgian cardiologist who has been studying gerontology for the past 12 years, is convinced that exercise is a major factor in longevity.

The natives of the regions studied by Dr. Leaf never heard of aerobics or jogging or other formalized systems; nonetheless their constant physical activity, scampering over their mountainous terrain, certainly improved their cardiovascular systems so that oxygen supply to their heart muscles was superior.

Dr. Leaf attended the International Association of Gerontology Scientific Congress in Kiev in July, 1972. He came away from the meeting with a feeling that very little said there bore much relationship to the old people he had seen. At the Gerontology Congress, Dr. Leaf said he caught himself day dreaming about Abkhazia. I had a similar experience attending a national conference entitled, "Alternatives to Institutional Care." The public relations director of the sponsoring institution, in a personal communication to me, said, "You have a doing thing, instead of a talking thing – I am most impressed."

I humbly suggest that perhaps our scientists and researchers might, for a short while, lay aside their white coats and expedite the turning on of some green lights. I am more than a bit amused that our Dr. Leaf, age 52, on his return to Massachusetts adopted a regimen of jogging.

Medicine in the United States has largely overlooked prevention medicine and the importance of motivation. On a recent trip to London with my wife, we visited Westminster Abbey where I noted an inscription to the remains of John Dryden whose lines have strongly dominated my life pattern.

> By chase, our long lived fathers earned their food,
> Toil strung the nerves and purified the blood.
> But we, their sons, a pampered race of men,
> Are dwindled down to three score years and ten.
> Better to use your muscles, for health unbought,
> Than fee the doctors for a nauseous draught.
> The wise, for cure, on exercise depend,
> God never made his work for man to mend!
>
> — John Dryden (1631-1700)

At a national conference sponsored by the Center for the Study of Aging at Duke University, I heard a story about two Hebrew seminary students who met on the streets of a small village and together lamented the state of the world. One spoke and said, "You know, it doesn't pay to live and grow old". His companion rejoined, "More so, it is better not to have been born", to which the first one answered, "But who can be so lucky?"

For over 5,000 years a prayer has been whispered and sobbed from all rows in orthodox synagogues during the day of atonement, Yom Kippur, — "AL TASCHLI-CHENU L'ES ZIKNU" — "Do not cast me away in my old age".

Our dream, our goal, is for a nationwide replication of our prototype programs in "Project Preventicare." We will not cast aside those who desperately need us; if we can help them curtail self-pity, encourage their self-discipline, enhance their self-image, then add a prescription of love, understanding, compassion and direction, the mission is possible.

CONCLUSION

One of the most important factors in adjusting to retirement is physical mobility, without which it is extremely difficult for the senior citizen to enjoy a long and happy retirement.

If we cannot cure aging, we can slow it down and inhibit its degradations by gradually changing improper habit patterns and by strengthening body functions through planned and sensible activity. Recognize those symptoms of aging — poor circulation, aching muscles and joints, arthritis, reduced co-ordination, chronic fatigue — and be assured that regular exercise can ameliorate these insidious changes.

Much preoccupation with rehabilitation or secondary prevention is directed to not much more than five percent of our elderly population, while habilitation, thus far insufficiently utilized, might improve the life style of the majority, physically, emotionally and mentally, thus putting off in time the degenerative processes inherent in aging.

The millions over 65 growing much faster in numbers than the population at large are those who have the least time left and who need us the most. We must therefore be concerned with primary prevention (habilitation) for that which we prevent will need no cure.

REFERENCES

Åstrand, P. and Rodahl, K. (1970) *Textbook of Work Physiology,* McGraw Hill, N.Y.
Leaf, A. (1973) *Nat Geo* 143, 93.
Mayer, J. (1968) *Overweight*, Prentice Hall, Englewood Cliffs, N.J.

Changing the Habits and Thought Patterns of the Aged to Promote Better Health Through Activity Programs in Institutions

Manuel Rodstein, M.D.

INTRODUCTION

The best way to promote better health through activity programs in institutions is to provide an active environment which includes activity of two basic types. In the first, the aged are involved as part of the audience for lectures, films, concerts, operas, theatrical performances and similar programs. In the second and more important type, the aged participate in a variety of activities provided by occupational therapy, reality orientation, literary, music, language and religious groups, games, sports and exercises specially tailored to fit the mental and physical capacities of the wide spectrum of age and functional capacity found in the population of any large institution for the aged.

Benefits of Good Activity Programs

The therapeutic milieu of the long-term care institution dedicated to such a multidisciplinary activity program has a number of beneficial effects including the engendering of motivation. This is the resurgence within the patient of the desire to participate actively, compared to a too frequent preadmission state of hopelessness, resignation, disappointment and apathy, compounded by the almost universal feelings of rejection experienced by any old person on admission to a long-term care institution and doubly compounded by the stresses of transplantation shock with its concommitant severe physical and emotional reactions in adjusting to a change of environment and life situation. Maddox (1963) has shown a clear trend between the relationship of activity and the degree of life satisfaction. Over a three-year period of observation, he found that old people whose activity increased tended to become better satisfied with life. Those whose activity fell off tended to become less satisfied.

Despite chronic illness and disability, a well designed activity program will result in a considerable degree of mental and physical rehabilitation for the patient. Even a partial victory is of value if the process of decline is arrested for an appreciable period of time resulting in some added satisfaction and meaning in living. Long ago, Cicero (106-45 BC) commented, "Exercise and temperance can preserve something of our early strength even in old age," and Joseph Addison (1672-1719) noted, "Exercise ferments the Humors, casts them into their proper Channels, throws off Redundancies, and helps Nature in those secret Distributions, without which the Body cannot subsist in its Vigour, nor the Soul act with Cheerfullness" (Adams, 1973). (See Chapter 2 for other historical aspects of the value of exercise.)

An activity program also provides a valuable by-product through stimulating the staff to overcome their physical and emotional strains and feelings of hopelessness and boredom, so often found among those providing long-term care to the chronically ill aged. For the physician caring for old people in institutions it expands his therapeutic armamentarium and options.

THE GERIATRICIAN'S ROLE

To begin with, how does the physician determine the need for physical activity? Second, what kind of activity and what controls and precautions are indicated? Third, what are the physiological benefits of an activity program, the duration after the program is discontinued, the limitations and the price in side effects?

Initially every aged individual should be thoroughly evaluated from general medical, cardiovascular and psychiatric points of view to determine whether he or she can withstand the physical and mental stresses not only of activity but even more importantly of inactivity. The stresses of inactivity have been well outlined by Wenger (1973). Inactivity such as bed rest causes a decrease of physical work capacity as shown by a decrease of 20 to 25 percent in maximal oxygen uptake even in healthy young adults at bedrest for three weeks, an increased heart rate response to effort and a tendency to orthostatic hypotension due to decreased blood volume. Increased blood viscosity due to a relatively greater decrease in plasma volume than in red cell mass, together with venous stasis, results in a greater incidence of thrombosis and embolization. Lung volume, vital capacity and serum protein concentration are all decreased. There is a negative nitrogen and calcium balance. Muscle contractile strength is decreased by as much as 10 to 15 percent for each week of inactivity. In addition, the aged at bedrest are more prone to bedsores, obstipation, urinary retention, accelerated osteoporosis and hypostatic pneumonia. The sum of these changes result in an increased susceptibility to falls and accidental injury.

The patient must be persuaded to accept the fact that apparently increased types of activities are really less strenuous than the alternatives, for example, that chair rest is less strenuous than bedrest and that the use of a bedside commode is less stressful than that of a bedpan, particularly with regard to strain on the cardiovascular system in terms of decrease of oxygen cost. Coe (1954) has shown that cardiac work is 23 percent less sitting in a chair than lying in the recumbent position.

Initial low energy activity should include self-care, such as feeding, shaving, the use of a bedside commode and active and passive extremity motion. Later, chair rest and progressive ambulation are introduced. Physical activity is avoided immediately after meals and interspersed with periods of rest. Isometric exercises are dangerous as they increase the load on the left ventricle and may provoke cardiac arrhythmias. Diversional activities such as music and watching television are encouraged. If chest pain, dyspnea, tachycardias over 120, ischemic electrocardiographic S-T segment depressions or arrhythmias develop or there is a fall in systolic blood pressure of over 20 mm., the level of physical activity must be decreased (Wenger, 1973). The Valsalva maneuver, which may be precipitated by straining on the bedpan, passing flatus, or pushing up on the bed, is dangerous as Benchimol et al. (1972) have shown a 72 percent reduction in coronary blood flow velocity during it. Dock (1944) has considered it to be a common cause of sudden death during early acute myocardial infarction.

For the normotensive, ambulatory aged without significant defects of the cardiovascular, pulmonary or musculoskeletal systems contraindicating such activity, regular daily walking, gradually increased in degree so as to accelerate the heart rate to 100-130 beats per minute, depending upon age and physical condition and after an appropriate warm-up period, will produce not only greater animation, self-esteem through a sense of well-being and attaining a more attractive body, but also achieve a lower heart rate at a given external work load together with an increased cardiac stroke volume at an unchanged cardiac output. Thus, cardiac work is reduced and cardiac efficiency, maximal oxygen consumption and work capacity are increased. The frequency of cardiac arrhythmias is reduced, body weight may be reduced and blood pressure lowered. (deVries, 1970, 1971; deVries and Adams, 1972; Rodstein, 1973; The Committee on Exercise of the American Heart Association, 1972; Terjueng et al., 1973).

Competitive sports, sudden bursts of effort, Valsalva maneuvers, isometric work and calisthenics which strain the lower back, knees and hips should be avoided. Strenuous jogging may further damage arthritic and osteoporotic backs, hips, knees, ankles and feet.

However, the program must be maintained as the benefits will quickly disappear in a short period of time once the exercise program is discontinued Supervision by qualified personnel, availability of appropriate resuscitatory equipment and careful initial tolerance are essential. The nature and degree of exercise for the aged must also consider their background and conditioning. In the present generation of aged in this country, less than half received some form of physical education during their school years and only seven percent received formal education in swimming (Report of President's Council on Physical Fitness and Sports, 1973).

The Committee on Exercise of the American Heart Association advocates a gradual five minute warm-up for the aged at the beginning of any single exercise program. They recommend that in the initial stages of an exercise program intensities of exercise should not demand more than 75 percent of an individual's maximal attainable heart rate. According to the tables in this monograph, this would mean a heart rate of 127-130 beats per minute for those 75 years of age and over. DeVries (1971) believes that exercise prescribed systematically and in moderation is not of undue concern for the cardiovascular system of healthy, normotensive elder men. (See Chapter 5.)

Among those over 75 years of age, clinical judgment must be employed in pre-scribing exercise as many cannot participate more than partially or at all because of physical and mental defects. Among the more than 1,000 aged institutionalized in The Jewish Home and Hospital for Aged of New York, ranging in age from 75 to 100 years with an average age of 84 years, over 40 percent have appreciable degrees of chronic brain syndrome, 80 percent have evidence of organic heart disease and 50 percent are in some degree of congestive heart failure. Even submaximal exercise testing of this group at 60-75 percent of maximal levels would produce a high percentage of ischemic electrocardiographic S-T segment depressions and/or signifi-cant arrhythmias. Strandell (1963) found in apparently healthy aged individuals that the incidence of S-T segment depressions with exercise increased from four to 38 percent with advancing age. In my opinion, heart rates of 130 or more would not be tolerated by many of this type of aged population without resultant angina and/or dyspnea.

THE ROLE OF THE RECREATIONAL AND OCCUPATIONAL THERAPIST

In addition to the medical aspects of activity and rehabilitation, The Jewish Home and Hospital for Aged of New York offers a wide range of recreational and occupa-tional activities in an attempt to provide something for everyone. There are weekly Fitness Fun sessions, attended by up to 50 individuals at each of our two major centers, open to all who wish to attend, whether ambulatory or wheelchair-bound. These one hour sessions begin with an initial warm-up period followed by mild exercises and games such as passing soft beach balls, interspersed with jokes, songs and stories led by the recreation leader. Light refreshments are served at the end of the session. Medical clearance is obtained for activities. A form of low effort bowling with light balls on a short alley is popular with male residents.

Occupational therapy and workshop activities are carried out not only in the main special areas but also on the floors. Reality orientation is an active program, par-ticularly among those with moderate to severe chronic brain syndrome. There is a unit staff team meeting weekly on each floor with participation by all involved in the care of the aged individual. Particular attention is paid to the role of the nurse's aide, the person with the greatest contact with the aged individual and the one most involved in his or her every day care.

For those with well-preserved mental function, there are courses sponsored by the New York Community College such as in psychology and the comparative cultures of Israel, Russia and China. A group of 40 aged individuals, attending nine weekly sessions, participated intensely. Dr. Muriel Oberleder, who conducted the course in psychology, gave the group a Rorschach test at the conclusion of the course and found them to be realistic, with good reasoning power, responsive, creative, with good abstracting and introspective abilities and not rigid. They were able to integrate new stimuli and had good emotional and behavioral aspect and controls (Taft, 1973). This is, of course, a self-selected supernormal group which demonstrates that, in old age, activity, good mental function and hygiene go together. For the large number of institutionalized aged with overt or covert depression, special efforts at detection, together with counselling and the use of the ataractic and mood elevating drugs, will help activate them.

In addition to these programs, there is a wide range of activities among which the most popular are concerts, lectures, theatre groups, opera groups, music and art appreciation, drawing, dancing (both folk and ballroom), choral singing, drama, nature study, outdoor activities, literature study groups, philosophy and painting.

An attempt is made from the date of admission to involve every person in activities to a maximal degree. Constant liaison is maintained with the medical department to set limitations in accordance with the condition of the individual. There are, of course, a number of the aged who are unwilling to become involved in any form of activity. Study of such individuals reveals that most have been loners all of their lives.

A remarkably successful program combining sensory stimulation (olfactory, tactile, kinesthetic, etc.) and reality orientation (date, person, place, etc.) has been used to activate aged individuals with advanced chronic brain syndrome (Sinz, 1973). This program is conducted by two occupational therapists for two and one-half hours a day on a floor with a census of 31 females with this condition. The daily program consists of first greeting each patient by name and encouraging recall of time, day and purpose for being in the room and a make-up session to encourage self-care and to reinforce feelings of positive self-esteem and cleanliness through grooming (i.e., combing of hair, putting on make-up and using a mirror to study the results). Exercise practice followed with use of the abacus, picture lacing board, peg board, letter work puzzles and coordination board to increase concentration, improve motor function and hand-eye coordination. Upon improvement, craft media are introduced to utilize residual or relearned skills such as table frame weaving, simple knotting, crocheting, simple embroidery, painting, tile mosaics,. etc. All patients engage in activities such as rhythm band, ball playing and cooking. The end products of cooking (i.e., cookies, biscuits and pizzas) are eaten by their creators. Touching, hugging, tactile communication as tokens of warmth, acceptance and affection from therapist to patient are emphasized. This form of basic communication is essential and successful in reaching the nonverbal patient and provides reassurance as to acceptability and lovability, and contributes to positive self-esteem.

After one and one-half years of experience, formerly nonresponding and nonverbal patients recognized the therapists and returned their greetings. Approximately one third learned to operate on a simple level in small groups and one third could do more independent work in groups of six to eight, the more rapid responders doing more complex work, some on their own without supervision. The artistic products of the group decorate the day room where the activities are conducted. Excellent cooperation by the nursing staff on the floor helped to create a general atmosphere of creative energy and positive activity.

In some institutions for the aged, sheltered workshops function as a form of activity with medical clearance and supervision. Contracts are obtained from industry for the packaging, assembly and distribution of small articles such as luggage handles, button display cards, poker chips or work on ladies' belts in need of fasteners. Workers are paid on a piece-work basis with a guaranteed minimum

(Shore, 1966). The workers benefit from the small supplementation of their spending monies and derive physical and psychological benefits from their activity.

However, a number of negative factors must not be overlooked. First, what are the safeguards against the aged residents becoming a source of cheap labor, competing with other community groups such as disabled veterans, the blind and other handicapped groups for remunerative employment? Second, how harmful are the pressures engendered by the need for meeting production schedules and deadlines? Third, there is the need for subsidization of the program and contract solicitation as well as the prevention of accidents.

CONCLUSION

Altering the habits and thought patterns of the aged in institutions for the promotion of better health through activity programs demands a continuous, organized, ongoing activity program since human beings do not like persistency. All members of the staff must be involved under the direction of skilled professionals. In this way, the physical and mental health of the aged will be improved, their relatives will be happier and easier to deal with and staff will show greater interest in their work and provide better care to their aged patients.

REFERENCES

Adams, C. W. (1973) *Am J Cardiol* 32, 127.

Benchimol, A., Wang, R. F., Desser, K. B., Gartlan, J. L., Jr. (1972) *Ann Intern Med* 77, 357.

Coe, W. S. (1954) *Arch Intern Med* 40, 42.

deVries, H. A. (1970) *J Geront* 25, 325.

deVries, H. A. (1971) *Geriatrics* 26, 94 and 26, 102.

deVries, H. A., and Adams, G. M. (1972) *J Gerontol* 27, 344.

Dock, W. (1944) *JAMA* 125, 1083.

Maddox, G. L. (1963) *Social Forces* 42, 199.

Report of President's Council on Physical Fitness and Sports (1973) *Aging* 226, 22.

Rodstein, M. (1973) *Mental Illness in Later Life,* American Psychiatric Association, Washington, D.C.

Sinz, M. (1973) Personal communication.

Shore, H. (1966) *Professional Nursing Home* 8, 14.

Strandell, T. (1963) *Acta Med Scand* 174, 479.

Taft, S. (1973) Personal communication.

Terjueng, R. S., Baldwin, K. M., Cooksey, J., Samson, B., and Sutter, R. A. (1973) *J Am Geriatr Soc* 21, 164.

The Committee on Exercise, American Heart Association (1972) *Exercise Testing and Training of Apparently Healthy Individuals. A Handbook for Physicians*, American Heart Association, New York.

Wenger, N. K. (1973) *Cardiology* 58, 1.

Developing Staff Capability for Physical Fitness Programs

Paul A. L. Haber, M.D.

INTRODUCTION

Physical fitness is more than the mere absence of disease or disability. It represents the ability of the human organism to maintain the integrity of its homeostasis in the face of environmental stress and a positive capability to return to a normal state after doing a certain amount of vigorous physical exercise more rapidly and with greater ease than comparable human organisms not in a state of physical fitness. The incorporation of programs to promote improved physical fitness, mental and social health, and well-being is an essential ingredient of any institutional program for the aging.

The Veterans Administration with a major commitment to the care of the aging and the aged veteran has recognized the value of such programs. It is very much concerned with the physical fitness of its patients and particularly of aged patients, who tend to remain in institutions longer than their younger counterparts. As a result, the VA Administration has developed an inclusive, comprehensive physical fitness program for the aged which is based upon a multi-disciplinary approach using the classical rehabilitation therapy techniques and other services. The success of such programs often revolves around the leadership; and, therefore, it is important to develop proper staff capability for fitness training programs in agencies and institutions – the theme of this chapter.

The Veterans Administration currently operates 171 hospitals, 86 nursing homes, 209 clinics and 18 domiciliaries. It services a population of about 85,000 people within its facilities and arranges and pays for the care of a total of about 165,000 people, 60,000 of whom are over the age of 65.

The design of all facilities for institutional programs for the aged, spanning a range of domiciliary, nursing home, intermediate care and day centers, includes the incorporation of physical space for exercise and calisthenics. Historically, these exer-

221

cises were based on a mandatory compliance. Today, of course, we shrink from any treatment or rehabilitation modality based on other than full voluntary compliance.

The range of comprehensive programs for the elderly now includes a variety of noninstitutional programs such as hospital-based home care, personal home care and outpatient program. We have begun to incorporate physical fitness programs in these various noninstitutional programs. Our basic philosophy in developing the comprehensive institutional program for the aging is twofold: (1) we wish to prevent institutionalization whenever possible and (2) we wish to remake the institutions so as to divest them of any depersonalizing attributes which may have crept in over the years.

A program of physical fitness is therefore essential to the development of both of these objectives. Underlying all of the programs is the profound conviction that care for the aged should not foment dependency and a program of physical fitness is therefore essential to a state of less independency.

REQUISITES FOR PHYSICAL FITNESS PROGRAMS

Total Commitment

One of the first requisites of a real physical fitness program is the commitment of the agency or the institution *in toto* to the idea of physical fitness. This means that no single service or professional discipline can claim to be the sole guardian of the physical fitness program in an institution. At every hospital the entire staff including the manager of the station of the director, the chief of staff and the professional and administrative staff must be dedicated to the idea of physical fitness. I remember quite clearly the failure of a program to curtail smoking among emphysema patients until the doctor who directed the clinic himself decided to forego smoking. The look of annoyance on the patients' faces as the doctor vigorously puffed on a cigarette while he extolled the virtues of a nonsmoking regimen was all too clear to ignore. And so it is with physical fitness.

The necessity for total commitment on the part of the staff to a physical fitness program appears obvious, but there are other more subtle reasons which relate to the problems of institutionalization. Too often, one of the most pernicious aspects of an institution is that the staff tends to assume a proprietary attitude towards the institution and, thus, towards the patients themselves. A program of physical fitness, insofar as it contributes a state of lessened physical (and therefore mental) dependency, can be an outward sign and symbol of staff willingness to permit greater independence on the part of the aging patient.

The fitness program cannot exist by itself. It must be developed in concert with a full appreciation of the complete aspects of psychological, social and physiological fitness which makes it of some moment of importance.

Along this line of total commitment for fitness, the Veterans Administration has developed a good institutional attitude towards the problems of smoking and alcoholism. It has successfully sought to curtail smoking in its facilities by discouraging the sale of cigarettes in canteens and patient service shops and has developed an alcoholism treatment program at about 45 of its stations.

One of the most significant programs in the Veterans Administration to enhance physiological fitness has been the conduct of an experiment on changing dietary patterns to reduce arteriosclerosis. This study of 300 patients and 300 controls on a diet very low in unsaturated fats was conducted for eight years. The results show an inconclusive but encouraging decrease in mortality from cardiovascular deaths due to arteriosclerosis among the tested patients and a very marked reduction in the number of cardiovascular accidents, such as myocardial infarctions and cerebral vascular accidents (strokes). The sample size would have to be considerably larger to be able to draw final conclusions.

The Rehabilitation Service

But, all of these foregoing ideas do not really do anything more than set the stage for physical fitness. Although no single service has a monopoly on interest in physical fitness, the service with the greatest interest is the Rehabilitation Service. This service, formerly designated as Physical Medicine Rehabilitation Service, was begun in the Veterans Administration at the close of World War II and, with the use of such outstanding consultants as Dr. Howard Rusk and Dr. Arthur Kessler, developed into a very well-organized Rehabilitation Medicine Service. It was deployed at all of our facilities and consisted of programs usually under the direction of a physiatrist who was assisted by a coordinator of the programs and a variety of therapists: corrective therapists, physical therapists, manual arts therapists, occupational therapists, industrial therapists and education therapists. The corrective and physical therapists probably have the greatest interest in the physical fitness program and it was to them that the great bulk of patients and staff turned for instruction in physical fitness.

The growing and special needs of geriatric patients have been recognized by those involved in occupational therapy and physical therapy education. New program "essentials" on the academic level for occupational therapy cover physiology dealing with the disorders of aging, and the clinical experience required stipulates that the student must work with an aging population as part of the total education and training program. Physical therapy follows much the same process.

There are in existence in the United States the following numbers of O.T. and P.T. programs at two levels; also shown are the number of 1972 graduates and the number of VA hospitals providing clinical experience for students.

	Educ. Programs	1972 Graduates	Clinical Training VAH	Trainees
Occupational Therapy				
Professional level	40	940	54	575
Assistant	36	570	16	93
Physical Therapy				
Professional level	63	1,740	53	784
Assistant	21	789	11	67

There are also a number of graduate level programs in both disciplines in which VA hospitals participate.

Preventive Maintenance

One particular program for preventive maintenance conducted at the VA Hospital, Brecksville, Ohio, demonstrates many of the points I have mentioned. At this facility, a diverse group, including the hospital director, the assistant hospital director, the management analyst, the chief of the psychiatric service, the chief of the rehabilitation medicine service, four staff physicians, dentist, the chief of medical illustration, the coordinator of the Rehabilitation Medicine Service, the chief of Pharmacy Service and many others enrolled in a class of concentrated calisthenics and running. Each participant was requested to sign a statement of consent to work in this program and to have a thorough physical examination which was then evaluated and approved by the chief of Personnel Health Service and the chief of Rehabilitation Medicine Service. The examination included pulse rate, blood pressure, and electrocardiogram recordings. Body weights were taken prior to the initiation of the exercise programs and were rechecked every two months thereafter. The age of the participating members ranged from 31 to 67 years (average 52) and the majority were considered overweight for their body build, height and age.

The exercise program, devised by Frank R. Coleman, Chief of Corrective Therapy, and enthusiastically supported by the hospital director, consisted of three basic parts which were performed three days a week. Each session lasted one-half hour. First, there were calisthenic routines — 5 to 20 calisthenic exercises geared for both muscle stretching and cardiovascular efficiency were performed on a progressive level. The number of repetitions increased from the initial six to eight, then to 10. As time went on, the cadence of the execution of the exercises was increased. Proper execution of these exercises was demonstrated originally and spot checking was performed periodically so that the maximum potential benefit from this phase of the program could be realized by the participants.

The second part of the program was running. A progressive series of running procedures were instituted in the gymnasium where one full lap around the floor was approximately 100 yards long and 20 laps equaled a mile. The participants started by running one-half lap followed by a walking period of one lap for three repetitions. After one week, this routine was extended to four repetitions, then to six repetitions in the third week and, in the fourth week, the men ran one complete lap. They walked one lap for every three repetitions and the cycle repeated itself. After approximately 17 to 18 weeks, the men ran the entire 20 laps continuously with safety and without undue fatigue.

The third part of the program was swimming. After the first month of calisthenics and running, it was decided to use swimming for a change of pace and variety. The planned swimming routines were instituted every other Friday for every sixth session. The swimming routines were organized to include both the good and poor swimmers, and the men were instructed to swim the laps of the pool in a variety of strokes, again on a progressive pattern. The poor swimmers were encouraged to participate with strict adherence to quality, but the number of swimming procedures varied.

The goals for those in the program obviously differed. Some were psychological: the will to prove a point, to enhance one's masculinity or to succeed in an area formerly beyond grasp. The physical goals were more obvious: the abundance of weight problems, shortness of breath, the feeling of lethargy, the will to improve one's physical condition in cardiovascular efficiency and an attempt to regain some of the vigor and resiliency of youth. These played a prominent part in keeping the men on the program, but initially brought only pain and often excessive fatigue to the performer. In six months, the majority of the men showed significant weight loss, especially those who were originally overweight and who definitely had the interest and will to improve themselves. EKG reports did not show any significant changes, but the duration of the program was too short to judge the results.

Thus, the entire effort demonstrated the commitment of the staff members of the Brecksville VA Hospital and did more to energize their aging patients to enroll in a comparable program than any other device. The demonstration of staff commitment and the will of the staff to keep physically fit was one of the key points in developing staff capability in the physical fitness program.

CONCLUSION

Physical fitness programs for the aging can be a vital part of any institutional program aimed at improving the health and well-being of an aged population. The most essential ingredient in developing a staff capability for such programs is a multidisciplinary approach and a sense of total commitment. The Veterans Administration has incorporated such a program of physical fitness in its comprehensive, integrated program for the aging.

Community Program for Tension Control

Nicholas G. Alexiou, M.D.

INTRODUCTION

Relaxation is a very vogue thing, but how to do it sensibly and safely is another matter. In the modern medical world, relaxation techniques immediately bring to mind the use of pharmacologic agents prescribed by the physician or purchased over the counter in pharmacies on the recommendation of TV commercials. So popular is the "pop a pill" concept that even school children have become involved, swallowing one pill to sleep or relax and another to pep them up. The medical profession is offered a vast array of choices in muscle relaxants, tranquilizers, sedatives, hypnotics or ataractics. Patients have also discovered that alcohol-containing cocktails serve as relaxants as well as social contact lubricants. College students have discovered marihuana and narcotics provide them with needed relaxation. Drugs however are not always necessary and certainly not the best answer. What else is available? As medical specialists in physical medicine, physiatrists offer several modalities to facilitate relaxation, including passive nonpharmacologic exercises, whirlpool baths, warm baths, saunas, heat pads and massage. Their active or passive nonpharmacologic exercises for muscle tension control embrace teaching muscle contraction and relaxation, strength-building exercises and flexibility exercises. Their effectiveness can be determined by measuring muscle tension with electromyographs.

Society, too, has discovered active and passive relaxation exercises in the form of dancing, Yoga, walking, swings, rocking chairs, calisthenics, stretching, isometrics and running. Some techniques in the realm of physical education, to some degree, are taught in elementary and secondary schools. Environmental change and music also facilitate relaxation.

All these techniques apply to the person over 50 years of age, as well as the young. In working with older citizens, it is important to be aware that people of all ages face frustration and tension and need to release accumulated tensions at regular intervals. Persons caring for older citizens should be familiar with specific techniques of training methods that can be employed to assist their tense, anxious clients to adjust to their frustrations and ease their tension (i.e., to relax). Some of these methods are discussed in this chapter and others in Chapter 27.

METHODS

Techniques

It is important that the proper technique is chosen and appropriately applied by a sympathetic and knowledgeable therapist for the patient to benefit. Most techniques discussed here are simple, familiar and inexpensive, but each can be rendered useless by inappropriate application in terms of timing, intensity, duration and environmental circumstances.

For most elderly and the severely chronically disabled, useful relaxation measures include heat, massage and passive exercise. For the less severely disabled and elderly, use of a rocking chair or swing is a beneficial form of exercise in addition to heat, massages and passive motion. For minimally disabled and middle-aged adults, walking is a very relaxing exercise. The time to start some active muscle stretching, which also facilitates relaxation, is when active exercises are begun.

Next in the progression from passive to active relaxation techniques comes exercise in the form of calisthenics and sustained physical activity, to the point of fatigue. "Fatigue is nature's inducement to sleep," stated the late Boston cardiologist, Dr. Paul Dudley White. "Brisk walking to the point of fatigue, like other forms of exercise, are ideal antidotes against emotional stress and, therefore, have a bearing upon the general problem of fitness. Exercise is the best tranquilizer in the world" (White, 1970).

Problems

The natural enjoyment of movement for sake of movement, as in dancing, is a pleasure of children and young adults, but unfortunately is gradually withdrawn with maturation because of society's standards of propriety. By middle or old age, movement of the body or motor action is too often discouraged or frowned upon. Opportunities for relaxing movements of exercises, minimal at best, are severely restricted in older citizens. Everything is done for the safety of the older patient, to protect him from injury or fall, even to the point of securely fastening him in bed and setting up side rails. A prescription for bed rest may be the worst news for the patient. The end results of such lack of movement may be muscular atrophy, poor coordination, skeletal osteoporosis, mental confusion and physical deterioration.

Kreitler and Kreitler (1970) report that older, inactive people (over 50 years) perceive their bodies to be broader and heavier than they are and experience body activity as increasingly strenuous. They quickly establish a faulty feedback system leading to more inactivity. A progressive restriction of physical exercise leads to corresponding alteration of body image, more clumsiness and fear of physical activity. Normal adults over 50 tend to be introspective. They explore the emotional and intellectual spheres and are more reflective. They tend not to indulge in physical activity as they did when they were younger. As a consequence, they have a tendency to build up tension. Their pent-up tensions and aggression lead to frustration, and manifestations of this may surface as a sudden release or acting out of aggression. Younger people, on the other hand, can act out without rebuke and thereby release their tensions, but this way is unacceptable in older people. In addition, many forces, ranging from social pressures to inner fear, tend to immobilize the person over 50 years of age and raise his tensions.

On the other hand, there is abundant evidence to suggest that regular body exercise provides profound emotional and physical satisfaction. It improves coordination, establishes a sense of security and appropriate body image, improves general body circulation, allows for release of aggressive tendencies and reduces tension. In addition, physically active people are socially more acceptable.

Rationale

How do relaxation techniques relieve tension? Generally, tension is produced by anxiety. The stimuli causing the anxiety, whether physical or emotional, are transmitted to the brain and, through the central nervous system, can affect many other body systems. The brain sends messages to the neuromuscular skeletal system which responds with muscle contraction. Prolonged muscle contraction leads to increased tension and symptoms of fatigue, pain, headache, muscle or joint aching and shortening of muscles. Hyperventilation and hormonal adrenergic responses are other response manifestations of anxiety. On the other hand, slow rhythmic motions and quiet sounds tend to transmit slow rhythmic stimuli to the brain which, in turn, responds with slow rhythmic messages to the musculoskeletal system and causes the muscle to contract at a slower rate.

The hypothalamus apparently acts as the control center for the autonomic nervous system to maintain homeostasis. It receives afferent fibers from the cerebral cortex directly and the thalamus indirectly. These afferent fibers form part of the ascending reticular activating system. The homeostatic mechanisms are affected by the type and number of afferent impulses. Low rate, low intensity, monotonous stimulation of peripheral afferent nerves brings about synchronization of the electroencephalographic waves and even sleep by decreasing the tonic activity of the ascending reticular activating system. It is possible to influence the hypothalamus by impulses through afferent somatic and visceral nerves. Dr. W. Bronk et al. (1936) showed that rhythmic variations in the potential in the hypothalamus sympathetic nervous system may be elicited and result from stimulation of afferent visual nerves. Pompeiano and Swett (1962) demonstrated electroencephalographic and behavioral manifestations of sleepiness induced by cutaneous nerve stimulation in normal cats.

The object of teaching relaxation techniques is to break this cycle of prolonged contraction and tension. The first step is to develop the subject's awareness of his tension symptoms and the circumstances that lead to the tension. Next, he is helped to identify muscle groups which respond most to the tension situation. Then, breaking of the cycle is necessary. Initially, this step may require active therapeutic intervention using heat, medication, massage and passive movement. The application of active or passive exercises, with slow rhythmic pace, reduces the frequency and intensity of proprioceptive and enteroceptive impulses so that the person relaxes. After these steps have been initiated and some relief obtained, the education of the patient begins, involving him in his own therapy.

Shavasan Technique

A simple technique that demonstrates this principle is the art of Shavasan, a Yogic breathing exercise. The subject is placed in a comfortable supine position and asked to slow his respirations voluntarily. He is then instructed to breathe in and out slowly at first. When he can do this, he is requested voluntarily to hold his breath slightly, at the end of inspiration, and to hold it slightly longer, at the end of expiration. K. K. Datey et al. (1960) reported marked relaxation and lowering of the respiratory rate and blood pressure in persons who learned this breathing exercise. They believe this exercise probably influences the hypothalamus through the continuous feedback of slow rhythmic proprioceptive and enteroceptive impulses and tends to lower the settings of the central nervous system response initiating centers, leading to the desired relaxation.

The element of concentration is very important in the instruction phase since extraneous thoughts and stimuli have to be "tuned out". Such concentration can be assisted by providing a quiet environment initially and directing the patient to focus on his breathing movements.

Change in Environment

Control of the environment also produces a therapeutic effect. Dr. W. Raab (1970), a pioneer in preventive myocardiology, advocated programs that remove an individual from his usual environment and treat him in quiet, natural, picturesque, rural settings. The remainder of his prescription for controlling tension, and incidentally heart disease, included regular physical training and avoidance of smoking.

The commonest objection to relaxation exercises is that they take too much time. A sound program, in fact, does take a one-half hour session several times weekly. Some individuals become so well-trained or conditioned, however, that they can achieve tension-relieving relaxation in a session of only 5 to 10 minutes.

Exercise may relax people better than drugs. In 10 middle-aged and older anxious or tense males. deVries reported the onset of action of the tranquilizer meprobamate was one-half hour with a peak level in one hour. The optimal relaxation of exercise appeared immediately and lasted up to one hour. The single meprobamate dose of 400 mg produced less muscular relaxation than a single dose of exercise consisting of a walk lasting 15 minutes at a rate which raised and sustained the pulse rate to 120 beats per minute (de Vries and Adam, 1972). He pointed to the relative freedom from toxic drug reactions in a physical exercise prescription for relaxation. The usual therapeutic dose of meprobamate may compromise coordination, reaction time and motor function in the elderly.

The Jacobson Method

The exercise and relaxation instruction program offered to the New York State Education Department employees is the method described by Jacobson (1938,

1957). This method is a direct and practical instructional technique which has been effective and rewarding. Each day following a physical exercise period of one-half hour, the program participants are required to lie supine on the gymnasium floor and rest 15 minutes three times weekly for 15 weeks. This technique is beneficial, safe and achieves the control needed, even in "middle-aged subjects" over 50 years of age. Under the watchful eye of a program coordinator, they are taught during this period how to recognize muscle tension in various parts and muscle groups of the body, and are asked to contract muscle groups and feel the muscle tension sensation. Then they are told to relax and become conscious of that sensation. Each participant is encouraged to repeat the process and practice the technique in his office, at home and while driving a car. Descriptive material is given to each participant for reading.

This fitness group is also taught to do "Shavasan" breathing as described previously. This technique works for many, assisting them to achieve a more complete state of relaxation.

CONCLUSION

The positive experience with the N.Y.S. Education Department program indicates that exercises for tension control, including change of environment, "Shavasan" breathing, walking and the Jacobson relaxation method as described in this chapter, are simple effective relaxation techniques highly suitable for "Fitness After 50" community programs.

REFERENCES

Bronk, D. W., Lewy, F. H., and Larrabee, M. D. (1936) *Am J Physiol* 116, 15.
Datey, K. K., Deshmukh, S. N., Dalvi, C. P., and Vinekar, S. L. (1969) *Angiology* 20, 325.
deVries, H. A. and Adam, G. (1972) *Am J Physiol Med* 51, 130.
Jacobson, E. (1938) *Progressive Relaxation*, Ed. 2, University of Chicago Press, Chicago.
Jacobson, E. (1957) *You Must Relax*, Ed. 4, McGraw-Hill, New York.
Kreitler, H., and Kreitler, S. (1970) in *Medicine and Sport*, Vol. 4 (Brunner, D., and Jokl, E., eds.), University Park Press, Baltimore.
Pompeiano, O., and Swett, J. E. (1962) *Arch Ital Biol* 100, 311.
Raab, W. (1970) *Preventive Myocardiology*, Charles C Thomas, Springfield.
White, P. D. (1970) in *Medicine and Sport*, Vol. 4 (Brunner, D. and Jokl, E., eds.), University Park Press, Baltimore.

Organization of Exercise Programs

Lloyd C. Arnold

PRINCIPLES OF AN EXERCISE PROGRAM

Objectives

The first step in organizing an exercise program is the development of a set of well defined objectives. Such objectives for a fitness program should include:

1. Improvement of cardiovascular function
2. Development of muscular strength
3. Development of endurance
4. Development of flexibility of joints
5. Provision for relaxation and release of tension
6. Delay of the aging process
7. Development of coordination and learn new skills
8. Development of an understanding of the role of exercise and physical activity in the maintenance of good health
9. Opportunity for social growth and development

The Exercise Program

The exercise session should consist of three basic parts: warm-up, peak work and cooling off.

Warm-up Period

The warm-up period is designed to prepare the body for the work to come. There should be a gradual increase of intensity as the warm-up progresses. Warm-up should be rhythmic and have a natural flow from one movement to another. A warm-up should be about 20 minutes in length, assuming fairly good conditions exist.

Peak Work

After the warm-up is finished, one moves in to the part of the exercise program which develops muscular strength, endurance and fitness. This part of an exercise program should include exercises for all major joint movements. It should maintain a high level of activity without creating local fatigue. This can be achieved by moving from one exercise (one muscle group) to another. For example, if the session requires 10 repetitions, give five now and five later. Don't work to the point where the participant has local fatigue. Do not perform swinging exercises against fixed joints as this puts undesirable strain on muscles, tendons and ligaments. It is better to do strength exercises in sets rather than constantly to exhaustion. Encourage the class to work at its own rate. Do not insist that members keep up or stay with the count. This is one area where we err most, because the instructor is overly conscious of how the class looks and counts cadence so that everybody is in line doing the same thing at the same time. The training program must be readily adaptable to individual needs while, at the same time, permitting a group approach. For example, in jogging around the room, some can jog in the middle where the distance is shorter and some can jog at different speeds. Offer opportunities and suggest ways that accommodate individual differences.

Interval training principle should be used (i.e., work, rest; work, rest; or work, recovery; work, recovery, using various speeds and various tempos). Exercise intensity should be individually controlled. In many YMCAs, the heart rate is often used as a way of monitoring the exercise intensity. The participants are taught to count their own pulses. Be alert to environmental problems such as heat and cold. Do not permit a competitive atmosphere to develop. Set an example and establish a class atmosphere which encourages everyone, regardless of the level of skill, fitness and motivation. This is difficult to achieve in this age of drive and competitiveness, but work at it. Be conservative. It doesn't take a lot of exercise for the untrained to get a training effect. Keep the activities varied and interesting.

Cooling Off Period

The cooling off period is designed to gradually return the body to a nonexercising state. Emphasize relaxing exercises. This period should be completed in five to 10 minutes, and the heart rate should be back to 110-120 beats per minute.

Leadership

Leadership can be divided into two categories, volunteers and paid leaders. Both have many traits in common. Critical in the selection and development of leadership is the recruitment of leaders who:

1. Believe in the benefits of the program and its contribution to a better life.
2. Set an example of healthful living, regular physical activity and weight control.
3. Reject smoking and excessive use of alcohol.
4. Are well informed and seek ways to share this information.
5. Like people.
6. Are sensitive to the needs of the participants.
7. Are enthusiastic, cheerful and warm.

A Philosophy for Success

Now, if you take these factors, the program which includes a series of objectives and the principles of how to run an exercise program, and add good leadership, then a philosophy for success must be considered. When one looks at the kinds of programs YMCAs operate and analyzes why people come, clues for such a philosophy become apparent. People come to the YMCA to exercise for some of the following reasons and many persons for most of them:

1. The doctor, the husband, the wife or a friend recommends it.
2. They desire to lose weight.
3. They desire to get into shape — to participate in other sports activities, recreation, or just to improve fitness.
4. They fear a heart attack.
5. They enjoy the fellowship.
6. They want to feel better, stronger and healthier.
7. A friend is already involved and says he enjoys it.
8. It's the "in" thing to do in our society today.

Motivation

How do you motivate people to keep active? Whitehouse (Chap. 13) has discussed this subject from a psychologist's viewpoint. As physical educators we have tried to separate these items and here are some of the things we believe are helpful. They are motivated if:

1. You show them results. In addition to feeling good, they are motivated if they see improvement, a lowering pulse rate or weight reduction or some other objective measure.
2. You make the activities interesting and fun.
3. You vary the activities.
4. You use music.
5. You create incentive kinds of programs such as long distance runs, with participants running across the country using a map with markings to show progress, or a 50-mile swim.
6. You educate the participants to activity and help them develop habits of exercise.
7. You begin to relate exercise to total health.
8. You recognize their achievements.
9. You give opportunities for leadership.
10. You give opportunities for service.

Involvement

One of the exciting principles of adult education, which is receiving more and more significance in the last few years, is based to a large extent on individual involvement. For years educators have said that you learn best those things you want to learn and those things you get personally involved in. Every person in a program of exercise must be involved to a high degree. Leadership in a program of exercise must be "people centered" as compared with "subject centered." Interested concern must center on that particular individual. The participant, programs and activities must be evaluated on the basis of meeting personal needs.

Individual involvement leads to individual commitment and then to higher levels of interest, learning and retention. Leadership training should be designed to minimize depersonalization and dehumanization. Leadership success requires compassion, love, enthusiasm and even missionary zeal as well as a philosophy of acceptance of others and a sense of responsibility for themselves and others. Participants are concerned with love, ego, fun, vanity, social growth and feeling better. Consider offering others the chance to share your leadership. Others may not be able to reach the standards of education and performance which you maintain for yourself but you will find that if you offer leadership experience, they will quickly respond to the challenge. This is a more sophisticated level of leadership. It's a harder technique than the typical standing-in-the-front-of-the-class leader. An old Chinese philosopher declared:

> A leader is best when people barely know that he exists,
> Not so good when people obey him and proclaim him,
> Worse when they despise him.
> Fail to honor people, they fail to honor you.
> But a good leader who talks little,
> When his work is done — his aims fulfilled,
> They will say — we did this ourselves.

CONCLUSION

It is important that each individual has access to the facts about exercise and an understanding and appreciation of its value. Galileo once said, "You cannot teach a man anything; you can only teach him to find it within himself."

The challenge is to help people find within themselves the need and the will to act intelligently and exercise diligently.

Popularizing Physical Fitness After Fifty Via Television

Maggie Lettvin

INTRODUCTION

Television is the way to reach millions of people of all ages in their homes with common sense and fun applied to self-care. Many people see television more often and for longer periods of time than they see the members of their own families. Television is especially suited to carry useful health and exercise messages to the aged needing self-care, those on the fringe and those headed in that direction. It is unrealistic to expect older people to exercise well in strange surroundings such as a gymnasium where strangers do strange new things to them with equipment. In this situation, the reassurance of home is lacking, and there is the further complication of embarrassment at one's body and plight. Furthermore, they cannot move or be moved easily. They should be treated gratis as they often have little or no money. To reach this large group of the elderly where they are — in hospitals, nursing homes, their own homes — television seems the obvious answer.

METHODS

Exercise for the elderly can often be done more easily and better in private. When nobody is watching, an elderly person can without embarrassment work through his clumsiness and mistakes with some hope of restoring function. The fitness problems of the elderly without serious disease are, for the most part, mainly the problems caused by long periods of "disuse" or "misuse". The methods by which they may be treated are not too different from those exercises used in less extreme cases of "disuse" or "misuse". But in the elderly the therapist must take into account the more fragile bone, muscle and connective tissue and the much longer time it takes to balance the systems that regulate the aged body. A slower start and a much more gradual progression will not only prevent injury, aches and pains, but will insure that each step taken will be small enough to prove totally successful. A little-used elderly body has habits that are going to be hard to break. To succeed in getting a new habit set, the small daily increments in movement will have to be so totally rewarding, so

237

constantly successful, so obviously restorative of systems thought to be lost as to be a sure thing. It is too easy, otherwise, to relax back into old comfortable habits, self-destructive or not.

Objectives of Exercise

The minimum necessary goals to strive for in the elderly are:
1. Getting in and out of bed
2. Getting in and out of chairs
3. Walking
4. Walking up and down stairs
5. Getting on and off the floor
6. Making use of the hands.

Each goal requires the development of adequate circulation, flexibility, balance, strenth and endurance, especially in the muscles of the lower back and legs. Many individuals can perform these minimal functions only by also using their arms and hands.

Individual and Personally Supervised Exercise

For individuals confined to bed with circulatory problems, the beginning exercises might be designed to improve flexibility and circulation. They should be done only for as many seconds at a time as the person involved feels comfortable. Patience, hope and cheerfulness rather than force and disapproval can accomplish much. Giving praise in the beginning for accomplishment is very encouraging to the bed-ridden patient's recovery. A progress chart listing the daily number of exercises done may be of immense help to the elderly. If one is used to living at a standstill, as many of the elderly are, an obviously visible, even though slight, progression showing a positive direction and improvement in mobility keeps one striving and also constitutes a source of pride and joy to the older person. There are too few such satisfactions in the life of the elderly as we all know.

Many people with disabilities cannot cope with their problems, not because they are incapable of varying amounts of recovery, but because the approach sometimes demands so great an effort that even the first step towards recovery is improbable or impossible.

To have one's body fail to follow one's commands is a terrible blow to ego and self-respect and a failure of a process upon which we have come to depend. It places the individual in a completely different category where both the person and the rest of the world suddenly or gradually come to see himself or herself as a loser rather than a winner. Winning and losing can become habits just as any other habits. Somehow that loser image has to be changed and changed fast. The damaged person has to be given tasks which are totally manageable — not to show up his or her weaknesses, but to improve those parts and supplement his strengths — to make him look, feel and be successful with each move.

It is of great help to both the exercise instructor and the participant to do each new set of variations together the first time. This allows the instructor to know that the exercise is really effective, to see that it is within the capabilities of the exerciser and to check the exerciser for correct positioning and possible jerking into or through a position because of lack of strength. Any exercise causing discomfort the first time it is done may mean that a slight change at this time will prevent more discomfort, maybe even pain, when done without supervision. In some patients, some pain is inevitable, but the rewards of successfully gaining ground and progressive movement should more than compensate for the discomfort. Small successes in number of repetitions must be praised and hope constantly given. Pain sometimes must be a part of recovery, but if there is a way to prevent it without stopping the progression from step to step, that way should be taken.

The doctor prescribes the number of exercises he thinks wise for each patient according to his condition. Any week's exercise can be repeated if necessary, but this is generally not beneficial. The person so treated feels he is being "left back" and tends to get discouraged. It is better to add a slight variation which covers the same ground rather than to repeat the same exercises (Fig. 1).

The progressions can be accomplished in many ways. For example, a few seconds of work in the morning with several hours rest afterwards usually will allow one to repeat those exercises in the afternoon, or to exercise some other part of the body. To do twice as much at one time may only discourage older people, making them ache or tiring them. It not only will be unsuccessful and produce a pattern of failure but also cause the individual to become more dependent on the instructor as the goader to push him into exercises against his wishes and feelings.

Charting Progress

An exercise progress chart, like the sample one in this chapter (Fig. 2), is helpful to motivate the elderly client to continue. Show the person how to make out the chart from the beginning (Fig. 3). Make him responsible for filling it in. The satisfactions gained when he is finally able to sneak a few privately done repetitions into the chart belong to both of you. In the final analysis, if you do not succeed in making him feel and be responsible for his own improvement in movement, you have gained nothing and neither has he. If it takes constant attendance from a second party to keep one moving, it's not going to be of lasting benefit. It is therefore of primary importance from the beginning of the exercise program to give the person the responsibility for his own life and his own body. You show him the route, applaud as he starts in the right direction, but let him do the driving. In patients where new learning at almost every level is gone, then and only then should improvement depend on another person.

This chart, preferably begun in the hospital with the cooperation of the doctor, will give each person the responsibility for his own progress and success. The trainee learns quickly from a nurse or aide how to check off the chart. This is also the time to talk over the exercises with him if he can't read. Illustrations help, too (see Chap. 23).

The patient's complete written record on the back is useful so that nothing is ever forgotten or misunderstood. With the complete record at hand, the doctor can

Instructions For the Homebound Exercise Program

DOCTOR'S NOTE TO PATIENT

You may exercise every _____ hours for _____ minutes. On the first day, you may do each exercise _____ times each exercise period. Each day do _____ more of each exercise each exercise break.

DO NOT MOVE FASTER THAN THE CHART ALLOWS. CALL YOUR DOCTOR IF YOU GET DIZZY, SHORT OF BREATH, OR HAVE ACHES OR PAINS.

Always put your name and the date and note on the back of every single chart if there's a special problem.

Keep the chart in whatever spot you can arrange to spend the most time. Fill in the chart as you complete each exercise.

If you're in good condition, do the exercise(s) that you can do comfortably once the first day, twice the second day, three times the third day, and so on. When you find you can do 25 of any one exercise, cautiously, move on to the next more difficult version of the exercise.

If you're in poor shape, or have a progressive disease, start with very few exercises and build up; don't do them too often. Do one exercise once a day for the whole first week, if only that much feels comfortable. During the whole second week do one exercise in the morning and do it once again in the evening. Add as slowly as you need to prevent any relapses. Never overdo! Exhaustion can lead to relapses. Increase the number of exercises gradually. Keep your doctor up-to-date with your progress and call him if you have any unusual symptoms.

If you miss one exercise period, "do not try to make it up by doing twice as much the next period. Continue as if you had not missed, or even slow down a little."

Check off each exercise period when completed for the doctor's information!

Leave an hour for rest after each meal, then continue. Suggest breakfast be eaten at 8:00 to 9:00 and begin exercises at 10:00. Lunch between noon and 1:00 and begin exercises again at 2:00.

Any person who does not take the responsibility for moving his own body is not going to do much more than move from one condition to another for the rest of his life. Putting oneself in the doctor's hands for a medical condition is all very well, but a doctor cannot save or prolong one's life unless one helps in recovery efforts.

Fig. 1. The exercise prescription and instructions.

EXERCISE	MONDAY	TUESDAY	WEDNESDAY	THURSDAY	FRIDAY	SATURDAY	SUNDAY
			(time of day) (number of times exercise is done)				

Fig. 2. Front sheet of exercise progress chart.

HOW TO KEEP THE EXERCISE CHART

Keep track of the times you exercise or the time you spend in position on the chart.

The far-left square is for the sketch or description of one specific exercise or position. The rest of the squares across the top of the sheet are for you to fill in the numbers you do that exercise each day......for a whole week.

You may want to write in the number of times you did the exercise in one day:

| 5 times |
| 4 times |
| 6 times |

— or the amount of time you spent doing the exercise in one day:

| 5 minutes |
| 15 minutes |
| 10 minutes |

— or the actual time you began and finished the exercise in one day:

| 8 - 8:15 AM |
| 12 - 12:05 PM |
| 6 - 6:30 PM |

Use the method that is easiest for you. MAKE SURE TO FILL IN THE INFORMATION FOR EACH TIME YOU EXERCISE......EACH DAY!!

NAME _____

ADDRESS (If this is the first visit)

_____

PHONE NUMBER _____

DATE

Fig. 3. Instructions for using the exercise chart.

(BACK OF CHART)

WANT SUGGESTIONS? SEND COMPLETE   (DOCTOR'S NAME-ADDRESS-
SYMPTOMS AND CHART TO: TELEPHONE NUMBER)

NAME: _____

ADDRESS: _____ ZIP _____

TELEPHONE: _____

PROBLEM: _____

DAILY RECORDING OF PROBLEMS, SYMPTOMS, PROGRESS, ACCIDENTS, ETC.
(Please be as complete as possible. This is the only way to see clearly how you are doing.)

DOCTORS NEED INFORMATION

Too often all troubles seem to disappear in a cloud of confusion just as we get to see the doctor.

You can help your doctor help you by giving him all the symptoms by which to judge what is wrong with you, every clue possible from which he can get a better idea!

> What part of you is bothered?
> Where?
> When did it start?
> When does it happen?
> How often?
> More often now than before?
> Mostly when you're in one position?
> Which position?
> Does the part look different to you?
> How?
> What kind of discomfort do you have?
> For how long?
> Does anything else tend to happen at the same time?
> For how long?
> How does it affect youu?
> What have you been doing for it?
> For how long?

Nothing is embarrassing to a doctor except a wrong diagnosis. Give him all the information he needs by writing it down ahead of time over a week or two unless your problem is more urgent. Certainly take enough time to write all the information down completely and clearly so that nothing is missed.

If your handwriting is poor, print or have a friend write it down for you.

Fig. 4. Back of exercise progress chart.

decide the importance of noted events. The top of the chart back supplies the nervous patient with an emergency number and his doctor's name if he gets rattled when faced with strange symptoms (Fig. 4).

The exercise program discussion covers a small sample of what every individual is capable of achieving at home with very little outside support. All the exercise material and much more have been sent out as supplementary sheets to the 53 public television shows "The Beautiful Machine" that TV station WGBH in Boston has distributed across the country. All this material was provided free for six years to anyone requesting it but rising costs have forced us to charge a small fee. Locally, we have sent out close to 10,000 sheets a year.

Letters of request for help with problems more extreme than those presented on the show were so common that I developed additional material, working with more disabled people. With such individuals, the easiest possible progression from one step to the next was carefully worked out to prevent injury, to be as foolproof as I could make them and extremely easy to understand.

Although the odds are against such phenomenal luck, as far as I know not one person has suffered injury or ill effects from the practice of these exercises. Part of this result, of course, stems from the fact that I try to get each individual not only to send me all symptoms, but also to have the exercise sheets I send approved by their doctors before they begin. Proper precautions are considered before the movements are designed and prevailing medical conditions and the time to be spent exercising are all taken into consideration.

The letters I received also lead me to suggest to people who write in that they consult neurologists, orthopedists, internists, and other doctors. The mail is staggering and the programs continue because of their success with the public at home watching and exercising with television.

CONCLUSION

Television can be a positive tool for better dissemination and use of health information of self-help, exercise and fitness after 50. There is almost no limit to what national television programs on preventive medicine and health can do for improving fitness after 50.

Section IV

Practical Exercise and Relaxation Programs

Principles of Exercise for Musculoskeletal Reconditioning and Fitness

Hans Kraus, M.D.

INTRODUCTION

The major part of our population lives under considerable stress and strain without an opportunity for physical outlet, let alone sufficient physical exercise. As a result, many people are generally underexercised and tense, especially the group that seeks a remedy in physical exercise. Current interest in such physical fitness has resulted in ever-increasing numbers of exercise groups and classes as well as numerous books about fitness and fitness exercises. Unfortunately, in most of these presentations, some basic principles of exercise are often neglected to the detriment of the exercise participant.

It is therefore important and worthwhile to outline these principles in this chapter and especially to appraise the minimum muscular fitness of participants in exercise programs.

KRAUS-WEBER MUSCLE TESTS

Test 1

This maneuver tests hip-flexing and abdominal muscles. The subject lies flat on his back with hands behind his neck and legs extended. The feet may be held down by the examiner or by a heavy object which will not move. The examiner directs the subject to: "Keep your hands behind your neck and roll up to a sitting position" (Fig. 1).

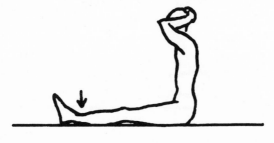

Test 2

This maneuver tests abdominal muscles. The participant lies flat on his back, with hands behind neck and knees bent. The examiner holds the patient's feet down on the table or floor; or a heavy object may be used to do this. The examiner directs the patient to: "Keep your hands behind your neck and roll up to a sitting position" (Fig. 2).

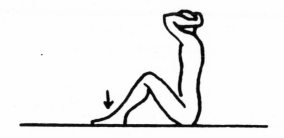

Test 3

This maneuver tests hip-flexing muscles. The participant lies supinely on his back with hands behind his neck and legs extended. The examiner directs the patient to: "Keep your knees straight and lift your feet ten inches off the floor or table and hold that position for ten seconds" (Fig. 3).

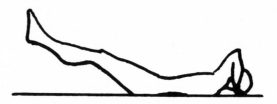

Test 4

This maneuver tests the upper back muscles. The participant is instructed to lie prone on his stomach with pillow under the abdomen and hands behind his neck. The examiner holds the patient's feet and hips on the table or floor and directs the participant to: "Raise your trunk and hold that position for ten seconds" (Fig. 4).

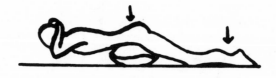

Test 5

This maneuver tests the muscles of the lower back. The participant is instructed to assume the same position as in Test 4, but this time the examiner holds the patient's shoulders and hips down on the table or floor. The examiner directs the participant to: "Lift your legs and hold that position for ten seconds" (Fig. 5).

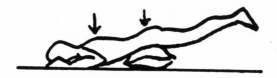

Test 6

This maneuver tests muscle tension or flexibility. The participant is directed to stand erect in stockings or bare feet with knees stiff and hands at sides. The examiner directs the participant to: "Put your feet together, keeping the knees straight. Bend slowly and see how close you can come to touching the floor with your fingertips. If you cannot perform this the first time, try it again. Relax, drop your head forward and try to let your torso 'hang' from your hips while keeping your knees stiff" (Fig. 6).

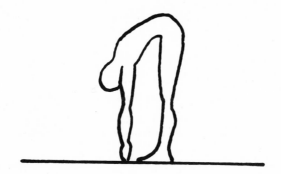

Interpretation of Basic Muscle Tests

Most people will pass the minimum muscular fitness test for strength of back muscles because these muscles are usually active as we sit. However, a certain number will fail the test for abdominal strength or hip flexor strength and will need special strengthening exercises for these muscle groups (Kraus, 1963, 1965). If a patient fails one or more of these tests, he should go through a gradual reconditioning period before he advances to aerobic work demanding an effort he cannot perform without exposure to muscle strain and sprains. Such strains and sprains are a frequent cause for drop-outs from fitness programs.

We can gauge the muscle stiffness of the patient by his lack of ability to complete the floor touch test (Fig. 6). If we ask a patient to "let go" instead of trying hard to reach the floor, we often see that he can reach down further than when he strains to accomplish the test movement. The difference between relaxed movement and un-relaxed movement provides a gauge of the patient's muscle tension. However, quite often tension is concentrated in neck and shoulder girdle muscles. Then the neck motion or ability to raise the arms completely to 170° or 180° helps to evaluate stiffness and relative tension in that area (Kraus, 1970).

THE EXERCISE SESSION

Relaxation

The exercise session should always start with a relaxation period which includes lying on the floor with the knees flexed, inhaling deeply and exhaling slowly, shrug-ging and relaxing shoulders and relaxing and limbering the legs. Depending on the individual's tension, this period should last from five to 10-15 minutes.

Warm-up

A warm-up period should follow and prepare the person for more demanding activ-ity. The warm-up period, initially started with the participant on the floor, should include exercises such as rolling over on the floor, simple flexion-extension of the knees and hips, lying on the back and lying on the side, hand-knee position and arching the back (catback), and lying on the back and bringing both flexed knees up to the chest. Some gentle stretching exercises for the hamstrings should follow, such as flexion-extension of knees and hips or straight-leg raise. Sit-ups with the hands behind the neck should precede the standing stretching period. If the patient is not able to perform this movement, he should do it with his hands at the side or, to start with, only bringing up the head and shoulder without a full sit-up. Sitting on a bench and bending forward to the middle and both sides is another excellent back limber-ing exercise. Only after completing these lying exercises should the subject stand up and start standing stretches of calf muscles and hamstrings and finally attempt gently to reach towards the floor.

Aerobic Work

Once all this is done, the person is finally ready for aerobic work. The most feasible aerobic work is jogging which should be preceded by a short walk and concluded with a period of walking. Depending on the ability of the group, the jogging period may later increase in speed and duration. In some instances, weight lifting can be added to develop strength, preferably starting with light weights, gradually proceeding to heavier ones and then returning to light ones as cool-off. A few repetitions of any one lift is preferable to the usual "10 reps". Changing to different forms of lift after three or four repetitions helps avoid muscle stiffness.

Cool-Off

Experience shows that if a muscle is left at the peak of exertion without cool-off, muscle stiffness very frequently results. Exercise lessons should therefore be a build-up from relaxation, proceeding to warm-up, culminating in workout, returning to cool-off, and finally winding up with relaxation.

To avoid muscle tension and stiffness, multi-repetition and speed exercises must be avoided. They have no place in a conditioning class, especially not at the beginning and should be reserved for well-conditioned young people who work for upper levels of fitness. With advancing age, the relaxation, warm-up and cool-off periods will have to increase in length. The workout will have to be on a lower level of effort and last longer to be effective. There is no such thing as a 10 minute fitness program.

We usually let our subjects repeat the exercises two to four times at most and keep changing from prone and supine position in the warm-up period to avoid muscle stiffness.

CONCLUSION

If the outlined proper exercise procedure is followed, the people will usually leave their exercise periods with a pleasant, relaxed and warm feeling in a state of well-being rather than stiffness and strain. They will return for more exercise not only because it is "good for them," but because they wish to experience again the pleasant feeling of well-being — the result of a properly conducted and paced fitness class.

REFERENCES

Kraus, H. (1963) *Therapeutic Exercise,* Charles C Thomas, Publisher, Springfield, Ill.
Kraus, H. (1965) *Backache, Stress and Tension*, Simon & Schuster, Inc., New York.
Kraus, H. (1970) *Clinical Treatment of Back and Neck Pain*, McGraw-Hill Book Company, New York.

Conditioning Exercise Programs for Normal Older Persons

Robert E. Wear

INTRODUCTION

Men and women of all ages should be able to attain and maintain a vitality for living by proper health care, regular medical checkups, concern about adequate and proper nutrition, sufficient rest and relaxation, and a regular regimen of challenging physical activity.

Dynamic health is the ability to move vitally, participate vigorously and be energetic and active. Most people, however, suffer from chronic disabilities (Cureton, 1965) or, as described by Kraus and Raab (1961), hypokinetic diseases brought about by insufficient exercise. After the middle years, a sedentary way of life may increase cardiovascular problems and heart disease (Fox and Skinner, 1964), and cause high blood pressure, low back pain and hypotonic abdominal musculature with poor posture, rearranged body weight and composition (Brozek, 1952), decline in muscular strength and endurance (Asmussen and Heeboll-Nielsen, 1962), and stiffening joints accompanied by degenerative changes and decreased range of motion (Chapman, deVries and Swezey, 1972; Wright and Johns, 1961).

Many signs and symptoms of the aging process represent a decrement in general health and it is important to test the correlation between psychological and physical effects of exercise against the indices of reduced functionality related to aging. This chapter reviews evidence supporting a positive correlation between exercise training and retarded age-related dysfunction, and suggests some practical exercise regimens that help maintain good physical health.

The search for conditioning programs that retard physiological aging (Karvonen, 1961; Bortz, 1960) and inactivity has been in progress for many years. One of the foremost researchers, Dr. deVries and his staff, working with retirees at the Leisure World Retirement Center in Laguna Hills, California (deVries, 1970; Adams and deVries, 1973), found that for men, ages 52 to 88, and women, ages 52 to 79, carefully conducted exercise training regimens improved general physical fitness.

Improvements in oxygen transport capacity of the body, vital capacity and systolic and diastolic blood pressure were noted in the older men after six, 18, and 42 weeks of vigorous conditioning. Likewise, after three months of graduated physical activity, the women showed improved physical work capacity and lowered resting heart rate.

PRINCIPLES FOR FITNESS PROGRAMING

My experiences with adult fitness programs at the University of New Hampshire and research studies at the University of Southern California have led me to make the following observations on planning and implementing physical activities for older men and women.

The participant must get a thorough physical examination, including some type of stress and performance tests to evaluate physiological status under maximal or submaximal work loads. If sanctioned by the referring doctor and the exercise leader, the participant may be given individualized exercise prescriptions to follow independently. Exercise workouts should be performed at graduated stages of intensity and regular intervals throughout the entire experience. Finally, the participant should be periodically reevaluated so that a new prescription for physical activity can be made to provide an individualized, gradual and judicious increase in the work load. Supervision is always important, but it is an especially salient factor in the early stages of one's exercise experience. Overenthusiasm and misdirected strenuousness of competition must be minimized to prevent discomfort and possible temporary or permanent injury.

The adult physical fitness director must remember that he is not a doctor but only a "paramedic" with extensive training and qualifications in physical education, physical therapy and/or adult fitness. His part in the program is concerned with the health and safety of his participants and must be conducted with medical cooperation, guidance and approval.

The Medical Evaluation

The medical evaluation of the participant by a qualified and interested physician is the first step on the road to dynamic fitness (Kasch and Boyer, 1968). Its primary purpose is to avoid future injury or illness of the participant when subjected to intense stress and reduce the liability of the exercise leader for not taking all proper precautions. Exercise is not without hazards when the body is not fit enough to take it. Only a qualified doctor can determine whether an older person can safely embark on such a conditioning program.

Medical forms providing information about any illnesses, weaknesses and restrictions relevant to the proposed intensity of the activity program should be completed. The examination itself should include a complete history and physical evaluation that identifies any orthopedic problems and rules out infections. Resting and stress electrocardiograms (a continuous monitoring of pulse, blood pressure and ECG during graded exercise on treadmill, step test or bicycle) may be obtained from local medical facilities or, under certain circumstances, may be performed by qualified clinical personnel under medical supervision (Kannel, 1972). Other data such as chest x-ray, serum cholesterol, blood lipids, triglycerides, urinalysis and tests of pulmonary function (maximum breathing capacity and timed vital capacity) are desirable so that the physician and the fitness director have a clearer picture of the individual's fitness status and capability.

Baseline Evaluations

Baseline evaluations include anthropometric measures, body fat percentage analysis and the assessment of muscle strength, endurance and joint flexibility. Some type of stress testing of work capacity is a further step for assuring the safety and security of the prospective participant. With older adults, submaximal stress tests are preferable, utilizing either the work bicycle, treadmill or the step test (deVries, 1974) if not previously performed in the doctor's office. These evaluations help determine the ability of the heart and circulatory system to respond to precise work loads for a given period of time. From these data, the individual's maximum oxygen consumption can be predicted and he can be classified as to fitness levels according to age and weight by internationally accepted norms (Åstrand and Rhyming, 1954). Individualized exercise programs regulating the intensity, duration and recovery from activity can then be prescribed.

In stress testing, it is imperative to begin with a light work load and progress only to submaximal levels to avoid overexerting an unconditioned individual. Maximal stress loading and overwork is unnecessary, potentially dangerous and may discourage the person being tested. Judgment is necessary to determine an appropriate level of exertion required of each participant, particularly one who has had long periods of relative inactivity (Fig. 1).

Work capacity tests and baseline evaluations let the participant know how he compares to the normal population and are thus a valuable counseling and motivational tool when they act as a measure of progress and change resulting from the exercise program (Golding, 1972). This type of testing should be repeated at regular intervals, preferably every three to six months.

An excellent physical fitness testing and conditioning format for the novice as well as the experienced physical fitness director has been published by the National Council YMCA (Myers, Golding and Sinning, 1973). It presents sound evaluative and administrative procedures and norms (for middle-aged males) that are economical in time, easily comprehended and simple to use.

EXERCISE CONDITIONING PROGRAMS

Goals and Outcomes

The primary objective of a soundly conceived, adult fitness program is to improve the physical capacity, vigor and energy reserves of the participants. Physical deterioration is prevented by strengthening muscle and ligament systems through flexibility and stamina exercises. Short-windedness, fast heart rates and early fatigue noted during beginning workouts are signs of ineffective cardiovascular fitness and are often dramatically reversed by timed fast and slow walk or jog-walk interval training and pulse rate monitoring. Finally, emotional and neuromuscular tensions

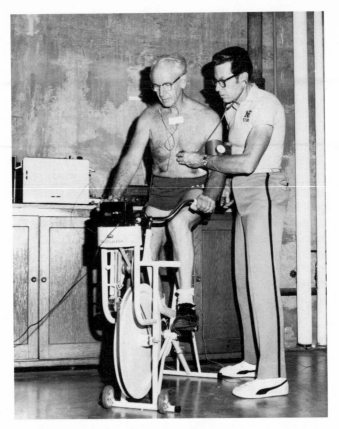

Fig. 1. Stress testing.

are usually counteracted through specific relaxation and stretching techniques (Jacobson, 1956).

The following general conditioning program is for adults who have been medically screened and stress tested as "fit to be fit." It is designed to improve their muscle and joint flexibility, muscle tone, cardiovascular function and vitality and emotional well-being. Specific exercises and conditioning routines are selected to enhance strength, endurance, circulatory and respiratory development and to stretch muscles and connective tissue for relaxation and relief of soreness.

The University of New Hampshire adult fitness programs for both men and women consist of a one-hour session three times a week over a three-month period. Class sessions include a 20-minute period of rhythmic calisthenic activities with stress upon flexibility and muscular endurance, 20 minutes of aerobic (with oxygen) endurance activity and a 10-minute cooling down period of static stretching and progressive relaxation. Occasionally the class will report to the swimming pool for an hour of water exercises, low intensity gutter drills, bobbing, sculling, easy lap swimming and informal games.

Rhythmic Flexibility and Endurance Training

Purpose

The rhythmic flexibility exercises are primarily designed to improve muscle tone and durability and to increase gradually the range of motion around body joints. Indirectly, they seem to promote better posture, alignment, balance and coordination.

Movement and Low Intensity

One secret of success in conducting calisthenics is to keep exercises simple, varied and fun, and the participants moving in continuous series of sequences. The intensity and the amount of work performed (the number of repetitions of an exercise per unit time) should start at a low level — as few as three to five repetitions — and gradually increase over a three-month period up to 10 repetitions during any exercise period.

The Warm-up

The first 5 or 10 minutes are spent in a graduated warm-up period of walking to music with a beat, slow-paced jogging and walking intervals combined with arm swinging, body bending and trunk rotation maneuvers.

Exercise Patterning

The warm-up session is followed by 15 minutes of slow easy stretching, pulling and swinging action. Rhythmic movement of muscles progresses from joint to joint and from head to foot. To avoid local fatigue, the exercise progression should include no more than one series of movements at a joint at a time. Joint areas to be exercised are the neck, arms and shoulders, trunk and lower spine, hip and thighs, knees, ankles and feet. No specific joint order is mandatory as long as the same area is not subjected to more than one pattern of activity at a time.

To induce greater stretchability and relaxation and to improve flexibility, rhythmic and slow tempoed activity that fully flexes and extends the joints through a full range of motion should be emphasized.

Avoid Arm Support and Isometrics

During the first few months, arm support exercises such as pull-ups, push-ups and bar hanging should be avoided to prevent overtaxing underdeveloped muscles and joints of the upper torso in poorly conditioned adults. Likewise, isometrics, where muscles are pitted against muscles or are contracted against an immovable object, need to be eliminated. Isometric contractions generally cause muscles to compress the arteries and prevent a free flow of blood through muscle tissues (deVries, 1974). Muscles need all the blood and oxygen they can get and blood flow is facilitated by rhythmic rather than static contractions during activity (Royce, 1958).

Work the Legs

During early training, greater emphasis should be given to increasing the strength, endurance and circulation of the legs in preference to that of the arms and shoulders. The upper body is generally weak and flaccid due to disuse and atrophy in many inactive adults. Furthermore, the massaging action of the leg muscles acting as a "muscle pump" upon the veins of the leg and thigh during strenuous activity promotes the pushing of venous blood flow to the right side of the heart.

Change Body Positions

The constant change of various body positions during the rhythmic activity period also contributes to gravitation forces acting upon the circulatory system and to relief from muscle tension (Kasch and Boyer, 1968). These "teeter-totter" movements might include such progressions as proceeding from a standing to a prone position, back to side reclining, legs high in the air in a shoulder support to a front lying attitude, and then back to a standing position.

Strength and Stamina Training

This preliminary period of flexibility training of the musculoskeletal system should gradually incorporate more strength and endurance components. Greater durability is achieved using the overload principle for movements that are moderately resistant to muscular contractions. The pace of the exercise might at times be increased. Strength and stamina of the muscles of the abdomen, arms and shoulders, and thighs and lower legs can be increased by raising the body weight against gravity at modified and graduated stress intensity levels.

Counteract Gravitational Forces

It is especially important to incorporate activities that strengthen the "antigravity" muscle portions of the body — the hip and lower trunk, knees and ankles (Wallis and Logan, 1964). Special muscle groups prevent these areas from collapsing and falling forward through the force of gravity and the weight of the upper body superstructure (head, thorax, shoulders and arms — all attached to the spinal column). Exercise routines should overload the following muscles of support: the sacrospinalis, which extends the back from the head to the sacrum; the abdominals on the anterior trunk acting as counter balance flexors; the gluteus maximus which extends the posterior hip; the four-headed quadriceps on the anterior thigh which extends the knee; and, last but not least, the gastrocnemius and soleus forming the calf of the leg, whose pull upon the tendon of Achilles lifts the heel and raises the foot at the ankle.

Swing Free and Do Your Own Thing

Older participants, especially, should avoid exercises that fix and stiffen joints (trying to touch the toes with locked knees) or increasing the flexibility of the lower back by performing jerking and bouncing movements against stiff-legged resistance. These movements may inflict undue strain upon ligaments, muscles and tendons, and result in cramping and soreness. Participants should be encouraged to "swing free", to bend their knees, flex hips, rotate at the trunk, and to swing arms in a natural and comfortable style. Exercise is more fun and enjoyable when individuals are permitted to activate at their own tempo and within their own limitations (Hornbaker, 1974). They need not keep up with other members of the class.

Keep Routines Progressive and Varied

Finally, the exercise leader should have in mind a general progressive routine that enables exercise sequences to move easily from one movement to another without loss of time or continuity. Much local fatigue can be avoided by creating a high overall activity level in smoothly shifting loads of work from one muscle group to another with few repetitions and then returning to the same joints with new movements.

There are no scientific exercise routines that produce unusual or special results. The choice of exercises and movement sequences is unlimited. Many excellent source books on the market provide a wide variability of selection (Royal Canadian Air Force Pamphlet, 1962; Kasch and Boyer, 1968; Cureton, 1965; President's Council on Physical Fitness and Sports, 1965, 1968 and 1973; Myers, Golding and Sinning, 1973; Swengros and Monteleone, 1971). The movements selected for older participants should be simple, easily comprehended, uncomplicated and graduated in stress intensity. They should permit freedom and enjoyment of individualized movement.

Cardiovascular-Respiratory Endurance Training

The cardiovascular-respiratory aerobic activity sessions range from 10 to 20 minutes for the beginning participant which the seasoned jogger may extend to 30 minutes or longer. Early workouts involve two to five minutes of warm-up after the flexibility exercises, 15 to 20 minutes of fast and slow walking or job-walking intervals, and a five-minute tapering off (cooling-down) period.

Purpose

The purpose of these activities is to improve the efficiency and capacity of cardio-respiratory functioning through a gradual increase in the amount of work performed by the body per unit time. Progress is made in easy stages through the use of interval training (Fox et al., 1973; Fox and Matthews, 1974) and the overload principle. In this way, performance is improved by increasing the amount of exercise (work load) to be accomplished, by intensifying the pace at which it is performed or by a combination of both.

The body, unlike a machine, follows the law of use and disuse — that is, energy initiates energy and inactivity leads to deterioration (Bortz, 1960). Physical capacity is developed only by the expenditure of energy that imposes stresses upon the system. In turn, the body specifically adapts to these stresses, permitting more effective performance of muscular tasks (Wallis and Logan, 1964). Unfortunately, this adaptation is reversible and the less one does, the less one can do. Wallis and Logan (1964) have developed the SAID Principle (Specific Adaptation to Imposed Demands) to explain how man can best achieve physical improvements. To receive the greatest fitness with the least amount of time and effort, one must impose specific muscular demands or stresses to achieve those adaptations (see Appendix A).

The Warm-up

The warm-up period for the endurance training portion is a continuation of the musculoskeletal flexibility activity session or a progression of alternate slow and fast walking intervals that increase the pulse rate and breathing and elevate the body temperature. The monotony of walking can be alleviated by including short intervals of backward stepping with high knee action and vigorous swinging of the arms. Other variations include side to side step hopping, "grape-vine twist" foot movements, slow skipping, fast heel-and-toe stepping and the high arm swinging action of "Australian" marching. These modifications must be used with caution as fast or unaccustomed movements can raise the pulse rate drastically and may overstress the poorly conditioned participant.

Choice of Conditioning Programs

During the first three months of conditioning, the older participant should follow one of three types of program: (1) a modified walking regimen, (2) an interval fast-walk and slow-walk routine or (3) job and walk interval intensities. Selection is based upon the evaluation of the medical and fitness profiles and upon collaboration between the instructor and the consulting physician (South Carolina Heart Association, 1969).

The Modified Walking Program

Those men and women who are greatly overweight, underexercised or have orthopedic, muscle-joint problems should begin with moderate exercises such as the Preventive Care Program (Hornbaker, 1974), swimming, bicycling or a modified walking regimen as outlined in Table 1.

TABLE 1

MODIFIED WALKING PROGRAM FOR ADULT FITNESS

Level I Mile Walk Program:

Pace: 1/4 mile in 5 minutes.
      1 mile in 20 minutes.

Level II Mile Walk Program:

Pace: 1/4 mile in 4 minutes.
      1 mile in 16 minutes.

Exercise Period*	Miles	Minutes	Exercise Period*	Miles	Minutes
1	1	20	1	1	16
2	1 1/4	25	2	1 1/4	20
3	1 1/2	30	3	1 1/2	24
4	1 3/4	35	4	1 3/4	28
5	2	40	5	2	32
6	2 1/4	45	6	2 1/4	36
7	2 1/2	50	7	2 1/2	40
8	2 3/4	55	8	2 3/4	44
9	3	60	9	3	48

Level III Mile Walk Program:

Pace: 1/4 mile in 3 1/2 minutes.
        1 mile in 14 minutes.

Exercise Period*	Miles	Minutes
1	1	14
2	1 1/4	17 1/2
3	1 1/2	21
4	1 3/4	24 1/2
5	2	28
6	2 1/4	31 1/2
7	2 1/2	35
8	2 3/4	38 1/2
9	3	42
10	3 1/4	45 1/2
11	3 1/2	49
12	3 3/4	52 1/2
13	4	56

Directions:

1. Warm up with slow and easy walking. Do rhythmic loosening up exercises.

2. Stride out the designated distance at the suggested time schedule.

3. Stop and monitor your pulse rate at the beginning, half-way point and end of workout for 10 seconds.

4. Keep your pace to approx. 120 heart rate level per minute (20 monitored beats in a 10 second period).

5. Definitely keep your pulse rate below 132 beats per minute (22 in 10 seconds). Never surpass twice your normal beating heart rate!

6. Slow down your pace or stop and rest when winded, fatigued or pulse rate is too rapid.

*7. Increase the distance walked a 1/4 mile each exercise period in the recommended time only if your monitored heart rate and body fatigue warrant the change. Otherwise, stay at the same intensity level.

8. Keep a careful daily record of your accomplishments on the *Walking Fitness Progress Chart.*

9. Additional distances may be added if advisable.

Enthusiastic fitness aspirants should not undertake three miles of walking in one hour the first day unless accustomed to that distance and intensity.

If the heart rate remains at the proper level and there is no excessive fatigue, the distance walked should be increased a quarter mile each following exercise period until the three miles can be achieved comfortably in one hour. Once Level I is mastered, Level II is undertaken by walking faster graduated quarter-mile intervals, eventually leading to a mile in 16 minutes and three miles in 48 minutes. This procedure is repeated through Level III where the participant steps up his pace to achieve a mile in 14 minutes (sometimes called the Boy Scout pace). The ability to walk four miles in less than one hour is a notable achievement for many individuals.

To obtain pulse rates for all walking and jogging programs the heart beat is monitored for 10 seconds at the carotid or radial artery and multiplied by six to determine the intensity of the work just experienced. A Monthly Walking Fitness Progress Chart (Table 2) permits daily charting of progress in distance walked, pace, total walking time and weight gain or loss.

Rule for Endurance Intensity Training

The guiding rule for endurance intensity training is to stress the body gradually. It is imperative to slow down or stop and rest when one is winded, fatigued or has a monitored pulse rate that is too rapid. In this way, the strength and endurance of

TABLE 2

MONTH										
Date	Walk Dist.	Pace	Total Time	Wt. Lbs.	Walk Dist.	Pace	Total Time	Wt. Lbs.	REMARKS
1									
2									
3									
4									
5									
6									
7									
8									
9									
10									
11									
12									
13									
14									
15									
Total Miles									

WALKING FITNESS PROGRESS CHART

muscles and joints are improved and soreness, stiffness and overfatigue are prevented. Many years of inactivity cause short windedness and abdominal softness. At least several months of intensified exercise are necessary to restore higher levels of fitness. The older participant still has years of more vigorous living ahead of him if he patiently allows his body to gradually adapt to increasing loads of work.

The Adult Fast and Slow Walk Fitness Program

The Fast and Slow Walk Fitness program (Table 3) is a more intense training for the poorly conditioned participant. Pulse rate monitoring is done at regular intervals by each individual during the 15- to 20-minute workout. The participant is instructed not to exceed his estimated age maximum heart rate (calculated by subtracting one's age from 220), a reference point which should be lowered by 15 or 20 beats during early months of training. In the sedentary individual, the heart rate should range between 110 to 120 beats per minute (the training heart rate) to avoid overstressing. As conditioning improves, the participant may move up to the

120 to 130 beat level, or 70 percent of his modified estimated maximum heart rate. higher ranges of heart rate (130 to 140 beats per minute) are reserved for the better conditioned walker or jogger.

An average resting heart rate should be taken several times at different intervals during the week with the subject in a sitting or reclining relaxed position prior to eating, drinking and smoking. The resting rate is a good reference point to evaluate before the workout and end point to approach at the completion of the exercise period. Monitored pulse beats should return to within 10 to 15 beats of the starting level at the end of the cooling off period (see Appendix A). Failure to return to this starting rate suggests overloading and the level of training should be reduced.

TABLE 3

ADULT FAST AND SLOW WALKING FITNESS PROGRAM

Name _____ Address _____
Age Maximum Heart Rate _____ Training Heart Rate _____
Average Resting Heart Rate _____ Body Weight _____ lbs.

DATE			
PRESCRIPTION			
H.R. 2ND MIN.			
H.R. 8TH MIN.			
H.R. 15TH MIN.			

Exercise Prescription for Fast and Slow Walk Program

Intensity Level	Minutes		Intensity Level	Minutes	
Special	Fast Walk 1/4	Walk 1	E.	Fast Walk 1 1/2	Walk 1/4
A.	Fast Walk 1/2	Walk 1	F.	Fast Walk 1 3/4	Walk 1/4
B.	Fast Walk 3/4	Walk 3/4	G.	Fast Walk 2	Walk 1/4
C.	Fast Walk 1	Walk 1/2	H.	Fast Walk 2-20	Walk 1/4
D.	Fast Walk 1 1/4	Walk 1/4			

Total time of interval training workout: 15-20 minutes. Cooling-off period: Minimum of 5 minutes. Slow walk. Easy rhythmic exercises and static stretching.

The Adult Jog-Walk Fitness Program

The Adult Jog-Walk Fitness Program (Table 4) is similar to the progressive pattern of the fast and slow walk procedure. However, the increased intensity of jogging will raise the heart rate index to levels above those of the walking program. The pulse rate should be kept within five or eight beats per minute of the training rate during the first three months of conditioning. Based upon medical and stress testing evaluations, the training rate is now a predetermined 70 to 75 percent of the subject's estimated maximum heart rate during this early training period. For all participants 40 to 60 years of age, heart rates should be kept below 140 beats per minute. Thereafter, the pulse rate level is maintained for better conditioned participants under 150. This restriction follows the Age-Target Heart Rate Scale proposed by the Scandinavian Committee on ECG Classification (1967) and the guidelines of the Committee on Exercise of the American Heart Association (1972) and the Tennessee Heart Association Physical Exercise Committee (1971).

TABLE 4

ADULT JOG-WALK FITNESS PROGRAM

Name _____   Address _____
Age Maximum Heart Rate _____   Training Heart Rate _____
Average Resting Heart Rate _____   Body Weight _____lbs.

| DATE |
| PRESCRIPTION |
| H.R. 2ND MIN. |
| H.R. 8TH MIN. |
| H.R. 15TH MIN. |

Exercise Prescriptions for Jog-Walking Program

Intensity Level		Minutes		Intensity Level		Minutes	
Special	Jog 1/4		Walk 1	E.	Jog 1 1/2		Walk 1/4
A.	Jog 1/2		Walk 1	F.	Jog 1 3/4		Walk 1/4
B.	Jog 3/4		Walk 3/4	G.	Jog 2		Walk 1/4
C.	Jog 1		Walk 1/2	H.	Jog 2-20		Walk 1/4
D.	Jog 1 1/4		Walk 1/4				

Total time of interval training workout: 15-20 minutes. Cooling off period: Minimum of 5 minutes. Slow walk. Easy rhythmic exercises and static stretching.

Exercise Intensity Control

In the fast and slow walk and jog-walk programs, each participant performs at his own comfortable pace level independent of other class members for prescribed time intervals. This is followed by leisurely walking. As the heart rate adapts to set stress loads of work intensity, as determined either by timed or distance durations, new stress levels are prescribed to keep the individual at a "training" and not a "maintaining" level of activity. Detailed instructions for both programs are presented in Table 5.

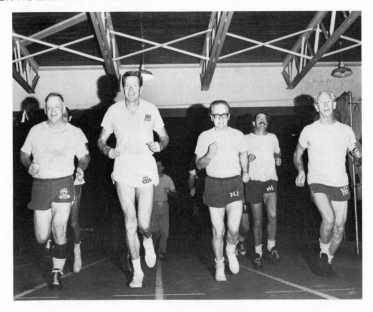

Fig. 2. Adult jog-walk.

TABLE 5

INSTRUCTIONS FOR THE ADULT FAST AND SLOW WALK
AND
ADULT JOG-WALK FITNESS PROGRAMS

1. Carefully monitor your pulse rate for 10 seconds immediately after jogging at approximately the second, eighth and 15th minute periods of your workout.

   a. Locate your pulse at the carotid artery of the neck (one inch below the jaw level) or at the radial artery on the thumb side of the lower wrist immediately after fast walking.

   b. Stop your movement and count your pulse beats for 10 seconds using a wrist or stop watch. Multiply this heart rate by six to determine your approximate heart rate for one minute at this intensity or work.

   c. Record this rate in the appropriate space on the chart.

2. Continue your fast and slow walking program for 15 to 20 minutes. Slow down your pace if your monitored pulse rate is above your *Training Heart Rate*.

3. Stop your workout and immediately contact your instructor if you have difficulty in breathing, chest tightness, dizziness or loss of coordination.

4. Progress to the next exercise intensity prescription level only when your recorded three pulse rates for a one day's workout are below your training level and with approval of your instructor.

5. Your workout has been too intensive if your pulse rate has not returned to 120 beats per minute or lower within three minutes following your last fast-walking session.

Three hours a week of rhythmic exercises, heart monitoring interval walking and/or jogging training, and cooling down periods seem to produce training changes in the unconditioned participant. Once a desirable level of fitness is attained, maintenance can be achieved in less frequent sessions of at least two per week on alternating days. However, exercise for dynamic health is a lifetime commitment since conditioning seems to deteriorate rapidly on return to sedentary habits.

Gauging Exercise Ability

The exercise leader must constantly warn participants to follow prescribed exercise dosages particularly at the early stages of training. The tendency is to go too fast and to be too competitive. Those who score in the lower levels of the preliminary stress tests should be required to participate only in walking, bicycling or swimming programs. Likewise, individuals with problems of obesity, hypertension or musculoskeletal weaknesses, and those showing adverse effects to regular exercise, such as breathing difficulties and high heart rate response, must be observed carefully and restricted in their activity. Any participant should be asked to temporarily interrupt the training program when an injury, infection or minor illness occurs that could be aggravated by exercise. "Working out" a cold or exercising when not feeling well is a poor policy. Likewise, those recovering from an illness should resume exercise at levels below pre-illness conditions (American Heart Association Committee on Exercise, 1972).

Warning Signs of Over-exertion

The instructor should also inform the participants about the warning signals of overexertion during their workouts. These include unusual fatigue during or after the activity period, persistent fatigue during the following day, persistent muscular aches and pains, and unusual restlessness during sleep or insomnia. Exercise at a markedly reduced level should then be prescribed until doses of activity can be handled effectively (Tennessee Heart Association Physical Exercise Committee, 1971). The heart rate following the completion of jog-walk interval exercise should return to 120 beats per minute or under within three minutes. Persistent higher rates may indicate that the participant has overworked and that following workouts must be curtailed.

Danger Signals for Stopping Exercise

Exercise must be stopped immediately and the participant referred to his doctor under the following conditions:

1. Fainting, light-headedness or dizziness.
2. Irregular heart rate.
3. Musculoskeletal problems aggravated by the exercise.
4. Nausea, vomiting or severe discomfort.
5. Any chest pain or pain referred to the arm, jaw, teeth or ear.
6. Loss of coordination.
7. Persistent fatigue.
8. Failure of the pulse to recover below the 140 level within five minutes after cessation of exercise (South Carolina Heart Association, 1969).

The Valsalva Maneuver

Exercise leaders should emphatically caution participants to avoid breath holding during rhythmic exercises and jogging sequences. Normal breathing or utilizing forced expiration during the contraction phase of each exercise movement is a basic rule. Regular respiration avoids the "Valsalva Effect" or "Maneuver" which increases intrathoracic pressure when the breath is held during heavy resistance exercise. Since increased intrathoracic pressure decreases venous return of the blood to the heart, resulting in lowered cardiac output, decreased stroke volume and decreased blood flow to the brain are noted with possible fainting or dizziness (Rosenblum and Delman, 1965).

The Cooling Down and Tapering Off Period

The cooling down and tapering off period, the third and final phase of any exercise program, permits the subject's heart rate, respiration and general metabolism to return gradually to preexercise level. The best activities for a good leveling off process are mild jogging, slow walking and light flexibility activities similar to those performed during the warm-up period. Rhythmic arm swinging and leg rotating exercises help to return the blood from the extremities to the heart. A most effective way to end the period is with five to 10 minutes of progressive relaxation techniques using the Jacobson method (Jacobson, 1956) or static stretching (deVries, 1962).

Static stretching, based upon Hatha Yoga techniques, is valuable for improving flexibility and muscle tone and is preferable to the bouncing, bobbing or jerky movements performed against stiffened or fixed joints. In the past, ballistic procedures have been considered the ideal technique for loosening up muscles and reducing tension. This is no longer true.

After intensive electromyographic evaluations in the physiology of exercise stress laboratory, deVries (1966) developed the following static stretching exercises. The technique is to place the body in nine different positions and to hold each position for one to two minutes at a time in an easy and quiet manner. This should be done several times a day to improve flexibility and facilitate the greatest possible stretch on muscles and related connective tissue. It is most effective in preventing and alleviating muscle soreness and fatigue and in achieving a full range of joint mobility in older subjects.

The nine static stretching positions are:

1. The upper trunk stretcher.
2. The lower trunk stretcher.
3. The upper back stretcher.
4. The upper and lower back stretcher.
5. The neck stretcher.
6. The trunk twister (Fig. 3).
7. The toe pointer.
8. The calf and shoulder stretcher.
9. The shoulder and biceps stretcher.

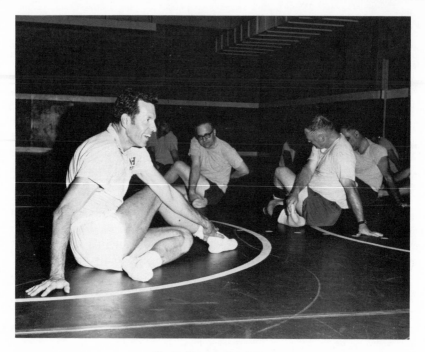

Fig. 3. The trunk twister.

These positions and the static stretching technique are thoroughly described and illustrated by deVries (1974).

CONCLUSION

The following practical ideas and techniques for implementing a conditioning program for older adult participants have been presented:

1. Older men and women can attain a greater vitality for living by taking care of themselves through proper medical evaluation, exercise and sound health practices.

2. Physical conditioning programs such as discussed in this chapter and book can counteract the effects of inactivity and physiological aging.

3. The primary goal of a soundly conceived and conducted adult fitness program is to improve the physical capacity, vigor and energy reserves of the participants.

4. Dynamic fitness is a means and not an end in itself to greater personal achievement. It is attained by using the basic principles of use and disuse, specific adaptations to imposed demands, interval training, regularity, overload and progression.

5. The basic elements of physical fitness include strength, muscle endurance, flexibility and cardiovascular respiratory stamina.

6. Physical fitness requires hard, regular and persistent work and is not achieved overnight. It is a lifetime endeavor that demands a dedicated scheduling of time, personal effort, facilities and equipment on a regular basis.

7. Guiding principles for conducting successful adult fitness programs include:
   a. Careful medical evaluation of each participant.
   b. Stress testing and physical capacity evaluations.
   c. Prescription of exercise dosage and carefully supervised conditioning programs under competent leadership.
   d. Retesting and reevaluation at regular intervals for motivation, assessment and improved levels of conditioning.

8. The exercise conditioning program should comprise:
   a. A warm-up period of loosening up exercises to prepare the body for more intense activity.
   b. Rhythmic flexibility activity to promote muscle tone, range of motion and endurance of the musculoskeletal system.
   c. Cardiovascular respiratory endurance training to improve the capacity of the heart, blood vessel and respiratory systems of the body.
   d. A cooling off and tapering down period to permit fast heart rates, respiration and metabolism to return gradually to preexercise levels.

9. Of foremost importance is the constant observation and control of exercise intensity to match the capability of the individual participant. Danger signals of overexertion and proper precautions for the safety and progress of the participant must be kept in mind.

REFERENCES

Adams, G. M., and deVries, H. A. (1973) *J Gerontol* 28, 50.

American Heart Association, The Committee on Exercise (1972) *Exercise Testing and Training of Apparently Healthy Individuals: A Handbook for Physicians*, American Heart Association, New York.

Asmussen, E., and Heeboll-Nielsen, K. (1962) *Ergonomics*, 5, 167.

Åstrand, P.-O., and Rhyming, I. (1954) *J Appl Physiol* 7, 218.

Bortz, E. L. (1960) in *Exercise and Fitness*, Athletic Institute, Chicago.

Brozek, J. (1952) *Federation Proceedings*, 11, 784.

Canadian 5BX and Canadian XBX (1962) *Plan for Physical Fitness*, The Royal Canadian Air Force Pamphlet 30/1.

Chapman, E. A., deVries, H. A., and Swezey, R. (1972) *J Gerontol* 27, 218.

Cureton, T. K. (1965) *Physical Fitness and Dynamic Health*, The Dial Press, Inc., New York.

deVries, H. A. (1962) *Res Q* 33, 222.

deVries, H. A. (1966) *Am J Phys Med* 45, 119.

deVries, H. A. (1970) *J Gerontol* 25, 325.

deVries, H. A. (1974) *Physiology of Exercise for Physical Education and Athletics*, Wm. C. Brown Co., Dubuque, Iowa.

deVries, H. A. (1974) *Vigor Regained*, Prentice-Hall, Inc., Englewood Cliffs, N. J.

Fox, E. L., Bartels, R. I., Billings, C. E., Matthews, D. K. et al. (1973) *Med Sci Sports*, 5, 18.

Fox, E. L., and Matthews, D. K. (1974) *Interval Training Conditioning for Sports and General Fitness*, W. B. Saunders Company, Philadelphia.

Fox, S. M., and Skinner, J. S. (1964) *Am J Cardiol* 14, 731.

Golding, L. A. (1972) in *Exercise and the Heart* (Robert L. Morse, ed.), Charles C Thomas, Springfield, Ill.

Jacobson, E. (1956) *Progressive Relaxation*, University of Chicago Press, Chicago.

Hornbaker, A. (1974) *Preventive Care, Easy Exercise Against Aging*, Drake Publishers, Inc., New York.

Kannel, W. B. (1972) in *Exercise and the Heart* (Robert L. Morse, ed.), Charles C Thomas, Springfield, Ill.

Karvonen, M. J. (1959) in *Work and the Heart* (F. F. Rosenbaum and E. L. Belknap, eds.), Paul Hoeber, New York.

Karvonen, M. J. (1961) in *Health and Fitness in the Modern World*, Athletic Institute, Chicago.

Kasch, F. W., and Boyer, J. L. (1968) *Adult Fitness Principles and Practices*, National Press Books, Palo Alto, Ca.

Kraus, H., and Raab, W. (1961) *Hypokinetic Disease*, Charles C Thomas, Springfield, Ill.

The President's Council on Physical Fitness and Sports (1965) *Adult Physical Fitness*, U. S. Government Printing Office, Washington, D. C.

The President's Council on Physical Fitness and Sports (1973) *America, Be Fit*, U. S. Government Printing Office, Washington, D. C.

The President's Council on Physical Fitness and Sports and the Administration of Aging (1968) *The Fitness Challenge. . . .in the Later Years: An Exercise Program for Older Americans*, AOA Publication No. 802, Washington, D. C.

Rosenblum, R., and Delman, A. J. (1965) *Am J Cardiol* 15, 868.

Royce, J. (1958) *Res Q Am Assoc Health Phys Educ* 29, 204.

Scandinavian Committee on ECG Classification (1967) *Acta Med Scand Suppl* 481.

South Carolina Heart Association (1969) *J SC Med Assoc, suppl* 65, 12.

Swengros, G., and Monteleone, J. J. (1971) *Fitness with Glenn Swengros*, Hawthorn Books, Inc., New York.

Tennessee Heart Association Physical Exercise Committee (1971) *Physician's Handbook for Evaluation of Cardiovascular and Physical Fitness*, Tennessee Heart Association, Nashville, Tenn.

Wallis, E. L., and Logan, G. A. (1964) *Figure Improvement and Body Conditioning Through Exercise*, Prentice-Hall, Englewood Cliffs, N. J.

Wright, V., and John, R. J. (1961) *Ann Rheum Dis* 20, 36.

The Y's Way to Physical Fitness (1973) (C.R. Myers, L.A. Golding, and W.E. Sinning, eds.) Rodale Press, Inc., Emmaus, Pa.

At-Home Television Exercises for the Elderly

Maggie Lettvin

INTRODUCTION

Many elderly tend to overlook and neglect the possibility of improving their physical and mental functions as they grow older. For this reason accurate information and sensible advice on how to perform simple exercises which help them to recover such functions give the elderly a reassuring sense of being able to help themselves. Television is the best way to reach the great numbers of the elderly confined at home.

My experience with at-home television exercises for the elderly has shown that television is a perfect instrument for the wide dissemination of knowledge, advice and reinforcement for exercise at home. The repetition of a program, the added reinforcement of an exercise sheet, a chart to keep one faithful and to show progress proving that one is moving in the right direction give surprisingly good results.

In this chapter I present information I have collected and collated from many sources dealing with human movement* and then programmed into the small steps necessary to develop better body movements in the elderly and the ailing, slowly and evenly, from one level of fitness to the next. These steps are summarized in these sample exercise and instruction sheets. Most of them are self-explanatory. These instructions used in my television exercise program have proven useful and practical.

MIRRORS

There is no better way to judge your condition than by looking at yourself in a mirror. Something may be weakening and sagging without your being aware of it. Your muscle tone may be slowly lessening, body fat slowly gathering over little-used muscles and without a mirror all you notice is that your clothing size is changing.

---

* I owe more than can be written here to my friends in the media who support and produce such programs, and to the authorities in the fields of human movement whose studies have helped me to design and assemble these programs and information sheets.

The extra weight which you could easily see with a mirror may be dragging you earthward; your posture may be bad but without a mirror you may not even be aware of it, except for your slowly growing discomfort, aches or pains.

Every one of us — no matter what our conditions — needs a full-length mirror. Whether we hate it or not, it tells the truth; we have to know the truth before we can change the situation.

To exercise properly there is no better way to judge how you are doing than to watch yourself while you do!

Since being able to do is what we are after, don't be satisfied with looking at yourself after the work is done. Watch yourself while you are exercising. For all you know, unless you have looked at yourself while you were practicing, you may have been performing the movement not quite perfectly. Just a slight change in position can change the results of an exercise.

Any drastic body alteration (such as an amputation or paralysis, a palsy or any other disability), can make you think you're moving one way while you're really moving in quite another. Without a mirror it is difficult to know how to change the way you're moving to "look normal." With a mirror, it is possible to see and make a move that "looks" normal and then accustom yourself to the way it "feels". Then constant practice is necessary until that new move becomes a habit and it no longer feels strange. From that day on, the new habit of moving becomes "normal"!

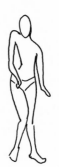

The best possible location of your mirror is at one end of your longest hall. Watching yourself move toward it several times a day will change your posture and your carriage faster than any other method.

Put a reminding message at the top of the mirror if there's some special part that you're trying to change. This is not narcissistic or vain but a very solid self-help method. Most of us tend to see our faults rather than our virtues. Seeing the problem is half the battle.

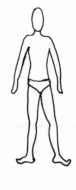

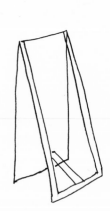

CAUTIONS

If you're just beginning to exercise, or if you suspect you're out of shape, be sure to get approval from your doctor before you begin to exercise. Be sure to do no more than your doctor advises.

Here are a few rules for beginners to help you get the most out of exercise whether you exercise "when you feel like it" (that is, not very often) or if you plan to exercise regularly.

1. Wear loose clothing.
2. Go barefoot when exercising.
3. Start each exercise period slowly; walk and/or use flexibility exercises. Use a hot bath, warm clothes or many (or electric) blankets if walking is impossible.
4. Breathe deeply.
5. Stretch or bounce gently, never hard.
6. Don't work too hard.
7. If you feel uncomfortable doing any movement, work very gently and carefully as you do it.
8. Once in a while everybody has a bad day; if you do, stop and start again the next day.
9. A little stiffness means that your body is building in all directions so don't stop; keep at it regularly.
10. Compete only with yourself; one more exercise or just one more of any exercise is an improvement.
11. Taper off slowly at the end of an exercise period; walk or do flexibility exercises.

Most people need exercise daily. If you follow these easy rules and exercise regularly, you will increase your strength without overwork or undue strain.

CURVATURES

For some strange reason, the general opinion is that exercises done in bed are of no use, but exercise is exercise no matter what position you're in when you move. Of course, some care must be taken according to the softness, hardness or sagging of the patient's bed.

The position of the person in bed can make the difference between comfort or pain and between improving or getting worse. Anyone complaining of pain while trying to sleep should investigate his bed, sleeping habits, general health, eating and postural habits. Changing the sleeping position of patients with scoliosis, kyphosis, and lordosis can lessen or undo some of the extreme curves and muscle strain caused by prolonged daytime standing or walking which accentuates the curves through gravity and impact. Some pain or discomfort in these conditions arising from pinched nerves or muscles in spasm can be alleviated. Certainly eight hours of correct sleeping posture can correct or at least improve many problems.

Lower back problems causing extreme discomfort when you try to sleep may sometimes be helped by placing one or two pillows the right way to relieve such distress. If you sleep on your back, try placing one or two small pillows under your knees. You may also need a small folded towel tucked under the lowest edge of your buttocks. Continue to use a pillow or even two under your head. The hardness or softness of the bed relates only to how you personally are most comfortable. Hard beds are not necessarily right. If you sleep on your side, place one (or even two pillows as necessary) between your knees to prevent one leg pulling at an angle from your aching back. Place another pillow under your head. Get your knees and nose carefully close together.

Extreme Lordosis Or "Sway Back"

The problem which is caused by a back which curves in too much just above the buttocks is called extreme lordosis or a "sway back" It can cause lower back problems. Other posture problems accompanying a "sway back" may include a flabby belly, sunken chest, round shoulders and knees that are locked back.

If the curvature or "sway back" is extreme, start with just two or three simpler exercises. Repetition of these exercises will in time strengthen your back muscles, make the back more flexible, and improve the curvature.

When your back is more flexible, you must strengthen the abdominal muscles to hold the spine easily in the proper position. This can be accomplished by adding these special breathing exercises:

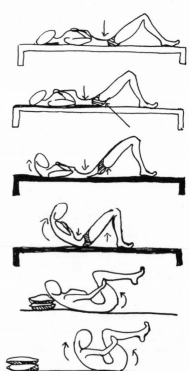

As you press your back down, purse your mouth and blow out slowly and completely.

As you slowly tighten your buttocks up purse your mouth and blow out slowly and steadily. *Do not lift your buttocks!* Let your buttock muscles do it! Slowly untighten them.

As you slowly lift your chin to your chest, purse your mouth and blow out slowly and steadily.

As you slowly roll up, purse your mouth and blow out slowly and steadily.

As you gently ease your knees up with your hands, purse your mouth and blow out slowly and steadily.

As you pull your knees and head up to try to touch, purse your mouth and breathe out slowly and steadily.

Exercise should not be violent. Gently and gradually increasing the stretch of the ligaments and muscles will slowly, day by day, bring your spine into healthier alignment and tighten the abdominal muscles to help it stay that way.

Be patient and consistent!

Be sure to change your walking posture also, or you'll be undoing your hard work.

Scoliosis

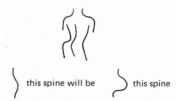

The scoliotic spine makes an S-curve, as in this picture:

One can be born with the problem, develop it after birth or develop it because of a short leg. Protecting oneself

this spine will be   this spine

from pain, deformed or deforming vertebrae and severe muscle spasms can also cause scoliosis. Poor postural habits and gravity also influence the curvature of the spine. A spine which is already sagging to the side will sag more under the pressure of gravity.

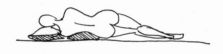

Unless a person has or is willing to develop the right habits to fight further changes, the scoliosis may become worse. One of the simplest methods of improving it can be accomplished during sleep.

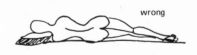

wrong

Lie on the side that bulges the most under your arm. Have the pillow under your head and another small pillow or folded towel under the bulge itself. These pillows will line your spine up better through the rib cage area. Then stretch your hip out along the bed to straighten the spine as much as possible. Reminding oneself to roll back into position when one rolls off the pillow soon gets a person into the habit of sleeping in a position that allows the spine to relax in a healthier alignment (position).

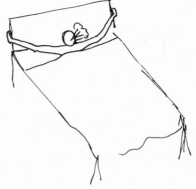

If your arms and hands are weak, begin holding onto the headboard and pulling down hard while breathing. Relax and repeat. *Start with one or two pulls* (morning and evening). Increase the number of times and the strength of pull. Fifty times in the morning and 50 times at night are not too much. When you can add on, try pursing your mouth and blowing out hard as you pull, inhaling as you relax.

If possible, hook your feet around the footboard of the bed, or tie something around the footboard to hook your feet through. This will help to stretch the spine. Pull with your feet in one direction as you pull with your arms in the other.

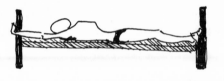

If you have lower back problems because of the scoliosis, put a small folded towel under the lower edge of your buttocks and pillows under your knees. If pulling with your feet causes pain, don't pull with them but pull from the headboard with your hands. *Do not do anything that hurts!*

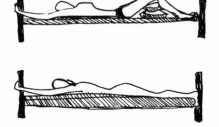

If you are not overweight, haven't a painful lower back and have no trouble lying on your abdomen, try doing the exercises in this position with your toes tucked in under the mattress.

Keep doing at least these few simple exercises if you cannot go on to other exercises or sports such as swimming. The only time your body will get significantly worse is when you stop trying to help it get better. When you do not exercise and/or you eat such a deficient diet that the body cannot repair itself or one that is too high in calories, adding weight and gravitational stress, your body will also get worse.

Kyphosis — Round Shoulders — Dowager's Hump

If you have round shoulders or a dowager's hump, you must stretch out the muscles across the front of the chest before you can shorten and develop the back of your shoulders, reshape shoulders, back and chest to look the way you want them and work the way they should.

One great time saver is to pin a folded face towel to the back of your pajamas where your back tends to bow out most strongly. While sleeping, remind yourself each time you roll over to roll back onto the towel again. (Do not use a pillow until your back is completely straightened up again, which sometimes takes months or years!)

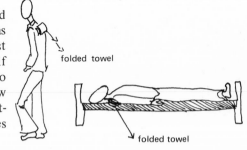

folded towel

folded towel

This position gently eases and stretches out the shortened chest muscles which pull the shoulders in and collapse the chest. Finally you should be able to easily stand with these muscles relaxed in the proper position.

In the morning, take hold of the headboard and pull down. This is a good exercise to use the important shoulder muscles while your back is still in the proper position from the flexibility gained from the sleeping position.

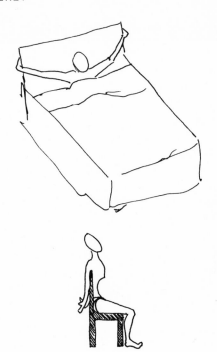

During the day, you can do other exercises to help stretch out the chest muscles and shorten the muscles in the upper back. These include the following:

Sitting in a chair or standing with your arms behind you (pelvis tucked under) hands clasped, palms out, thumbs up and *chin always up and in*, stretch your arms down gently and firmly behind you — don't just hold it! Repeat the move relaxing and tightening, time after time.

ABDOMINAL EXERCISES

Neither age, poor condition nor old abdominal surgery should prevent some work on the abdominal muscles. Poor tissue condition, in general, or other physical conditions and medical considerations may discourage surgical mending of hernias but the long-term results of weakened belly muscles should be seriously considered. It is important to regain the balance between back and belly muscles that is needed for balance in walking, for healthy lower backs, for ease in defecating and coughing, to support abdominal contents, to improve abdominal circulation and, most important, to improve self-image. A protruding belly really tires one out! The only possible excuses for lack of daily exercise of the abdominal muscles are inguinal or midline hernias. The exercises may have to begin with only blowing out all air from the lungs through a pursed mouth while lying on the back with knees bent, head on a pillow.

How To Do a Sit-up

Read the following cautions and suggestions and then, working steadily a little more each day, begin to move forward on the variations. When you want to and are capable, begin to do the exercises on your bed or on the floor. This set of exercises can also be done, if it is confortable for you, by sitting with your back a little away from the wall on the floor. Go on to chair or wall sit-ups.

What This Exercise Does for You

This exercise develops and strengthens the rectus abdominus, the pair of muscles which are like straps connecting from the top at the middle of your ribcage to your pubic bone or hip. This pair of muscles, about three inches long at the ribcage, has added strength by being connected over a reasonably wide area and to several ribs. The muscle is not just one long, unbroken line but has, above the navel, three insertions of connective tissue, or lines, across the muscle. From the navel down, there is one rather long, unbroken length of muscle which is more difficult to get really hard and flat. There are some other methods to reach this area which we will cover later. This area in women tends to have a natural covering of body fat which is difficult to get rid of without losing weight to the point of being gaunt; it is considered (and has been throughout history) a mark of beauty and femininity. Gauntness is not!

There is no necessity to sit on the floor. If you know that you cannot get down onto or up off the floor easily, sit right up on a wide bed to do the sit-ups instead. Have the sides protected so that, if you lose your balance, there is something to prevent you from falling on the floor.

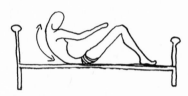

If your problem is just a matter of having bones that hurt when you roll them on the floor, try a thick rug or mat or a bunch of towels under you. This is such a useful exercise it should not be discarded except for medical reasons. If you have a medical problem, your doctor should be advising you on your exercising.

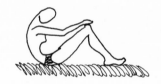

Beginning Sit-Ups

If you happen to be in very poor condition, you may prefer to do your beginning sit-ups in a chair. A pillow on the chair is allowed if your bottom is bony. Sit on the outside edge of the chair with your feet on the floor. Put your chin on your chest and let your lower back sink back toward the back of your chair, and with your arms out in front of you, roll back. If you fell back rather than rolled back, you will find it easier if you move your

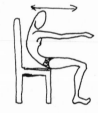

bottom a little farther back in the chair. If your feet came up off the floor, you may also need to sit slightly farther back. If your feet don't stay down because they don't quite touch the floor in the first place, put a cushion under them or a box, anything that allows you to keep your feet firmly planted. As you improve, move your bottom out farther and farther toward the front edge of the chair. Put your arms out straight in front with your knees bent just a little. Sit as close as you need to the back of a chair or wall, roll smoothly, not too slowly.

In a sit-up, the body should rise, rolling forward first from the head, then from the shoulders. Keep rolling up *without arching the back from the floor* until you're sitting up on the back of your pelvis, not way forward on the tips of your bottom bone with your back arched. Keep your chin on your chest at all times. Keep your ribs in front as close to your hipbones as possible by curling forward. Keep your knees bent and your feet on the floor without your feet being held down by anything. Curl back down to the chair, wall or the floor, one vertebrae at a time, keeping your chin on your chest as long as possible.

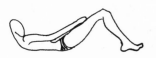 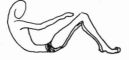 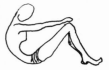

Try not to use momentum, especially when you are just beginning. The act of throwing yourself forward can be enough to give you little problems if you are not in very good condition, especially through the neck, shoulders, upper back and lower back. If your shoulders ache afterwards, and you know of no other reason why, it is likely that you are using momentum without being aware of it. Watch yourself carefully. Make sure that there is no point in your smooth rolling up where you suddenly jerk forward. The point where you may jerk forward is usually when your lower and upper back (almost to your shoulders) are still on the floor; this is when you are most likely to try to arch your back. Don't let that happen!

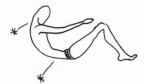 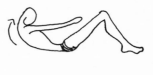

Be careful to continue to breathe out smoothly as you roll up, because your body needs more oxygen when moving. If you catch yourself holding your breath, remember that this will not only push up your blood pressure, but will also tighten the muscle over a forced-out belly wall, giving you a strong, but bell-shaped belly. Letting go little catches of breath from the back of your throat is also wrong and will lower your intake of oxygen, interfere with your blood pressure and make less than perfect a really useful exercise. This would prevent your being able to do as many sit-ups as you would otherwise be able to do. Resting after a certain number of any exercise allows the body to recover very quickly. Either rest completely or rest by doing an exercise which uses an entirely different muscle group and then return to doing sit-ups, or move back to an easier version instead of quitting completely.

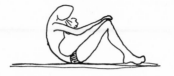

FLEXIBILITY OF HIP JOINT

Hip flexion is necessary for sitting, going up and down stairs, getting up off the floor (if you get there by accident), getting down onto and up off the floor (if you have the foresight to realize that someday you may fall in the street in front of a truck or get mugged on a deserted street). In any case, arthritic, inflexible hip joints prevent our walking as freely or as comfortably as we wish. Stiff joints and brittle bones, from a lack of movement, account for a large number of falls and other accidents among the elderly.

Hip Flexion (Being Able to Bend Your Thigh up Towards Your Chest)

There are several different ways to improve hip flexion. Try whichever ones give you the least discomfort, that are not too extreme for your condition and that you can best keep your balance with. Don't force the hip to flex beyond the point it can easily get to each day. A constant, steady practice of the right movement will often allow flexion to slowly return. If at any time while you are practicing hip flexion your lower trunk or legs go numb or tingle, do not continue with the exercises. *Report to your doctor.*

FIRST: exercises you can do in bed. Lie on your back with your hands under one knee. Pull one thigh gently up close to your chest and let it down gently. Then do the same with the other knee. Do the most flexible side first and use it to judge just how far the other side should be able to flex.

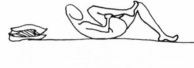

Crosswise on the bed (crosswise, so if you roll over you're still on the bed!), roll over onto your knees or climb up crosswise onto your bed on your knees.

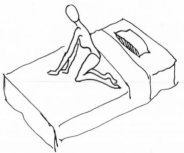

With your hands on the bed in front of you, lean forward. Then let yourself gently down to try to sit your buttocks on your heels. Lift your buttocks up again and lower gently again and again. With repeated tries, the hip joint will become less tight. Do not force it!

SECOND: chair exercises for hip flexion. While sitting in a chair, first lift the easiest thigh as close to the chest as possible with your hands under your knee. Then repeat the same move with the hip that needs to have better flexion. Another good hip flexion exercise is the swinging leg exercise. Stand on one foot on stairs or a phone book. Let your leg swing like a pendulum from the hip joint. A hip joint that is painful when you swing your leg may be less painful if a small weight (one-half to one lb.) is wrapped around each ankle. Swing the leg more gently until you get a feel for the exercise with the weight attached.

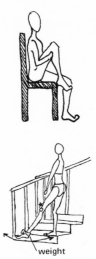

weight

KNEE FLEXIBILITY AND THIGH STRENGTH

Knee flexibility is one of the prime requisites for ease of walking. The knee is essentially a hinge joint and, though front to back flexibility is necessary, overstretching of the hamstrings can result in a sudden uncontrolled locking back of the knee while the person is in motion. Side to side flexibility of the knee should be discouraged. It should come from the foot and ankle, not the knee!

One of the most serious problems is the improper strengthening of the thigh muscles by lifting the leg after putting a weight on the ankle. This can only apply a shearing stress on the tissues of the knee joint which is presumably already in trouble. Attaching the weight just above the knee relieves all stress from the joint itself while safely increasing the strength of the thigh and improving the action of the knee. Starting with small weights is only sensible as weakened muscle invariably will have, as a consequence, weaker connective tissue attachments to the bone. A slow steady increase is conducive to a steady recovery of strength with no setbacks. At any age, setbacks tend to invite an end of the exercise routine.

In any case, even a slight detachment of connective tissue when the tissues are already weak increases debility and prolongs recovery.

Knee Flexibility

When you can't get the proper amount of bend at your knee, all kinds of problems arise. You can't squat. It is difficult to climb stairs and put on shoes and socks; it's difficult to walk. This condition often results from arthritis, other diseases, and accidents. It is important to begin work on knee flexibility while knee movement is still possible.

Start with no weight on the leg, no forc-
ing of the joint and natural movement.
Sitting a little further forward (or back)
on the table may make the difference in
how comfortable this exercise will be for
you.

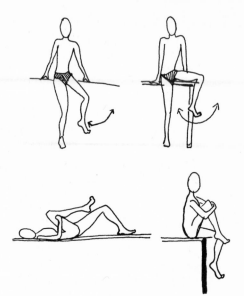

Make it comfortable! A pendulum-like
movement will increase circulation and
lubrication of the knee and should be
done as often as possible. If the knee
does not seem to be increasing in the
amount of back and forth movement it
can make, try these with just gentle pressure completely controlled by your
hands. Add just a little more pressure
each day. Do not cause yourself pain.

At the same time, begin the exercises in the next section to build the thigh
muscles while not involving the knee.

STRENGTHENING THIGH MUSCLES

Note: This method of strengthening the thighs puts no shearing action on the knee
joint since the weight is above, *not* below, the knee. Strong thigh muscles help to
protect the knees.

If for any reason you cannot stand and walk, your thigh muscles will begin to
weaken and the bones in your lower back and legs will begin to weaken by losing
calcium and probably other minerals. It is therefore important to keep the thigh
muscles strong enough so that when you are ready to stand and walk again, you are
also capable of doing it. Be aware of your other problems. If you have a hip
problem, the following exercise may give you discomfort. If it does, discontinue and
ask for or decide on a better or different exercise for your problem with your
advisor.

Sit on the edge of a chair with a
weight above the knee across the thigh (a
long bean bag weight), not too heavy to
begin with. Be sure there is no discomfort.

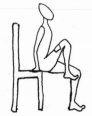

Lift and lower your thigh with your knee bent and bring your foot back to the floor each time (preferably with your leg straight but according to what is pain-free). Turn the foot *in* for some of the lifting or *out*, or both if it gives you no discomfort. This helps to get more muscles involved in the lifting. Begin with just a few (three) lifts an hour with little weight (one to three lbs.) and add one more lift (four) to each hour the next day. Continue this way for a week or until it seems to be too much time spent. Then lower the number of times and add a little more weight to the bean bag. Thigh muscles can be very strong! As long as you have no pain, discomfort or other problems, you can increase the weight you lift.

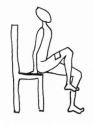

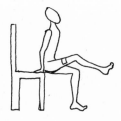

GETTING OUT OF CHAIRS

One of the more debilitating habits we pick up with age is helping ourselves up out of chairs with the use of our arms. This habit may have to do somewhat with chairs that we cannot put our feet under to get the proper leverage to help us get up. With such chairs, the aid of your arms becomes absolutely essential if you are ever to stand again. Once the thigh muscles have weakened, it is important to rise in any way you can, preferably without the use of your arms and, if possible, without the momentum of suddenly throwing yourself forward. When you are this weak, a little extra momentum can carry you too far forward and onto your face. If you have other muscle weaknesses or imbalances, the sudden movement can do other various kinds of damage. If getting up is totally impossible without the use of momentum, it is important that a sturdy table be right in front of you to prevent your toppling forward.

Again, it is necessary to advance slowly. Sit on two or three cushions as long as it takes to make getting up from the chair easy. (There is a built-in disgrace to having to "go back" to an easier exercise.)

This brings up a good point and that is the importance of starting at a level that is too easy! Immediate success, no matter how easy the exercise, pays big dividends in pride and encouragement. Added failure at a time of weakness cannot be condoned. It is the fault of the person advising the exercise, but it will be suffered by the person attempting it.

Start by sitting on two or even three cushions in a sturdy armchair facing a table. *Without using your hands* and without leaning too far forward, sit down into the chair and get up again. Throw yourself up if you need to, but do it carefully! The table will give you something to grab hold of if you have problems. Repeat this exercise several times the first day. Keep increasing the number of times until you can do 30 a day with no hands and no throwing.

Take one cushion out and start with a few repetitions the first day working your way up to 30 times again.

Take the last cushion out and start with few repetitions the first day. Work your way up to 30.

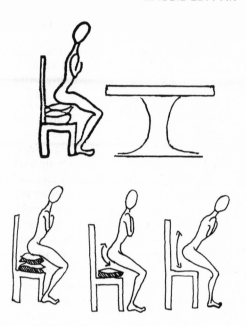

ACHING LEGS FROM VARICOSE VEINS, STANDING, LYMPHEDEMA

It is important to take great care if you are just beginning to move because of circulatory problems. If your feet and legs are swollen because of poor circulation of blood in your veins (which tends to make feet and legs deep red or even blue) or because of poor circulation of lymph (which leaves the foot swollen), the beginning treatment is to drain the affected limb by lying down and raising the leg up, resting it on a pillow or the head or foot of the bed until drainage either improves the size or the color, or both, of the troubled part. Still in the same position, gently tensing the calf muscle from five to 15 minutes will increase drainage.

Then bring the limb down to bed level and continue a steady tensing and relaxing motion for as long as seems comfortable. This exercise should be continued every hour or as often as the limb seems to need attention. The collection of blood or lymph can swell the foot to the point that the skin becomes stretched and very delicate, tending to split when the weight of the body is put on it. If the skin on your feet is very delicate, a piece of lambswool or a woolen scarf or blanket wrapped around the pillow helps prevent your skin from splitting or breaking. Do not use nylon, orlon or other synthetic fabrics which tend to cut into the skin. Only wool should be used when feet are in very poor condition. Walking against a pillow covered with lambswool, placed at the foot of the bed, after the limb is drained can give the needed movement without (in most cases) causing any trouble with the skin. In between periods of bed walking, the feet can be rested on top of the pillow for a comfortable period of time to aid drainage.

The more often the limb is drained by these methods early in the condition, and the more movement instituted immediately after each draining, the faster will be the return to the normal condition. Normal movement should be substituted for bed exercises and drainage as soon as possible. Rocking in a rocking chair, pulling the front of the feet up each time you lean back will help with the return to walking without putting the full body weight on the still delicate feet. Wool socks should be worn to protect the feet from scratches, other injuries or the cold. Cotton will not keep the warmth in. Keep shoes off to encourage better circulation. Socks should be slightly loose. Do not use colored or stretch socks.

Try not to let the tissues stay swollen. The longer they stay that way, the more likely they are to remain stretched out of shape even after recovery of normal lymph flow.

To keep the limb(s) from swelling, sleep with the limb or limbs that tend to swell resting on a pillow, slightly elevating them over the rest of the body.

The best place to start an exercise program after an acute problem with the circulatory system is in the hospital with the doctor or a nurse in attendance. All inflammation, irritation, or fever, or acute liver or kidney disorders, must be carefully watched and evaluated by the attending doctor. Then, a slow, steady, careful increase in movement may be added as needed. Strong or sudden exercises should be avoided since they increase blood pressure and body temperature. Overload is very likely to injure those muscles and joints unused to exercise, but, complete bed rest is just as wrong. Once the doctors prescribe movement, the first exercises must start slowly. A little exercise done slowly and for just a little while will rarely exhaust the patient, push his blood pressure up too far or cause discomfort or pain. If any shortness of breath, pain or aches develop on beginning to exercise the doctor must be alerted.

Legs aching right now?

Lie down. Put your legs up above your heart. Rest your legs on pillows.

Begin pulling the front of your feet up firmly toward your knees time after time while your legs are elevated.

Still aching?

Start massaging them from the foot toward the knee, still pulling the front of your foot up, time after time. Do both legs; even if only one aches, they're both in trouble. Make sure you massage from the foot toward the knee.

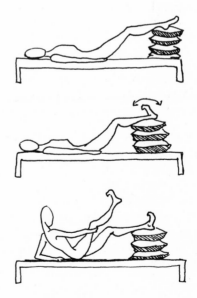

When the color of your feet is much improved, do not sit with legs hanging over the edge of your bed! Stand (no shoes) at the side of your bed, hold on and shift your weight from foot to foot.

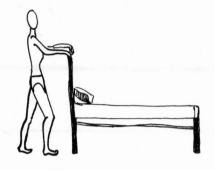

Move back and forth from this position to feet-elevated-in-bed position for several minutes each, several times every day, or rest several times during the day if you need, and if you can, with your feet elevated. Work your feet until your feet and legs stop aching and then rest with them up a while longer. Sleeping with them elevated will help. Don't keep them up longer than is comfortable for you. The massage and pumping action of the feet help to "milk" the blood back up toward the heart; the elevation of the legs allows gravity to help the process.

With your feet still up, you can pump them against a pillow as if you're walking, if you'd like to for a change.

When you are on your feet again, it is important to wear loose clothing and flat, comfortable shoes as much as possible. Do away with anything that slows circulation or prevents your moving freely. That includes girdles.

It is important for you to:

(1) remain as active as possible when you are on your feet;

(2) rock when you are sitting or twist first one foot and then the other, round and round;

(3) keep your weight normal to prevent too heavy a load on your circulatory system;

(4) walk;

(5) move all furniture out of the line of toe-stubbing (from this day forward, care and prevention must be a part of your life);

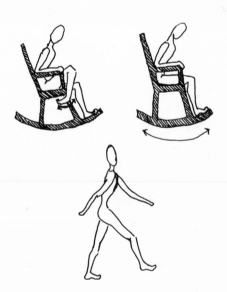

(6) wear only very soft, pliable leather or cloth shoes with plenty of ventilation, especially sandals;

(7) shift your weight from foot to foot when you must stand;

(8) come up onto your toes and down;

(9) roll your feet out and in; and

(10) walk with your feet against the pillow the last thing at night and the first thing in the morning.

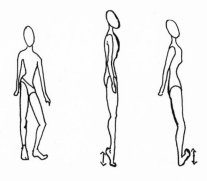

Never sit with feet down and still. Never wear any shoes longer than you must. Never do leg swinging exercises. Centrifugal force tends to drive blood and other fluids to the feet. Never stand for long periods, especially without moving as this tends to allow the blood and other fluids to pool in the feet because of gravity. Try to keep fluids from forming! Your body parts can get into bad habits, too. Remember, the only way to break a bad habit is consistently to prevent it. As soon as you see or feel any swelling, lift the affected part to drain. At the same time, start a pumping action or start pushing against something to help the drainage.

STIFF, PAINFUL OR PARTIALLY FROZEN JOINTS IN THE FEET

We tend to laugh at the old custom of binding women's feet in China, little realizing that our own customs of footwear are only one step removed. The 26 bones, the many joints, muscles and varieties of connective tissue are there for a purpose. To cut off the many possible delicate nuances of balance by encasing our feet in anything but the most pliable of materials shows a lack of serious attention to their design. The flexibility of the joints, the shock absorption of the arch, the ability of the foot to mold itself around small obstacles or to distribute the weight of the body in different ways, the help that a healthy metatarsal gives us in clutching with our toes for a faster take-off, the sensitivity of a foot to recognize what it is coming in contact with and to determine how to deal with it are all lost the moment we begin to wear shoes.

What we gain from shoes are corns, calluses, deformed toes, athlete's foot and poor balance; from worn-down shoes, aching knees and lower backs; from high heels, lordosis, weakened belly muscles and an inability to walk very far; from shoes too small, cutting down of circulation and a constant pained expression.

And then we hear from misinformed shoe salesmen that our feet will spread if we go barefoot! Just like the Chinese women's did? Your foot will spread only as far as it should have spread in the first place, if you're lucky!

For the toes soak feet in warm water first, if possible. Use your hand to straighten and bend the toes until you can bend and straighten them easily without using your hand.

FEET

If your feet are under the care of a doctor, or if your bones tend to be fragile, get approval from your doctor before you begin these exercises.

Sitting in a chair:

(a) Toe-heel, walk
(b) Up onto both toes and down
(c) Up onto one toe and down — then other

Then, do them standing:

(a) Toe crawl sitting in chair or on floor
(b) Same, standing
(c) Walk with marbles held under toes
(d) Pick up marbles

(a) Walk, toes turned in, heels out, up on outsides of feet
(b) Sit in a chair, knees together, feet turned, heels out and toes under

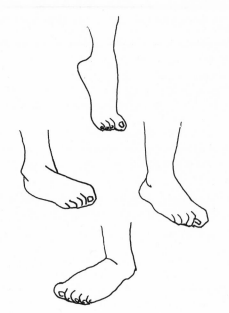

WALKING

After an acute circulatory problem only a very small percentage of older people will ever take up running or jumping rope or any very active sports unless they were inclined to be active before. A more normal and much more satisfying type of activity all can indulge in is walking. Forget swimming, bicycles, or anything that costs money. Walking, going up and down stairs and getting in and out of chairs will keep most normal, rather sedentary people in better condition than they enjoyed for the largest part of their lives.

Walking is a natural exercise that is good for everyone who is capable of walking. It uses every muscle and can be managed by almost everyone. It is the nonviolent exercise *par excellence*!

Most of us don't really move as much as we think we do! Try this. *Count* how many minutes you spend on your feet moving. Write it down. Then look at it and, if you find it unbelievably small, move a bit more tomorrow! It's so easy and pleasurable to change! All it takes is walking!

If you're going to go for a walk outside and, for any reason, you doubt your ability to return safely, take a friend with you. Or go for a walk, in place, behind your chair. If you feel or show any signs of sickness, stop. Start again when you're better. *Never* walk when you have a fever or a headache. But try not to postpone walking for more than a day unless you're sick.

To facilitate walking many elderly people needing bifocal glasses for failing vision should consider using two pairs of glasses for near and far vision instead of bi-focals. Balance is badly affected, falling occurs more often and walking is curtailed when bi-focals are first used and with each adjustment.

People with balance problems should also consider using a long sturdy umbrella that essentially provides a "third leg", without the embarassment of a cane. Even people with slight balance problems tend to discontinue walking rather than to endure the problems that come with walking. The use of the umbrella might give that extra little assurance which just might help to get them started again.

Consider flat, soft-soled shoes, preferably with an Oxford look to them, for those who have trouble with balance, but who have to "look" right. However, reduce heel height gradually! An immediate two-inch drop in heels can be disastrous to little used, brittle ligaments.

Consider nonstretch white wool socks as common household wear. They contain no dyes, won't cut off the circulation of the blood, are warm, provide good circulation of air to prevent infections and leave the foot entirely free to move as it should.

Balance is improved immediately or after a few hours practice. Don't be surprised if the feet ache a little for the first few days. Unless you are used to going barefoot around the house, try walking in place, barefoot or wearing socks, a few minutes at a time, holding onto the back of a sturdy chair if necessary.

Even a slight amount of stirring of the circulation is more than a lot of sedentary people get. Any encouragement is good. Consider using rocking chairs. Music in the background, if it is enjoyed, to keep time to is very helpful and needs only to be very low to get people unconsciously rocking in time with it. Disuse problems of long duration almost always carry with them balance problems as a side effect. Rocking increases circulation without the added worry of falling.

Walk outside if you can. Walking outdoors takes us out into an interesting world of ever-changing experiences, sights, and smells. It is best of all at dawn when there's dew on the grass and everything is quiet. Do you remember how it felt to walk barefoot in the grass? Try it; the ground is bumpy and uneven and the grass is a natural cushion. Such soft, pliable, uneven surface will get you used to the unexpected. That's what life is all about, isn't it, being ready for the unexpected and getting used to it? Go barefoot as much as you can; your feet, if they're "normal feet", work better if you do. Wear pliable shoes with air holes if you can't go barefoot. If your feet get sore or you begin to get blisters on your feet, cover and protect them immediately to prevent them from getting worse.

Bare feet, of course, can't "run down at the heels" so heelless shoes or bare feet are best. Your toes contract more when you are barefoot and your foot can roll forward freely and naturally. It's simple enough; your feet support your body, push you forward and give you a built-in set of shock absorbers, your very own arches!

Really stretch out! Walk fast and hard for a few minutes. You'll soon hit a natural stride and pace. And trying a bit harder than usual is a good way to gauge just how much you can do. Your body will fall naturally into whatever pace is comfortable for it.

Walking speeds up your heart beat naturally. Your lungs fill and empty. Your blood courses through the blood vessels. Your muscles stretch and contract. Your bones twist and turn naturally in their joints and sockets. Every body process is speeded up in a comfortable way. A good daily walk will, in time, lower your blood pressure, your pulse rate and your weight. Try to consciously relax while walking. Does this sound funny? Once walking has become a natural thing for you, it is natural to relax. Until then, think about it and do it purposely. Don't overdo! Wear comfortable clothes! Listen to your body! Again, you must be the final judge. Soon after you have walked, you should feel not tired, but elated! After you have been at it a while, you will be able to sense very small differences in your body.

Our children largely learn how to live from our example. So walk with and for them! What better way to spend time together, improving their health, having fun and a little adventure! Walking doesn't cost any money and you'll be building habits that will improve your life, their lives and the lives of their children, a real legacy anyone can give!

SCIATIC PAIN

So-called "sciatica" develops when the sciatic nerve in the back of the hip and leg becomes irritated and painful. Any pressure on the sciatic nerve along its course can irritate it causing the painful symptoms of "sciatica". Some conditions which can irritate the nerve are:

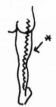

(1) carrying hard or lumpy objects in your hip pockets
(2) sitting on chairs with raised edges
(3) sitting on lumpy seats
(4) sitting on cold concrete
(5) overstretching too quickly
(6) buttock muscles so loose and underdeveloped that they flatten out
(7) too little muscle or fat to pad the bottom
(8) sitting too long on a toilet seat or straining to have a bowel movement
(9) cutting down the local circulation and applying pressure by crossing the legs
(10) extra weight
(11) lower back problems

If your bottom is flabby begin to build it up by clenching and unclenching the muscles of the buttocks time after time. Don't hold the clench; keep the circulation up by keeping it moving. If your bottom is bony from being underweight, put on weight and muscle by eating a good high protein diet.

Sit on warm and soft surfaces. Stand or rock rather than sitting still. Keep your bowels regular. Keep your legs uncrossed. Take walks.

Start an exercise program slowly and work up gradually. The exercise for lower back problems combined with a gradually increasing walking program seems to work best in relieving sciatic pain. Physiotherapy may also be helpful.

Walk until just this side of the point of pain, then rest and repeat at intervals during the day. Sometimes it takes weeks or even months for the pain to finally disappear completely. You will find that you can walk a little farther each day before the pain begins. If your doctor has given you other instructions, be sure to ask his advice about these suggestions.

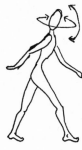

Being overweight will undo your efforts. Lose extra weight! It's worth the effort! Be patient!

SHOULDER JOINTS

Not to be able to use your arms and hands because of pain without thinking about them forces you to feel sorry for yourself. You can do nothing for or with anyone when bursitis or a painful shoulder joint prevents you from reacting normally.

It is extremely important to keep total flexibility. Keeping a painful shoulder still to prevent pain after the first few days is the worst possible thing you can do to yourself! When a joint is injured, calcium tends to deposit at the site of the injury, sometimes unbelievably quickly! To prevent freezing of the joint and to relieve the problems already existent, shoulder movement must be reinstituted as soon as possible using no muscle at all if possible. The shoulder joint is built with great flexibility and, when in good condition, can safely be extended an inch or more within the socket. This same flexibility leaves it vulnerable to injury. Muscles and ligaments surrounding the joint safeguard it and keep it securely within its natural confines. When the joint is injured, the spasms in these same muscles pulling the joint together can cause excruciating pain.

The best positions in which the shoulder joint can be moved reasonably freely without pain are illustrated below.

Even in this most conducive position to prevent use of the muscle, it is important to make certain the patient relaxes completely across the table and that the movement is only pendular and uses no lifting efforts. Supporting the arm in a pain-free position is very important. Any further irritating of tissues (indicated by the presence of pain) will prevent, or slow, recovery. Comfortable sleeping positions are also of great importance.

Stiff or Painful Shoulder Joint

Shoulders should be dealt with in this way:

Lie across a sturdy kitchen table from your hips to your head, competely relaxed, with the aching arm and shoulder hanging over the edge. Turn your head slowly towards that shoulder. Using no force, let your arm swing loosely like a pendulum, forward and back for a while, in under the table and out for a while, around in a circle in one direction, then around in the other direction. If any move is painful, hold a weight or some heavy, small object in your hand. Let it *feel* heavy! Let the shoulder joint hang

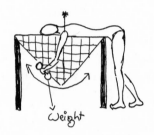

loose. Keep it loose and heavy and let it swing like a pendulum. When this causes no pain, move back to not using a weight. Do this exercise as soon and as often as the shoulder begins to hurt.

In the meantime, do not lift, carry, throw, catch, push or pull with that arm. Irritating the tissues will just keep the shoulder painful longer. Support the arm and shoulder by looping your thumb into your belt. (Wear one especially for this purpose or tie a scarf around your belt, leaving a large enough loop to put your arm through to the point that makes it least painful to you. Make two loops if that's better.)

For some, it is necessary to hook a thumb inside the open shirt or, for women, under a bra strap. It is important to keep the shoulder from hurting if it is at all possible.

When sleeping on your good side, support the painful side on a pillow placed in front of you.

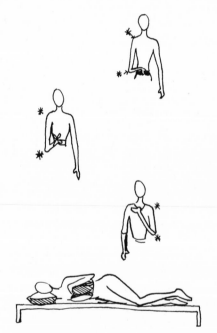

When sleeping on your back, wedge an extra pillow under the painful shoulder in such a way as to relieve the discomfort by pushing the shoulder forward. Let the elbow rest on another pillow or across your body, whichever is most comfortable.

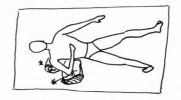

FOR LYMPHEDEMA OR SWELLING IN THE ARMS

Sleep on your back with your arms overhead, resting on a pillow.

Place pillows on either side of you to keep your arms at your sides, raised to the elbow — with hands across your belly.

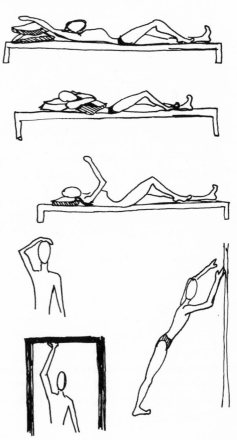

For faster drainage, clench and unclench your hands repeatedly. Then raise your arm, elbow bent overhead, over and over.

Do not do arm swinging exercises or let arms hang at your sides for long.

During the day, frequently rest the forearm on top of your head while tightening and relaxing the muscles of your whole arm, time after time.

Do pushups against the wall, with your arms from the elbows to hands high up the wall above shoulder level.

If you can, push your hands up against the roof of your car, or up against the top of doorways, over and over again.

BALANCE PROBLEMS

Mobility-limiting diseases of long duration including diseases that cause vertigo or dizziness almost always produce balance problems as a side effect.

But, whether the balance problem is of long or short duration, it is important for the person to accommodate to the problem. The chronic sufferer who looks normal evokes little sympathy and he may as well just get used to dealing with the world through his personal tilting or whirling view of it. It is probably easier to deal with an unremitting dizziness than sudden bursts of it. One problem is the nausea that is sometimes too overwhelming to deal with. Drugs should be suspect until all side-effects from them have been eliminated. Sometimes drugs delay recovery by causing depression or sleepiness. You should consult your physician to determine the exact cause and nature of your balance problem in order to get proper treatment. Also see sections on *Walking* and *Dizziness* for additional suggestions.

DIZZINESS

Dizziness is not the worst thing that could happen to you and there is a strong possibility that you can learn to accommodate to it, or "get used to it". It is possible that you may remain dizzy in spite of anything you may try to relieve it. Certainly you don't want dizziness to stop you from living. It doesn't have to prevent you from living a normal life unless you choose to "suffer" with it instead of dealing with it. Consult your doctor to determine the cause of your dizziness and get the proper medical treatment. Then, you may find these suggestions will also help you to get better accommodated to the condition if it persists.

Dizziness creates an obvious balance problem so you must begin getting used to the dizziness from a position in which you cannot fall — lying down!

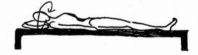

Lie down on a bed, in the center so you feel secure, on your back. Legs apart and arms out a little from your sides (even gripping the sides of the bed) will increase your feeling of safety. Now turn your head slowly from side to side. If it makes you dizzy, stop a minute to let the dizziness pass and repeat the move.

When you can without too much of a sick feeling, turn your head a little faster. Stop when you need to. When you're used to this move, try moving your head up and down, stopping when necessary, speeding up when you can take it.

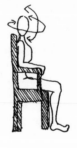

The next step is to sit in a sturdy arm chair placed in front of a table. Hold on the arms tightly and begin again to turn your head first left or right slowly, stopping when necessary, speeding up when you can.

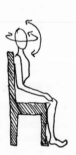

Then move your head up and down slowly, stopping when necessary, speeding up as you can.

When you are very sure of yourself, try the same exercise without holding on. Keep the table in front of you for safety's sake.

Next step:

When you are safely able to stand behind a sturdy chair, hold on and do the same set of exercises. If necessary go back to the chair exercises for a while.

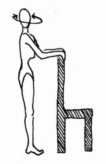

Move back to this exercise when you feel more sure of yourself.

Rest your hands more and more lightly on the edge of the chair until you can remove them completely.

Continue the exercises.

Next step:

Start walking, using a cane or umbrella. When you can, start doing these exercises slowly and gently as you walk. Don't do too many at a time or progress too rapidly to the more sudden turning of your head. The cane or umbrella can give you a much greater ability to balance when you are taken off guard by sudden dizziness.

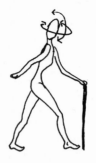

Next, practice your new balancing act in a little less restricted area. Pull a sturdy kitchen table out into the center of the room. Now, with one hand on the table, start walking around it. When you're ready, begin nodding your head a little. When you're handling that well, begin turning your head and continue to walk around the table. Change the direction that you're walking around the table from time to time. Some of you will find it much easier to turn in one direction than another. If so, try turning much more often to whichever side makes you feel least sure of yourself until you become somewhat accustomed to it.

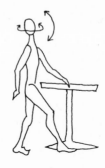

When you're ready to try your wings solo, without props, be sure to start on a well-carpeted floor if you can. Slippery or waxed floors should not be in any home, let alone yours.

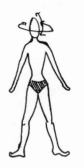

Now you're ready to practice, and practice is what it takes. No one retains the use of any ability that he doesn't keep in constant use.

Become a busy person for your health.

Become a busy person on your feet. The more you move, the less you will tend to notice your dizziness unless you are consciously trying to or don't have enough to do. Abrupt changes in amount of dizziness will always call themselves to your attention. Or it may take you a few minutes every day to become accustomed again to going in one direction while your head seems to be going in the other. The more you use your hands, the better your judgement of where to reach for something will become. Again, it will take constant and regular practice.

Use bi-focals only if your doctor insists. They tend to give you more trouble with balance. Two pairs of glasses for near and far vision make it easier to deal with balance problems, especially on stairs.

Live actively and you will live better.

Stair climbing is next and must be undertaken only where it is possible to hold onto railings, preferably two, one on either side. It is only sensible to always hold onto at least one railing for the rest of your life or as long as the dizziness lasts.

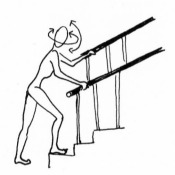

Nothing is too much for you to handle! Keep after it! You can be in control!

INCONTINENCE – WETTING YOURSELF

Incontinence will always deter people wishing to or needing to move around in the world because of the necessity to stay close to a toilet. In the long run, incontinence may lead to a myriad of other "loss of movement." Your doctor should be consulted for possible medical or surgical treatment to relieve symptoms of incontinence.

Quite often, wetting yourself when coughing, sneezing, laughing, etc., can be due to slight infections which need a doctor's help.

Whether you wet yourself a lot or a little, consult your doctor to find out just what is causing the problem. If your problem stems from a lot of weight pressing down and stretching the sphincter muscle open, which weakens it, from a pregnancy which does the same thing, from a general laxness of muscle tone even when this weakness is from a neurological disorder, then complete or almost complete control can be recovered in most instances.

There are times when simply building up the strength of the sphincter muscle will relieve symptoms of incontinence. These exercises should be done by everyone who has been catheterized, suffers from cystitis, and those with "undetermined cause" incontinence. Reregulating the insulted or weakened muscle by exercise is extremely important for the person's whole future.

In spite of the many causes for incontinence, most leakage problems seem to be from simple weakness of the sphincter. Practice and exercise may help strengthen the sphincter or increase control over it.

From this day forward when you pass water, never forget to stop and start *several* times. The stopping should be as complete and as sudden as you can make it! In the beginning, the weakness of the sphincter will make you feel as though you might not be able to start again, but never fear! Day by day, the stopping and the starting will get easier and easier. If it is difficult to start again, lean your belly in against your thighs. Sometimes pushing the hands in on the lower belly at the same time helps. Tightening up of the sphincter can be practiced all day long no matter where you are. Just don't do the letting down part until you need to.

Don't quite practicing when you've improved. This is a daily habit that can only serve you well!

CONCLUSION

These instruction sheets are a small sample of those sent to television viewers of all ages whose desire to rehabilitate and improve these physical conditions impels them to write for help.

Many problems can be helped by exercise. Finding the right movements and exercise for the specific problem helps greatly to reacclimate oneself to one's world. Although proper practice is the only way to achieve this, few will practice without hope and encouragement. And that's what we offer — the art of self-help, together with the necessary advice, confidence, and competence to extend these methods to other problems of people.

No one completely recovers from progressive illnesses, but exercises that improve circulation and muscle strength can often slow down the progression and the disability caused by the disease. Learning to use auxiliary surrounding muscles to a much greater degree effectively improves the body's balance, function and fitness.

Daily presentation, via television and repetition and practice by the housebound patient will incorporate these exercises into the mores and life style of people of all ages. With exercise and the better fitness attainable through exercise, the older person acquires a greater ease of movement which gradually becomes a learned and habitual response, opening up a new way of life leading to greater independence, health and happiness.

Gerokinesiatrics—A Pharmacopoeia of Exercises for the Elderly

Lawrence J. Frankel and Betty Byrd Richard

INTRODUCTION

These instructions have been developed specifically for instructors involved in teaching and implementing the Preventicare Exercise Program, as designed and developed by the Lawrence Frankel Foundation of Charleston, West Virginia. For best results, they should be followed precisely as described. The exercise program should be performed no less than three times per week, preferably one hour before mealtime. All exercise groups should be performed in their entirety (unless unusual or special circumstances prevail) because they were designed to involve the total musculo-skeletal system. There is sufficient variety and diversification among the exercise groups to allow, if necessary, modification for the severely debilitated, homebound or bed-bound. Participants should be taught that they must never hold their breath during exercise, and to *always exhale with effort*. Floor exercises are most comfortably performed on a mat, rug, or carpet.

The general design and plan of this pharmacopoeia of exercise maximizes mobility of the musculo-skeletal system and emphasizes peripheral circulation. Those few exercises that strengthen the cardiorespiratory function are so planned that target heart rate should not exceed 110 to 120 beats per minute. When significant medical problems are present, the patient's physician should be contacted for medical clearance to perform these exercises.

PREVENTICARE PHARMACOPOEIA

A. **Stretching** — For improving flexibility of hamstring muscles and the lower back. The hamstrings are the muscles behind the knee. Start with 3 repetitions and increase one each week for a maximum of 6. Starting position is on floor.

    1. Sitting in erect position, legs apart, slowly reach forward, bringing forehead as close to knee as possible, keeping head between arms. Hold on to the calf, ankle or toes (depending on beginning flexibility). Knees must be held flat to

floor. Bounce gently (refrain from fast jerky movements). Count — 1-2-3-4 and hold 2-3-4; 2-2-3-4 and hold 2-3-4, etc.

2. Sitting in erect position, legs apart, slowly reach forward as far as possible, keeping head between arms, knees flat to floor. Bounce gently to count of 1-2-3-4 and hold 2-3-4 and up ... 2-2-3-4 hold 2-3-4 and up, etc.

3. Sit in erect position, legs together, follow same procedure as above.

B. **Neck Exercises** — Improves the function and range of motion of the muscles and joints of the neck.

1. *Head Back and Forward*
Slowly bring head back as far as possible and then forward, chin on chest. 5 times each direction. Count — back and — two and 3 and etc.

2. *Ear Toward Shoulder*
(Keep shoulders perfectly still) Move head to side, the right ear toward the right shoulder and then the left ear toward the left shoulder. Count — one and (to the left) two (to the right) and (to the left), etc. 5 times each direction.

3. *Turn Head to Look Over Right Shoulder, Then Left Shoulder*
Turn head slowly — look over right shoulder, then look over left shoulder. 5 times in each direction. Count — one and — two and, etc. Important: Do not move shoulders or upper part of body while performing the head and neck exercises.

C. **Shoulder Exercises** — To enhance and improve range of motion in the shoulder girdle.

1. *Shrugs*
Arms at sides, shrug shoulders up toward the ears, 10 times. Count — up and — two and — three and, etc. The 'and' count is the downward motion.

2. *Rotations*
Shrug and rotate shoulders forward, slowly, 5 times, then rotate shoulder backward, 5 times. Count — one and two and — etc. The 'and' count is the completion of rotation.

3. *Arm Circles*
Extend arms horizontally sidewards, palms down, stretching with elbows not bent, head in good posture. Rotate arms from the shoulders, making very small circles, 10 times forward and then 10 times reverse. 1-2-3-4-5-6-7-8-9-10 and reverse 1-2-3-4-5-6-7-8-9-10.

D. **Hand, Wrist, and Finger Exercises** — To improve range of motion and flexibility. Often ameliorates arthritic conditions in this area.

1. *Hand Rotation*
Grasp right wrist with left hand, slowly rotate right hand, keeping palm facing down. 10 times clockwise and then rotate hand counter-clockwise 10 times. Repeat same procedure with opposite hand.

2. *Finger Stretching*
With right hand, palm facing down, gently force fingers back toward fore-arm, using left hand for leverage; then place left hand on top of right hand and force fingers down. 5 times each hand.

3. *Finger Flexion and Extension*
   Arms extended forward, close fist tightly − then extend fingers. Flex and extend 10 times. Count − flex and extend − two and − three and − four and.

E. **Ankle Exercise** − Improves range of motion and flexibility of the ankles.
   1. *Circles*
      Cross right leg over opposite knee and rotate foot slowly 10 times to outside, then reverse. Repeat procedure opposite foot. Count − one and − two and − etc. The 'and' count is the completion of rotation.
   2. *Ankle Flexion and Extension*
      With legs extended, stretch ankles forward − then backward, flex and extend 10 times. Count − flex and extend − two and, etc.

F. **Thigh Exercises** − For the abductors and adductors. To tone and strengthen the muscles inside and outside the thighs.
   From sitting position (floor, chair or couch)
   (A) Start with knees bent and together, hands on outside of knees, separate knees against resistance of hands to slow count of 5.
   (B) Place hands on inside of knees, with the knees widely separated. Bring knees together to slow count of 5 against hand resistance. Repeat 5 times − each direction.

G. **Abdominal Exercise** − To strengthen the upper and lower abdominal muscles which are the keystone to a healthy back.
   Half Sit-Ups (Supine Position)
   From position lying on back, legs extended, arms behind head, reach up and forward to touch fingers to beginning of knee caps. Hold this position for count of three and return to starting position. Important: Exhale forcefully with the effort − never hold the breath. Start with no more than three repetitions, gradually increasing by one each week to a maximum of 10 repetitions. Count − up − 2-3-4 and hold − 2-3-4 − 2-2-3-4 and hold 2-3-4, etc. (For those who may have some back problems, it is acceptable to perform this exercise with knees partially bent.)

H. **Specific Exercise to Stretch Hamstrings**
   From back lying position, legs fully extended, arms at side, raise right leg up and backward as far as possible and return, 10 times. Repeat 10 times with left leg. Count − up and − two and − three and − four and, etc. (For those with minor back problems, perform this exercise with knees bent just enough so the back is flat to the floor.)

I. **Back Relaxation Exercise** − To relax the muscles of the lower back.
   1. From back lying position, grasp right knee with both hands and pull toward chest, at the same time, bring chin toward the knee, very slow and easy cadence and then return to starting position. 10 times.
   2. Repeat same exercise, bringing the left knee to chest and then return to starting position. 10 times.

3. Grasp both knees and bring to chest as closely as possible, bringing chin toward knee and returning to original starting position. 10 times. Count — one and — two and — three and — etc. On the 'and' count the body is in a supine position, with arms at side.

J. **Back Arch Support** — Strengthens the upper back muscles and firms back of upper arms.

Start from sitting position, upper body erect, hands behind and slightly to the side. Raise hips from floor until body is perfectly straight with head back. Return to starting position. Repeat exercise 3 times, increasing one repetition each week until reaching a maximum of 10 repetitions. Count — up — 2-3-4 and down — 2-2-3-4 and down — 3-2-3-4 and down — 4-2-3-4 and down, etc.

K. **Side-Lying Exercises** — To strengthen and improve flexibility of the thighs, hips and muscles at side of the waist.

1. Lie on right side with head resting comfortably on extended arm — the other arm and hand to the side in front of waist for balance, the back slightly arched. Raise left leg up as far as possible. Do not bend the knee. Count up — and — two and, etc. The 'and' count is down. Repetitions: 10 times.
2. Kick legs in scissor fashion, fast cadence — 10 times. Do not bend knees.
3. Raise both legs and upper body simultaneously, looking over shoulder and back toward heels. Repetitions: Start with 3, increasing one each week to 10. Repeat these exercises on opposite side of body.

L. **Hyperextension Exercise** — Strengthens upper and lower back and improves flexibility of spine.

Start from front lying position with arms and legs fully extended and head down. Raise arms, legs and head simultaneously, arching the entire body without bending arms and legs. Maintaining this same arch position, extend arms sideward — then extend arms forward — holding momentarily and return to starting position (head down). This is a four count exercise — up — side — forward — and down — 2-2-3-4 3-2-3-4 4-2-3-4 5-2-3-4, etc. Repeat exercise 3 times adding one each week until reaching a maximum of 10.

M. **Gluteal Exercise** — Improves circulation in rectal sphincter.

Front lying position, resting head on arms, legs fully extended — put toes together and heels out To a slow count of four, tighten gluteal muscles, bringing heels together and then hold, then relax. Count — 1-2-3-4 hold . . . and relax 2-2-3-4 hold . . . and relax 3-2-3-4 hold . . . and relax, etc.

N. **Posture and Flexibility Drills for Shoulder Girdle**

A. *Broomstick Drills*

1. Using a 24-inch portion of a broomstick, raise broomstick forward and upward from knees to shoulder level and return. Repetitions: 10 times. Count up and 2 and 3 and 4 and, etc.
2. Reach forward and upward over head — keeping arms close to ears — stretching hard and return to knees. Same count as 1. 10 times.
3. Bring broomstick to chest level. Vigorously push forward and backward to chest. 10 times. Same count as 1.

4. Bring broomstick forward, upward vertical and behind neck. (Start with broomstick on knees and return to knees after each repetition.) Same count as above, 10.
5. Keep broomstick behind neck and twist from waist — right to left. 10 times. Same count as above. 10 times.
6. Hold broomstick at shoulder level with arms extended, grasping tightly. Roll stick forward 10 times and reverse 10 times. (Excellent finger exercise.)
7. Holding broomstick vertically, grasping tightly, wring slowly and vigorously. 10 times. (Has often ameliorated arthritic conditions of the fingers.)
8. Holding broomstick out at shoulder level, cross right arm over left arm and then left arm over right arm. 10 times. Same count as above. Do not bend arms.

B. *Dumbbell Drills*
If 2 pound dumbbells are available, they may be used in place of the broomstick drills. All dumbbell exercises should be performed from sitting position and lying position on floor. These dumbbell exercises may also be performed by those confined to a bed but who are able to sit up.
1. Raise dumbbells alternately with hands passing each other, bringing only to shoulder level. Count — one and two and three. Repetitions: Minimum 5 — optimum 10.
2. *Double Arm Stretching Toward Vertical* — Raise dumbbell forward and upward to vertical position, arms perfectly straight, stretch hard so that insides of arms are close to ears. Same count as above. Repetitions: Minimum 5 times; optimum 10.
3. *Punching* — Vigorously punch dumbbells alternately forward and backward so that hands pass each other. Same count as above. Repetitions: Minimum 5 times; optimum 10.
4. *Arm Circles* — Extend arms horizontally sidewards — palms down — stretch hard — make small concentric circles, first forward, then backward. Same count as above. Repetitions: Minimum 5 times; optimum 10.
5. *Semaphore* — Stretch one arm vertically close to ear, other arm horizontal sidewards, palm up.
   Alternately change position — left to right — same count as above. Repetitions: Minimum 5 times; optimum 10.
6. *Arm Flings* — Extend both arms horizontal forward, palms facing each other and vigorously swing dumbbells backward as far as possible (without bending arms) to horizontal sideward position. Always maintain arm position at shoulder level. Same count as #1. Repetitions: Minimum 5 times, optimum 10.
7a. *Dumbbell Exercises From Supine Postion* — From supine (back-lying position), start with arms vertically over chest. palms facing each other at shoulder width. Bring dumbbells down sidewards to the floor and return. Do not bend the arms. Same count as above. Repetitions: Minimum 5

times; optimum 10.

7b. From back-lying position, arms extended forward on the thighs, palms downs, bring arms backward stretching hard until back of hands touch the floor or mat — keeping arms close to ears — then return. Same count as above. Repetitions: minimum 5 times; optimum 10.

8. *Arm Circumductions* — From back-lying position, arms on thighs, crossed at wrists, palms down — reach sideward and backward behind head, keeping arms straight and close to floor to make complete circles. This exercise should be performed slowly and rhythmically. Repetitions: minimum 5 times; optimum 10. Then, reverse the rotations. Effort should be made to stretch all muscles toward the full range of motion.

C. One-pound vegetable cans may be used for each hand if dumbbells are unavailable. The counting and repetitions would be the same as those of the dumbbell exercises.

O. **Quadripedal Exercises**

A. *Cat Exercise* — This exercise improves the flexibility of the spine and tones the abdominal muscles.

Support weight on hands and knees, keeping arms straight and head up. Lower head toward chest, then s-l-o-w-l-y pull stomach muscles toward backbone to count of 5. . . then relax to original starting position. Repeat exercise 5 times. Count — 1-2-3-4-hold and relax 2-2-3-4-hold and relax 3-2-3-4-hold and relax, etc.

B. *Knee Flexion, Extension and Scale* — This combination exercise alternately acts to firm lower abdominals while relaxing the low back, then adds to kinesthetic awareness and balance as it helps to strengthen the upper and lower back. (A good gymnastic combination for the elderly.)

Support weight on hands and knees, flex knee to chest with chin toward knee, then extend the same leg backward and raise head simultaneously, . . extend opposite arm forward and upward — this final position is called scale. Alternate 5 times each side. Count — flex — extend — scale and change.

P. **Standing Exercises**

A. *Leg Lunging* — For coordination and strengthening and firming the muscles of the upper thigh.

Stand alone with hands on hips *or* hold hands with a group in a circle *or* maintain balance by holding on to back of chair. Lunge forward as far as possible. The thigh should be parallel to the floor and the back leg straight. (Upper body should always be vertical. *Do not lean forward.*) Return to starting position. Repetitions: Start with 3 on each leg, increasing one a week until 10. Count — one and two and three and, etc.

B. *Knees to Chest Exercise* — Improves balance, relaxes low back and firms abdominals.

Raise right knee to chest slowly 10 times. Repeat with left knee. Same count as above.

C. *Half Knee Bends* — Strengthens the thigh muscles while avoiding overstretching the front of the knee. Stand with heels together, toes pointed outward, squat to a half knee bend, keeping hands on hips or holding hands in a circle, or holding to back of chair for balance. Back must be perfectly straight. Same count as above. Repetitions: 10 times.

D. *Rag Doll Exercise* — A relaxing exercise for the muscles of the lower back, inhibiting tension and slightly stretching the hamstrings. Stand with legs approximately 12 to 14 inches apart. Bend slowly from the waist (do not bend knees). The head must remain between the arms. Drop as far as possible without effort — utilizing only the pull of gravity to move you forward and down, just as if you were a rag doll. Swing arms loosely and hold for a count of 5 and return to starting position.

E. *External Oblique Exercise* — Improves the flexibility and strengthens the sides of the waist. Standing with legs together, arms at side, step out with the right foot with the right arm circling overhead, the body leaning towards the left as far as possible. Return to starting position (legs together and arms at side) and then repeat opposite side. Count — one and two and three and, etc. (The and count is in the erect position.) Repetitions: 10 times.

F. *Windmills* — Enhances range of motion and circulation in the shoulder girdle. Holding hands in a circle or individually, rotate arms in large forward circles and then reverse. 10 times each direction. Fast cadence.

G. *Arm Flings* — Improves the flexibility of the scapular muscles (shoulder blades) and relieves tension in those areas. Standing, in erect position, raise arms to shoulder level, then fling outward and backward as far as possible, then fling arms forward *crossing the right arm over the left* and then fling outward and backward again, then fling arms forward crossing the left arm over the right. Count — one and two and, etc. Repetitions: 10.

APPENDIX

Musical rhythmics for coordination and mild acceleration of pulse. — Soft and pleasant music has a beneficial affect on mood and performance. With a planned cadence, it can have a therapeutic effect on the function of the heart and lungs. (See Alley Cat material.)

As people grow older, their sense of balance decreases and they suffer a preponderantly high degree of falls and broken bones. Incorporation of *balance exercises*, such as on the beam, could be very useful for group activities.

Medicine ball — Because of a sense of isolation and depression, the elderly seem to derive much pleasure and release from use of the 6-pound ball which can be used individually or in groups.

For those able to benefit from *cardiorespiratory exercises* and for whom no medical contra-indications are reported, the use of *interval training*, utilizing the 10-inch step stool, straddle strides or running in place, etc. routines, done in cycles, are excellent. For a few, the skills and benefits of rope skipping may be added. It is permissible in the beginning for some individuals while performing the cardiovascular exercises to hold onto the back of the chair until balance and confidence are optimal. It is advisable to get medical clearance before elderly patients are permitted to perform such interval training.

ALLEY CAT ROUTINE

With the weight on your left foot, move your right foot to the right side and back (short steps to music) *two times*. (Count: one and two and.) When your right foot comes back on the AND count the second time, *immediately* put your weight on your right foot and move your left foot out to the left side and back two times. When your left foot comes back on the AND count the second time, *immediately* put your weight on your left foot and move your right foot backwards (two times) and repeat with the left foot. Remember that these are short, fast steps and that changing weight from one foot to the other quickly is important so that you can keep step with the music. Next, bring your right knee up and down two times and then your left knee up and down two times . . . then, bring your right knee up and slap it with your right hand . . . then bring your left knee up and slap it with your left hand. . . then, clap your hands and then either make one quarter of a turn (if standing in a circle or standing in a straight line) *or* hold hands if standing in a circle. (This can be done holding hands in a circle if there is some danger of an elderly person losing his balance). The Alley Cat *could* be performed from a chair.

For those with very slow reflexes the count could be: Four steps to the right — four steps to the left — four steps back with right foot — four steps back with left foot, etc.

> *Counting:*　One and two and (Right foot out to side and back)
> 　　　　　　　two times.
> 　　　　　　Three and four and (Left foot out to side and back)
> 　　　　　　　two times.
> 　　　　　　One and two and (Right foot back and forward)
> 　　　　　　　two times.
> 　　　　　　Three and four and (Left foot back and forward)
> 　　　　　　　two times.
> 　　　　　　Right knee up twice.
> 　　　　　　Left knee up twice.
> 　　　　　　Slap and slap and clap and hold (or turn).

Music used for this routine to improve cardio-respiratory fitness is from Lawrence Welk's record titled, *Myron Floren's New Sound* (Ranwood Record.)

Exercises for the Elderly

Herman L. Kamenetz, M.D.

The human organism, different from the machine, improves its functions by working. Exercise maintains the flexibility of the joints, improves blood circulation, increases breathing ability, and maintains the strength of muscles necessary to keep the spine in proper position and to maintain the usefulness of all moving parts of the body. Most of all, exercise helps keep the heart in shape.

Age and illness impose some limitations on the normal daily activities, the good 'work out' the body gets even without engaging in special exercises. There are ways to make up for it, to get the necessary 'work out' despite these limitations. The following describes some of these ways, designed to make the elderly *feel less elderly*.

THE GROUND RULES

Exercise and overexertion are two different things. Overexertion is bad for the young and even worse for the elderly. The purpose of the exercise is to *get rid of muscle pain*, not to increase it; to *create relaxation*, not anxiety; to *train the lungs*, not to exhaust them; to *improve circulation*, not to tax the heart. Therefore, remember these ground rules:

• Do the exercises regularly, daily. It's a matter of *building up* your capabilities, not to put them to a test.

• Don't rush. Start slowly, do things at your own pace, *feeling comfortable* doing it. You may allow yourself 15 minutes to an hour to do your bit.

• A little heart pounding and panting after an exercise is normal as long as it doesn't continue for longer than a couple of minutes following the exercise.

307

• Exercises are best done two times each day: on arising in the morning and before going to sleep for the night. The morning exercises can begin while still in bed (lying position exercises) and they go along well with 'morning stretching.' They take the stiffness out of the joints and the sleepiness out of the muscles. The evening exercises will put a little fatigue into the muscles which enhances relaxation and helps set the stage for a restful sleep.

• As much as you're physically able, try any and all of the exercises described below, then choose the ones you prefer (either for fun or because they help you most) and do them every day.

Here's where the fun begins. However, in your first session do the following exercises (and possibly not all of them) only once. With more practice you can increase the number of repetitions.

Lying Down Exercises

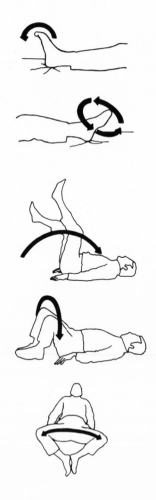

Toe Moving. Curl (flex) all toes as far as you can and then straighten them out as far as you can.

Foot Circling. Make a circle with your foot keeping your heel on the bed (later off the bed), first in one direction, then in the other. Exercise with each foot separately, later with both feet at the same time.

Bicycling. Turn on your back. Raise one knee up to your chest. Then lower it and raise the other knee at the same time. (Feel how the abdominal muscles become tight).

Twisting. Bend both knees as much as you can, your feet flat on the surface; let the knees fall together to one side while keeping your back flat. Repeat on the other side.

Knee Spreading. From the same position with bent knees, let them fall away from each other. When the knees are wide open, the soles of the feet are flat against each other. Relax while you keep this position three minutes.

Rolling. Raise your *right* arm over your head and reach up as far as you can while reaching down with your *right* heel; keep up the stretch and roll to your *left* side. Return on your back. Do the same with the other side.

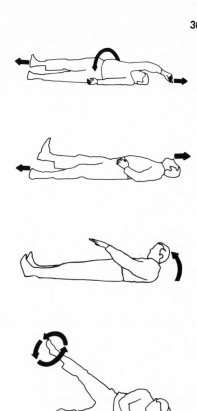

Stretching. Flat on your back, stretch yourself from head to feet, reaching down the bed with the heel (not toes) as far as you can; left heel, then right heel.

Chest Raising. Flat on back, legs straight, *inhale* deeply. Then, while you *exhale*, pull your abdomen in, lift your head for one second and return it slowly to the pillow while continuing to exhale. (With increasing training, prolong your expiration and lift head and shoulders. After practice you might try to lift head, shoulders, chest and entire trunk to sitting position.)

Leg Circling. Lie on your left side, make a circle with your right foot; forward, up and back, keeping the knee straight. Repeat on the other side.

Breathing and Knee Bending. Face down, arms to side, breathe twice deeply, feeling how your back bulges from the inhaled air. Bend knees alternately, trying to get heel close to the buttock.

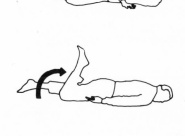

Sitting Up Exercises

Arm Circling. Raise your arms forward and upward as high as you can, then open them wide and return them to the side. Reverse the motion.

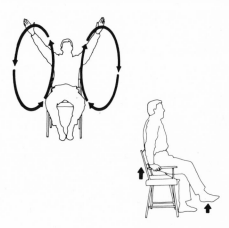

Pushup. (This exercise requires a wheelchair or chair with armrests). Hands on armrests. Push down on your hands, so that your elbows straighten, lifting your entire trunk and raising your buttocks off the seat. Then take one foot off the ground.

Trunk Bending. Stretch your back while you bend your trunk forward with your arms down. Go as far as you can, but only if there is no dizziness, redness of face or other discomfort. Then bend your trunk backward, and to either side.

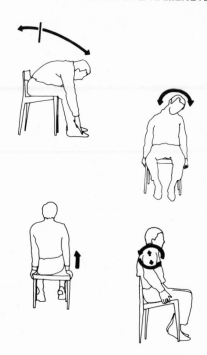

Neck Bending. Now stretch in particular your neck, without raising your chin. While you keep up the stretch of the neck, bend it forward, bringing your chin to your chest. Then bend it backward, then to one side and the other side.

Hip Hiking. Lift one buttock after the other up from the chair, without moving your head away.

Shoulder Circling. Shrug your shoulders and continue their motion backward, downward and forward to a full circle.

NOTE: Do not change directions fast and go very slowly, avoiding dizziness. It is also good not to do all neck bending exercises together but rather to intersperse them among the other exercises. (This applies to all exercises which might result in dizziness, particularly head circling, trunk circling and — more than any other — breathing exercises).

Standing Exercises

Lower Limb Swinging. While you hold on to a piece of furniture with one or both hands, swing one leg forward and backward; then sideward from left to right; then circle the limb. Try to increase these motions gradually. The motions that count are those in the hip joint.

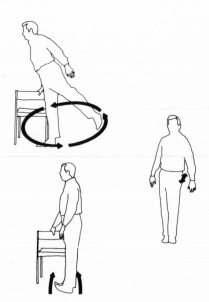

Pelvic Twisting. With feet together, move one side of your pelvis forward, then the other side, with as little motion as possible of the knees or the shoulders.

Toe and Heel Raising. 1. Raise yourself on your toes. 2. Come down on your heels. 3. Resting on your heels, raise both toes and feet.

Knee Bending. Take a secure support with both hands and make a knee bend which you make deeper according to your comfort. If you can, do this exercise in two ways: on your toes as well as on the entire sole of the foot.

Trunk Twisting. With legs apart, turn trunk to one side, as if you want to see what is behind you. Then turn to the other side. Keep your pelvis straight while you twist your trunk.

Arm Circling. Stand comfortably. With each arm make a circle which gradually increases to become as large as possible. Do this with both arms at the same time, first in one direction then in the other.

Trunk Bending. Stand securely with your legs about two feet apart. Bend your trunk forward, then backward, then to each side. Go very slowly and stop before getting dizzy.

Pelvic Tilting. With feet slightly apart, move your pelvis from side to side, then forward and backward. Try not to move your shoulders.

Walking and Jogging. You can do this indoors or outdoors. Walk easily, first slowly, then briskly, and add a few jogging steps if you are ready. The feet roll off from heel to toe.

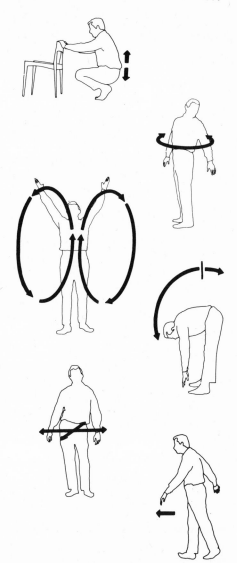

After this workout you should feel refreshed, not exhausted. How you feel will be your guide as to how much to exercise the following day and how much of other activities you may undertake (golfing, bicycling, dancing, or whatever pleases you).

Courtesy Armour Pharmaceutical Company

Rehabilitation Exercises for Home-Bound Patients

R. H. Cress, M.D.

INTRODUCTION

In 1969 only one in 7 men and one in 9 women over the age of 75 reported no chronic medical conditions, and although one-third of the women and one-sixth of the men reported conditions which interfered with normal activities (Cowdry and Steinberg, 1971), the majority remained noninstitutionalized. It can no longer be assumed, however, that sons and daughters will provide physical and financial care for their aged parents, and the state in many instances is saddled with the responsibility. As a result, the father, mother or elderly relative may spend the remainder of his life in a state institution, nursing home or other custodial facility.

The problems of institutionalized and homebound men and women are too often ignored by our youth- and future-oriented society even though the number of such patients increases annually. The elderly are seen as out-of-step, unattractive and meddlesome.

Those who would help this group of homebound men and women by rehabilitation must not only be aware of these problems; they must make intelligent choices. They must decide where the patient can best be treated, how much rehabilitation is possible and what exercises are appropriate. Rehabilitation should be considered a medical program designed to lessen the effects of inactivity, minimize disability and train the patient with residual permanent disability in the techniques of overcoming handicaps (Abramson, 1955). It includes prevention, correction and training, and the success of the rehabilitation depends upon the patient's ability to learn and remember. Rehabilitation is a learning process. Directing these decisions is the physician, whose role in the rehabilitation process is paramount. It is he who must win the confidence of the patient, educate the family, involve other professionals, keep informed as to the patient's progress, and act as sympathetic guide and counselor.

HOME VERSUS INSTITUTIONAL CARE

Far different environments may be the setting for the treatment of patients with virtually identical disorders (Rossman, 1971). An elderly patient with atherosclerosis, controlled congestive heart failure, moderate stiffness from Parkinsonism, mild organic mental syndrome and episodic nocturnal confusion may be treated in his home, a hospital, an extended care facility or nursing home or a psychiatric institution, depending upon his physician, his family and availability of community facilities. All too frequently, the environment for patient care is selected without proper consideration.

In most cases the choice of the hospital is not defensible except for diagnosis and complex surgical and medical treatments. The quality of the extended care facility or nursing home ranges from good to bad. Too often it appears to function as a repository for incapacitated patients without an alternative source of custodial care and a haven for incompetent medical and nursing personnel. The ability of some patients to adapt to these settings is a tribute to their flexibility and defenses! Despite these drawbacks, however, the basic importance of nursing homes in our society was indicated in the 1970 census, which counted their population at a million, far exceeding the hospitalized elderly population.

Although patients are usually homebound because of their limited physical capacities, psychological factors or economic resources, the selection of the third alternative, home care, depends heavily upon the family. In 1969, about 14 percent of those over 65 were bedfast, homebound or limited in mobility at home; 13 percent of those over 65 lived with children or other relatives. Obviously, whatever the age of the homebound individual, his family members will be involved, whether they are wives, husbands or children.

As a physician, I believe the following criteria should be met for a patient to be cared for at home, regardless of diagnosis: The patient must be able to walk or at least transfer from bed to chair with reasonable safety and without having to be lifted. He must have normal or nearly normal control of his excretory functions and be able to care for part of his personal needs, such as eating, dressing and toileting. His mental condition should be adequately clear, although not necessarily completely clear. Patients who require intensive care (more than one physician visit per week) should be hospitalized until their condition stabilizes. Patients in need of intensive rehabilitation effort are not candidates for a homebound program and should be placed either on a rehabilitation ward of a general hospital or in a rehabilitation center.

THE REHABILITATION TEAM

Rehabilitation teams have existed since the dawn of time, the original team having consisted of the witch doctor and his patient. Fortunately, some progress has been made since then and some patients may benefit today by well-organized programs which care for them in their homes and bring to them teams of a doctor, nurse, social worker, physiotherapist, occupational therapist, home health aide and homemaker. These teams, providing medical care in a familiar setting, utilizing the family as a medical resource, and decreasing the number of patients transferred to nursing homes or institutions, are said to reduce hospital stay and lower medical costs. There are, however, only about 100 such hospital-based teams in the United States, and the average physician, be he a physiatrist or specialist in gerontology, usually commands no such resources. His best team at a minimum consists of himself as physician-instructor, a learning patient and a learning family member. Other most commonly available team members are visiting nurses, visiting physical therapists, public health nurses and public health physical therapists. There may be only one or two of these professionals in a county or city, and they are instructors or educators at best. Although more private practicing physical therapists are available than formerly, money or some expectation of payment is usually necessary before this team member goes into action.

THE PHYSICIAN-PATIENT RELATIONSHIP

The relationship between a homebound patient and his physician is established when either the physician makes a house call, or the patient is brought physically to the physician's office. The latter way is more rewarding, because such a visit frees the patient from the situation of being absolutely homebound. Furthermore, in the office a nurse and secretary can assist and help marshall community resources where they exist and perform a great deal of administrative work. If the physician practices alone or in a nonideal rehabilitation setting, referrals to welfare or other assistance programs may be necessary. The assistance of a social worker is helpful, but when such assistance is unavailable, arrangements must be made by the secretary or office nurse. To arrange such programs the physician must gain the trust and confidence of the patient and his family and must elicit basic social information on the dwelling, economic circumstances, bathroom facilities, the patient's prehomebound personality and mobility level, and other factors usually not included in the regular medical history. Once these preliminary steps are underway, the key to continuing success is communication, in person, through the written word and/or by telephone. Many papers and many forms must be filled out. If they are not completed, the chances of seeing the patient again or of getting paid are diminished.

During the initial visit, the physician must do a careful history, physical and neurological examination. The laboratory work may be minimal, omitted or arranged for at a future visit, depending upon the results of the examination. An accurate diagnosis consists of 60 percent history, 30 percent physical examination and 10 percent "sixth sense" or "God knows what." The examination must include an evaluation of the range of motion of the joints and function of the musculoskeletal system, including some estimate of muscle strength at least in those muscles necessary for mobility. Balance, seated or standing, should be tested and evaluated. If the patient is ambulatory, his gait on level ground and stairs must be studied, and his stability and safety determined. If ambulatory aides, such as artificial limbs, walkers, crutches or canes, are needed in walking, they should be available for evaluation purposes. If possible, the physician should observe the patient's attempt to dress or undress. Such observations give valuable information as to the patient's ability to perform complex activities and remember learned acts as well as actually dressing and undressing himself.

After this initial examination, the physician should get answers to four basic questions: (1) Can the patient learn and remember? (2) Does this patient have sufficient functioning muscles to achieve a reasonable realistic goal? (3) Is this patient's disorder stable or rapidly malignant and progressive? (4) Does he have sufficient cardiopulmonary reserve to tolerate an active exercise program? Affirmative answers to all four questions are the basic requirements for any candidate for rehabilitation.

During subsequent visits, the physician can accumulate additional data by taking time to listen to his elderly patients and by being available between visits, even if only by telephone and for a limited time. Older people need to be wanted, loved, productive and to belong. They reveal their inner psychic conflicts by their answers to questions about dependency, authority figures and psychosexual functioning. They should be able to discuss death and other painful subjects. The old as well as the young need to make long-range plans and set goals. The physician should allow his elderly patient to dream, remember, plan and pursue.

EXERCISES, TRANSFER ACTIVITIES AND ASSISTIVE DEVICES

Types of Patients

The physician will commonly see three types of homebound elderly patients: (1) the well elderly patient who may only be semi-homebound because of economic, transportation or other minor problems; (2) the semi-incapacitated patient with mobility disorders combined with other chronic disorders but no significant psychological deterioration. The mobility disorder may be partial or completely remediable by rehabilitation or other techniques if sufficient time and effort are given to the patient's problems, and (3) the completely incapacitated patient, who is not a candidate for a rehabilitation program and will not be discussed here. The age of the elderly homebound patient normally tends to place the totally incapacitated patient in an institution such as a nursing home or extended care facility. If the family wishes to care for its totally incapacitated elderly member at home, they should be encouraged and all effort made to support them.

For the well elderly homebound patient, the physician first determines the reason he or she is homebound and attempts to diminish or alleviate it, if this is a reasonable goal. Some situations, however, should not be changed. If the patient is to have a certain degree of mobility and minimum capability, joints must be moved, muscles used and mind exercised. Open to this type of patient are three approaches to an exercise program. Sports and athletics; activities around the house such as gardening, cleaning, daily walking and stair climbing; and prescribed exercises that should be utilized as much as indicated. Remember that such patients may have round shoulders, tight hamstrings, short heel cords, a catch in the shoulder, low back pain, neckache and other minor problems. Emphasize the need for a modest amount of carefully planned, consistently performed and carefully executed exercises, but minimize complaints. Physical activity will provide emotional relief, diminish anxiety and tension and lessen discouragement (Goldner, 1973).

The physician must be prepared to demonstrate specific remedial exercises (Kottke, 1971; Kraus, 1963; Jebsen 1966). The services of a registered physical therapist, if easily available, should be utilized. When instructing patients in exercises, demonstrate the exercise to the patient and have him perform it with you and for you. Teach no more than three exercises at any one time, avoid complex written instructions, use simple diagrams and follow the patient at limited intervals as necessary. On each return visit, have him demonstrate the exercises and, if indicated, add additional ones. Walking, occasional running or swimming, mild calisthenics and sex are excellent forms of physical exercise to prevent social decline and maintain the musculoskeletal system in the best possible condition. Finally, patients should be advised to keep a daily diary of the time spent and the exercises performed.

The second type of homebound elderly patient who is semi-incapacitated due to a mobility disorder and other disorders without significant psychological deterioration presents additional problems. The evaluation process is the same for this patient. The mobility disorder must be clearly defined and the cause identified since the exact nature of the diagnosis affects the prognosis for functional restoration. The most frequent mobility disorders in this group, often combined with other chronic diseases, include stroke, fractures, osteoarthritis, amputations, Parkinsonism, spinal cord injury and other disorders usually of a neurological nature. The physician must also know about the patient's home environment since the ability to function depends upon the physical facilities in which the activity is to be performed.

Mobility and Exercise

Mobility disorders may be divided into four groups (Stalov, 1970). In the first group, a patient may perform completely an activity such as ambulation or stair climbing with independence and safety. In the second group, he can physically perform a given activity such as walking but not consistently or safely. In the third group, he can physically perform most but not all of a given activity such as walking. He needs partial physical assistance, either because of his environment or his disability or both. In the fourth group are patients for whom physical activity is absolutely impossible or who can perform no part of it themselves with any degree of safety.

In the elderly, the degree of independence and mobility is not necessarily fixed. Improvements can be made with training, exercise and instruction in the proper use of adaptive equipment. The elderly adapt poorly to changes in their physical condition or environment and their physical restoration decreases with age. Altering the physical environment of the elderly is also difficult because of emotional ties to familiar surroundings and reduced financial means. Changes can increase dependency or mental complications, and the physician should be alert to them. The elderly can learn to do familiar activities in new ways, but they take longer to do so.

To provide mobility and to prevent contractures, joints must be moved through a range of motion two or three times a day. When they are done for the patient by someone else, they are termed passive exercises. They can be taught to the most inept family member, provided the physician or another trained individual is willing to spend sufficient time to do so. In addition to these passive exercises, instruction in proper bed positioning, skin care and bowel and bladder control should be initiated. Later, instruction can be carried out by visiting nurses. Organizations, such as the American Heart Association and others, provide free pamphlets with illustrated instruction on bed positioning, passive exercises and skin care.

If it is necessary for the patient to remain in bed, ideally he should be permitted to do so for no more than half a day since this position invariably fosters contractures of the hips and knees, a short heel cord and adduction flexion contractures of the hips. If possible, he should sit or be assisted to sit in a comfortable chair, of the right height and in which he has some control of sitting balance. Sometime during the day, he should lie on his abdomen to prevent hip flexion contractures. If this is not possible, the patient should be placed on his side several times a day and the hip placed in an extended position. His tolerance to the seated position would be increased daily.

The patient's ability to be mobile and independent in bed can be fostered by helping him to move and raise his head and limbs and to turn in bed. Such movements protect him from decubitus ulcers, phlebitis and hypostatic pneumonia. The ability to rise to a sitting position at the edge of the bed and to maintain seated balance is important. Sitting balance comes before standing balance, and for this purpose overhead trapeze bars on hospital beds are useful. It is better, however, for bed turning to develop the patient's ability to press his arms into the bed and to develop activities where he can sit erect in a regular bed, utilizing his uninvolved extremities. The uninvolved muscles in a mobility disorder must function against a load if they are to develop strength. In other words, resistance is indicated. If these muscles are stressed 35 to 65 percent of their capacity, they will gain strength more rapidly.

Transfer Activities

Transfer activities — moving from bed to wheelchair or to a regular chair, or from the wheelchair to a toilet, bathtub, shower or car, or to assume a temporary standing position — require only normal strength or better in one side of the body and the ability to learn and remember. The ability to transfer lightens the load of the family member or other individual caring for the homebound patient.

The utilization of a properly prescribed wheelchair increases the patient's mobility and opportunity to exercise. The minimal requirements for such a wheelchair are that it be lightweight, collapsible, have removable desk-type arms, brakes, detachable swing-out foot rests, heel loops and foot pedals. Patients with only one good arm and leg, provided they are on the same side, can propel a wheelchair without assistance. Wheelchair activities or exercise embrace transfer activities into and out of the wheelchair under all circumstances. They require sitting balance, coordination and normal motion in at least one side of the body. They include propelling the wheelchair safely, without bumping into other people or objects, as well as doing push-ups with the upper extremity or extremities when indicated while in the wheelchair. The family member or other individual who teaches the semi-incapacitated patient to perform bed mobility, transfer and wheelchair mobility activities should praise each gain in mobility as a major triumph and a step upon which another stage of independence can be built.

Endurance exercises are exercises involving many repetitions of moving a low load against low capacity muscle strength. Coordination exercises involve strengthening weak muscles in the areas involved by numerous repetitions of the activities involved, as the patient observes his own movements. Improving coordination is like learning to drive or doing any other semi-automatic act that requires constant repetition.

Over 400 muscles can show weaknesses in various mobility disorders, and the physician must be selective in choosing those to be strengthened or treated. In the lower extremity, the most important muscles in standing and ambulation are the hip abductors, hip extensors and knee extensors. The dorsiflexors and plantar flexors and medial stabilizers of the ankle are less important. In the upper extremities, the muscles necessary for transfer activity and for utilization of crutches and other assistive devices are the shoulder girdle depressors, the elbow extensors and the wrist and forearm flexors. Notice that in the upper extremity we have not emphasized strengthening the biceps muscle.

In the usual sequence of events, the semi-incapacitated homebound elderly patient will progress from bed mobility to transfer activities, to wheelchair activity, to free-standing balance and, if bipedal, to ambulation with or without assisting devices such as walkers, crutches or canes. In other words, each activity of the mobility spectrum depends upon a preceding one, once again indicating that rehabilitation is a learning, training program and requires the ability to learn and remember. The patient may stall or stop at any stage because of insufficient follow-up or failure of his physician to maintain interest in the exercise program. His failure may also be due to the delay of his physician in completing the necessary papers or communications that keep the third party paying the other team members and providing the transportation necessary to transform the homebound patient to an outpatient. The patient may also fail or stall because he lacks sufficient musculoskeletal function to achieve the goal the physician has set for him.

The physician, if left to his own resources, may not be able to instruct and train the patient and his family or other individual in the necessary exercise techniques to overcome the deficiency. The physician or other family member working with the patient may lack ingenuity required to translate cans of beans, boxes of Jello, clothesline rope, pulleys and pillow cases into resistive exercise apparatus or other equipment. Any of these problems requires reevaluation, reassessment and, if necessary, a lowering of goals to a lower stage in the mobility process until it is successfully completed.

Assistive Devices

Some general rules should be followed in using assistive devices for mobility and walking (Bonner et al., 1968). Even a healthy individual, given a pair of crutches with a casted lower extremity and required to ambulate two or more city blocks, wonders why the foolish physician did not at least attempt to train him how to negotiate the curb and the traffic light and avoid bumping into the people on the street, much less carrying a brief case or providing some relief for his aching shoulder girdle musculature. In other words, proper instruction in their use is essential.

Another of the physician's problems, and not the least of these, will be knowing how to obtain the necessary equipment from various agencies such as Medicare or Medicaid, and where and how to order them and on what form. Again, the advice and suggestions of a helpful secretary, office nurse, visiting physical therapist or visiting nurse must not be neglected.

The assistive devices must be properly prescribed. A cane should be used for balancing rather than weight-bearing. If pain or weakness exists in one lower extremity, the cane should be used in the opposite hand. If a force greater than 30 to 40 pounds is carried on a cane, a forearm crutch or Lofstrand cane is necessary. If stability of the shoulder or shoulders is a particular problem, proper sitting axillary crutches are the best choice. If ambulation is slow and one hand must bear much weight, a broad-based, four-legged cane may be preferable. However, these are difficult to manage on stairs and over curbs. The walker or walkerette is more stable and may be the best means of ambulation for the patient with a fractured hip or the elderly amputee. All these assistive devices must be properly fitted and the patient and his family trained in their uses before they can be of any value.

CONCLUSION

The proper prescription for rehabilitation of the homebound patient requires the collection of a comprehensive medical and social history, physical and neurological examination, and an accurate diagnosis. It also involves a decision whether the patient is a candidate for rehabilitation and an analysis of what mobility disorder is present. Part of the rehabilitation program requires properly prescribed and executed exercises designed to lessen or contain the disorder, the procurement of assitive devices such as wheelchair, crutches, canes and the like, and training in their use. Finally, rehabilitation requires the availability of a humane, personal physician, who is interested in the patient as a human being, who listens to him and who advises him about his general problems of keeping more healthy and fit despite his illness. This key individual must keenly appreciate the over-all needs of older patients, and in addition to treating physical impairments, respond to the intangibles that color and sustain the lives of the elderly. This broad approach to rehabilitation also involves collaboration with physical therapists and other physicians, social service workers, priests, rabbis and ministers.

Family support is essential, and the position of the older patient within the family, his background, working career and living arrangements must be clarified in order to evaluate his status accurately. All these efforts, time-consuming as they are, are worthwhile, to maintain independence and mobility so essential to improving the aging, homebound patient's mental and physical health and fitness.

REFERENCES

Abramson, A. S. (1955) *Can Med Assoc J* 72, 327.

Bonner, C. F., Hofkash, J., Jebsen, R. H., and Newhauser, C. (1968) *Patient Care* 2, 16.

Cowdry, E. V., and Steinberg, F. U. (1971) *The Care of the Geriatric Patient*, C. F. Mosby, St. Louis.

Goldner, J. L. (1973) *South Med J* 66, 857.

Jebsen, R. H. (1966) *Northwest Med* 65, 724-747, 834-838, 1952-1953.

Kottke, F.J. (1971) in *Handbook of Physical Medicine and Rehabilitation* (Krusen, F. H., Kottke, F. J., Ellwood, P.M., Jr. eds.) W.B. Saunders, Philadelphia.

Kraus, H. (1963) *Therapeutic Exercise,* Charles C Thomas, Springfield, Ill.

Rossman, I. (1971) *Postgrad Med* 49, 215.

Stalov, W. D. (1970) *Postgrad Med* 47, 229.

Tension Control Techniques to Combat Stress

John A. Friedrich, Ph.D.

INTRODUCTION

In his book, "Future Shock", Alvin Toffler (1970) emphasizes the importance of being able to cope with the kinds of tension resulting from rapid changes in our life style. It is imperative that we learn to combat such stress-induced tension — and thus be able to adapt to "future shock".

The emotional stress that gets us down is the kind that makes it difficult or nearly impossible to relax. Intense and persistent anger, fear, frustration or worry bottled up inside of us can threaten our health. It is this undue emotional stress which leads to trouble.

According to Haughen et al. (1958):

"... Tension is largely just a habit, it should be possible to change it just like any other habit. If anxiety is simply an essential part of a normal homeostatic adjustment of a tense animal, learning relaxation should reduce or obviate it."

Proper techniques of conscious relaxation can significantly reduce various kinds of tension. Such techniques can be and are taught in many physical education classes. Dr. Edmund Jacobson, perhaps the leading authority in the area of relaxation techniques, believes that tension control can help children learn better (Jacobson, 1970) and that educators should teach relaxation techniques in schools. His extensive research in Chicago area schools substantiates this claim (Jacobson, 1967).

Fatigue breeds tension and, in turn, tension breeds fatigue. Relaxation can help break this vicious circle. Regular daily exercise, along with relaxation, will improve an organism's ability to withstand emotional stress through hormonal effects on the nervous system.

Individuals who are relatively inactive and sedentary in their work often develop significant muscle tension. A research study in the Psychology Department at Lehigh University found that, during concentrated mental effort, tension seemed to

323

flow over the muscular system in waves. Tension in one muscle is rising while it is subsiding in another. Tension is likely to develop in the arm muscles. Inability to relax and continued tension may cause physical changes in the small blood vessels of the body. Hypertension can develop into a lasting abnormality or disability.

Although sleep and rest are not necessary for the muscles, they are necessary for the brain and the central nervous system. Chronic fatigue may be related to a sleep deficit (Mackey, 1970). In effect then, if we can cut down the number of impulses coming into the central nervous system through relaxation, we can assist the body to renew itself.

Relaxation can be learned as a result of training just as any skill can be learned. William James, the psychologist, once stated, "If muscular contraction is removed from emotion, no emotion is left." What he is saying is that the brain and musculature are so closely allied that they cannot be regarded separately.

When the brain stem of a dog is transected between given landmarks, all the voluntary muscles contract, making the legs rigid enough for the dog to be placed on all four feet. This condition is known as "decerebrate rigidity". What happens is that the brain's suppressing effect on musculature is removed from control. A similar situation exists when a human develops a psychotic state, such as catatonic schizophrenia and assumes a rigid positon, (for example, with arms outstretched) for hours. This suppressing effect of the brain may be improved by training, which first involves the recognition of tension, then concentration on its removal.

Although the need to relax is recognized by many people, the ability to do so is often limited. The late physiologist, Dr. Arthur Steinhouse, presented a unique approach to the problem when he said:

> "We take coffee to wake up, pep pills to stay awake, and barbituates to fall asleep. With vitamins, we increase our appetite, with special tablets we shut it off, and slenderellas make up the difference in the calorie bookkeeping. With uplifts and girdles, we keep shape up front, with arch supports, we hold up our feet. We steer with power, drive with buttons, and tune TV with remote control from our easy chair. For pleasure, we smoke something up front. We drown our worries in alcohol, we reduce our tensions with tranquilizers, and deaden our pains with aspirin."

There is a real need to establish a dynamic balance between tension and relaxation. Regular activity, coupled with proper dietary, rest and relaxation practices, can more effectively and more easily accomplish desirable tension control. As Haughen et al. (1958) note,

> "Training oneself in relaxation to an effective degree is nowhere near as difficult as learning to be an expert pianist — on the other hand, it is not something that can be accomplished in a week after three easy lessons."

WHAT IS RELAXATION?

Emotions may be defined as mood responses marked by total nervous system action in which the vegetative system predominates (Jacobson, 1967; 1970).

Relaxation provides the body with much needed relief from stress. It enables the body to normalize and undo some of the stress-induced damage. Relaxation is defined by Webster as a less firm or tense state (abated in severity, or remitting a tension or effort). In terms of body movement, relaxation is getting the most results with minimum energy expenditure. In effect, body reactions are minimized; heart and respiratory rates slow down and nervous system messages decrease. Relaxation is not the same as sleep. A person can sleep and not be relaxed (Jacobson, 1938). The good athlete is tense when he moves; between movements (in the course of activity), however, he is relaxed. Complete relaxation within muscles at rest would be the absence of contraction. The muscle would be loose and limp and the nerves would carry no messages. One could not exist if he were completely relaxed. Various stages of relaxation are desirable for different times and different people. Although modern labor-saving devices tend to decrease physical drudgery, they have increased nervous strain and tension correspondingly, and thus made it important for an individual to know how to control voluntarily the tension in his muscles.

The term, "local relaxation" is specific for a certain body area such as the face or arms; "general relaxation", on the other hand, relates to the total body (Jacobson, 1929).

TENSION

What is Tension?

It is obvious that tension opposes relaxation. When a muscle is tense, it is in a state of contraction, a state of nervous anxiety and corresponding muscular rigidity. Tension, as we view it, is an increase in muscle tonus at a time when the increase is not related to activity needs of the muscles. Thus, tension may be seen as wasted muscular energy which produces many harmful effects.

Causes of Tension

The causes of tension seem numerous. Thoughts and desires, in addition to the varied pressures of living, certainly play a role (keeping up with the Joneses, vying for new positions, economical status, the winning of friends or spouses, lack of faith, failure to keep up with studies, etc.). Generally speaking, however, personal inadequacies or imagined inadequacies are usually involved. Some tension is undoubtedly helpful since it drives people on to greater achievement; undue tension over long periods of time which is not relieved is harmful, however.

Tension is caused by stress which may be mental, emotional or physical. Stress can be the spice of life or it can be harmful, depending upon the type and degree of stress and the manner in which the organism adapts to it. Stress may cause anxiety which may take the form of cognitive anxiety (anxiety in the mind) or somatic anxiety (stress related conditions in the body). Continued anxiety and tension can poison the body. The difficulty is not so much with the problems and fears we face, for to have problems is normal and desirable, but rather, the difficulty lies in our reaction to these problems. The tension cycle of worry → tension → more worry → more tension must be broken. It is necessary to break the worry habit and this takes time, effort and sometimes outside intervention. You can't always do it by yourself.

The hundreds of millions of dollars spent annually on "mood" or "happiness" pills in an attempt to escape our problems is certainly not the best answer. Facing our problems and using constructive ways of overcoming stress-induced tension is a wiser approach.

In the so-called "rat race" of present-day living, there are many causes for excessive emotional pressures, including worry over problems that are not ours to solve or cannot be solved, frustration and lack of self-confidence, and acceptance of responsibility for which we are not prepared. Many emotional problems due to an unrealistic approach to life tend to be common among college and university students. All these emotional pressures may cause tension which may be relieved in various ways, including physical activity.

Results of Tension

Stress-producing tension affects the body's automatic controls (Jacobson, 1967). Tension is the normal reaction to anxiety and, in turn, anxiety is often a normal reaction to danger or fear situations. This basic stimulus causes a reaction of muscle tension and organ-glandular readiness which, if released, produces a comfortable feeling but, if unreleased through activity, relaxation or otherwise, increases tension. All emotions involve stress to a certain degree. Fear prepares the body for either fight or flight, either of which demands some sort of body movement. An individual who is afraid or angry experiences a whole series of physiological reactions within his body. The pituitary secretes more ACTH hormone which, in turn, stimulates the adrenal glands and, this raises the blood pressure, causes more blood to be made, increases the blood sugar and the blood-clotting agent fibrinogen. Digestion slows and more acids are secreted into the stomach. If no physical body involvement takes place at this time, certain other uncomfortable symptoms may develop, including pain, irregular heart beat, stomachache, fuzzy vision, clammy and tingling hands and feet, insomnia, loss of appetite, depression, headache and muscle tightness. The most undesirable type of emotional stress is the kind that makes it difficult to relax. Fear and worry threaten our health. Properly expressed emotions, on the other hand, lead to relaxation and are beneficial for us. Undue emotional stress can be bad, but by understanding emotions we can help control stress.

A chronic worrier who has developed the bad habit of being anxious (which incidentally often develops at an early age) often cannot relax completely, even while sleeping. At times, he may be caught in a vicious circle similar to the following sequence of events. Fear causes a mental and physical reaction in him, often producing more fear and concern for his physical condition. This, in turn, leads to additional stress and anxiety. Unless this chain is broken, a pattern of chronic tension may be established. Such a tense and anxious individual often is also bothered by guilt feelings, an inferiority complex, lack of confidence and hostility, apprehension, mood disturbance, irritability and depression (Jacobson, 1967). In some cases, a siege of bad luck or illness aggravates the situation. For some people, tension may be a source of power which enables them to overcome many of their problems. Some people attempt to rid themselves of tension by "taking it out" on other people. Such responses are unhealthy and unproductive.

Today's physicians are well aware of the relationship and significance of emotions to health, since emotional reactions often lead to many kinds of illnesses. One study at the outpatient clinic at Yale University found that 76 percent of the patients had illnesses caused by emotional stress. Failure to control unpleasant emotions may be painful. The muscle tightness usually accompanying disagreeable emotions may cause pain in the back of the neck, chest, stomach and upper and lower back. Tension which contracts the muscles controlling blood vessel constriction often results in headaches and other similar pain. Many people neglect their tensions to the point that they build up to a state where control is diminished and nervous disorganization sets in (Jacobson, 1967; Rathbone, 1957).

The end product of tension of too much severity or too long duration may be physical or mental illness. Prolonged emotional stress, according to the American Medical Association, is related to over half of the ailments of people seeking medical treatment. Such prolonged tension, if repeated frequently, can alter body chemistry and lead to insomnia, ulcers, colitis, essential hypertension, high serum cholesterol, back pain, constipation and similar psychosomatic ailments which can disable and even kill. An individual under stress may even suffer foot problems related to stress since such a person tends to assume a constricted walking gait which places undue stress on vulnerable areas of the feet and may result in fallen arches, flat feet or bruised heels. These real illnesses often leave the victim incapacitated.

According to Dr. James Watt, former director of the National Heart Institute, most cases of coronary occlusion are related to a preceding pattern of stress, involving fear, anxiety and other emotional tensions, which lead up to the heart attack. Emotions tend to shorten the coagulation time of blood, thus probably setting the stage for the attack. In the opinion of many investigators, the key to understanding sudden death heart attacks relates to physical and emotional stress. The strain, regardless of its source, also produces arrhythmias in the vulnerable heart.

If skeletal and internal muscles remain tense for a period of time, pain may result. Such pain is often felt in the neck, upper back and chest. Repeated and continuous tension of this type may cause muscular rheumatism or fibrositis. Approximately 50 percent of the patients who complain of ulcer pain have an "emotional muscle pain" of the stomach caused by tension from the muscle of the stomach "squeezing down hard". Similar muscle tension pains are common in the areas of the intestine and the gall bladder. Tension also causes contraction of the muscles in the walls of the blood vessels resulting in headaches, skin eruption and other vascular problems. Pain is not only a symptom of muscle tension, but may also be a cause (Rathbone, 1957).

According to Dr. Hans Selye who has become famous for his research on stress, "unpleasant emotions are particularly effective stressors which may stimulate any or all of the body hormones." Such stimulation often produces undesirable results.

TENSION REDUCTION METHODS

Strengthening the body's defenses against stress and relieving tension and reaction to stress can combat stress diseases and tension problems. At least three basic approaches may be used to cope with the problems of stress (1) change our stress-producing society, (2) change our reaction to stress, or (3) treat the symptoms of overstress. The first approach is not too practical; the second is useful, but takes time; the third can yield effective results in a reasonable amount of time. A new course "Tension Control Techniques" recently established at Duke University provides a variety of useful techniques including autogenic relaxation, meditation, progressive relaxation, bio-feedback measures, centering, and other methods which proved most successful in helping the participants to become more aware of their tension and how to control it.

Psychological Methods

The person with a pattern of undue anxiety and worry may experience difficulty controlling and correcting this situation. Such individuals, who are seriously handicapped, should seek psychiatric help. However, the average individual with average tension can overcome much of his tension problems by following the suggestions in this section:

> Learn to live with a certain amount of tension, so that it is beneficial and not detrimental to you.
> Have a regular physical examination to dispel any fears about your health.
> Face your problems, identify them, and do something active to solve them. Running away from them only breeds more tension.
> Talk to someone about your worries.
> Analyze your assets and liabilities, and above all, count your blessings! Don't try to be too much of a perfectionist, since it can often lead to undue tension.
> Find some form of diversion and avoid idleness.
> Attempt to tune yourself down, know and accept your physical and emotional limitations.
> Get plenty of rest, recreation and exercise and make use of good relaxation techniques.
> Alter your environment.
> Change your ambitions.
> Use massage.
> Take lukewarm baths.
> Take proper medicines.
> Select proper moments for rest.
> Don't wait for fatigue (rest when you are tired).
> Make and follow a "to do" list.
> Remind yourself to keep relaxed.
> Take a rest at noon or before the evening meal.
> Be aware of tensions as they build up.
> Make it a habit to relax periodically throughout the day.

The concept of "centering" which involves feeling the center of your body (below the navel) and sinking to the center of your body may be helpful in handling tension.

The developing of an inner stillness, a calmness and feeling of body harmony can be useful for some people. The confident, competent person who is satisfied and interested in his work tends to be more relaxed. However, if he is afraid of failing, is frustrated by his own inadequacy, disinterested and uncomfortable, he will be tense. Anxiety and non-purposeful activity may increase his tensions.

Drs. B. K. Smith and R. Mines of Seton Hall College of Medicine recommend the following six techniques for relieving the tensions related to anxiety:

1. Use up the extra energy (caused by increased adrenalin and blood sugar) you often develop when you "tense up". Use it in a controlled manner and right away if possible.
2. Divert your nervous tension into such creative and productive activities as hobbies and sports.
3. Substitute something else for the object causing nervous stress. Hitting a golf ball instead of your professor or pulling weeds instead of pulling your room apart would typify this reaction.
4. Avoid continual disappointments by realistically planning to achieve life goals.
5. Work at self-organization. Organize your day. Set a priority on and plan your activities, but not so rigidly that you are continually frustrated. Include "vacuum hours" in your schedule (15 min. per hour) to catch up on your work.
6. Be yourself in your relations with other people. Trying to "keep up a front" increases tension and makes you insecure. Such insecurity often results in projecting onto others the fears we have about ourselves.

Other well-known tension relieving procedures (some are more effective than others) include:

Warm baths (sauna bath)	Snacks
Sleep and rest	Alcohol
Crying	Drugs
Laughing	Tranquilizers
Deep breathing	Hypnosis
Sexual expression	Yoga
Massage	Meditation
Sports and exercise	Hobbies

It seems sensible to take preventive steps before a serious tension situation develops. Such measures include avoiding high stress loads, particularly of a psychological origin and scheduling enough time off to relax, and get regular recreation and exercise. Other prophylactic means to reduce tension include talking out your troubles, doing something for others, trying to do just one basic thing at a time and not expecting and seeking perfection in all things. Basic to all these measures is faith and a belief in yourself and a commitment to a cause which is significant and meaningful to you.

Various forms of meditation may also assist relaxing (Rathbone, 1957). In his book, "The Relaxation Response", Dr. Herbert Bensen (1975) suggests some simple, yet effective techniques for meditating.

Sports and Exercise

Most people would be wise to participate regularly in sports and follow some recreational activities from which they can gain enjoyment and satisfaction as well as relief from tension. This is perhaps one of the most enjoyable and desirable techniques for minimizing tension in daily living. According to a study by Dr. O. E. Byrd of Stanford University, 92 percent of 400 physicians surveyed recommended walking, swimming, golf and bowling (in that order) as prime tension easers. Walking for fifteen minutes can be as effective as a tranquilizer.

Stress causes biochemical changes within the body and undue stress on the unconditioned body may eventually cause failure of the endocrine gland system. Failure to keep endocrine glands conditioned, ready and able to react and adapt to stresses is one of the main reasons they may not continue to function effectively. Lack of physical stimulation tends to cause them to shrink and become less responsive. According to Dr. Carl K. Schutz of New York, "muscular exercise appears to be effective in the restoration of a deranged cortical hormone balance". Exercise can have preventive value in that moderate regular exercise actually provides the adrenals with a mild type of stress which helps to condition and fortify them so they can handle severe stresses more effectively. They would be less likely to become worn out or deranged by serious stress situations. Dr. Hans Selye found that animals exposed to sudden great stressful situations sometimes developed heart lesions.

It is generally accepted that the physical and mental aspects of man are inseparable and affected by each other. As a result, tension should disappear if the musculature were relaxed. This is the principle of progressive muscular relaxation promulgated by Dr. Jacobsen and others. Progressive muscular relaxation techniques are usually more effective than any of the foregoing methods. In this technique, the individual first learns how to identify physical tension and then how to release it from voluntary muscles. This simple method can be learned like any physical skill. Some people may take longer than others to develop the skill of relaxing, but, once attained, it should never be forgotten (Rathbone, 1969). It is sound advice to learn to relax and prevent serious complications that may arise from tension.

Regular attention to relaxation can improve health. A conscious effort is sometimes necessary to induce a state of relaxation; however, activity of a vigorous type also aids significantly in bringing about the type of relaxation which the body requires.

How to Recognize Tension

The first step in progressive relaxation is to be able to recognize tension. It takes time and practice to get the feel of it and the ability to voluntarily control muscle tension is no different from learning other voluntary muscular skills. However, the average person does not have this skill and he needs much practice to learn how really to "let go" or "go negative". The removal of "residual tension" is essential to relaxation. Too much effort to relax may cause more tension (Jacobson, 1970).

Learn to relax the large muscles in the arms and legs first since tension is easier to recognize in them. Special emphasis is given to relaxing the muscles of the eyes and mouth since tension here is clearly related to thought processes. The use of biofeedback equipment which can enable an individual to identify levels of tension can often be helpful for the individual who has difficulty becoming aware of tension.

For effective use in daily living, muscular relaxation should become a habit, something done regularly, like eating, sleeping and exercising.

Some signs of tension are quite obvious whereas others are not. Look for such telltale signs as frowning, twitching, rapid, shallow breathing, tight mouth and nervous swallowing. Indications of muscular tension during examination include resistance to movement and inability to let the body parts be moved. Tense people usually have rigid posture. By trying to hold still, they tend to increase their tension. They don't move gracefully and have limited joint flexibility (Rathbone, 1957).

It takes just a moment to recognize tension in certain parts of the body.

1. Bend your foot toward your face, notice the tension in the leg just below the knee. Now bend the toe downward and notice the tension in the calf.

2. While lying on your back, lift your leg and observe the tension in your thigh. This procedure can be followed to establish a pattern throughout the body.

Jacobson's Relaxation Technique

Kinesthetically, it is necessary to "get the feel" of relaxing before much progress can be made. Willingness and eagerness to take the time to properly learn to relax along with the ability to perceive and reproduce the kinesthetic sensations determines success in this area of endeavor (Rathbone, 1969).

Jacobson's (1957) technique involves conscious relaxation of various muscle groups throughout the body executed in a progressive pattern. The best position for achieving such relaxation is flat on the back with legs straight and arms at the sides. This relaxation technique can be used in attempting to relax in going to sleep at night or when tension develops during the day. In this method, muscles are contracted and relaxed two to three times, each time exerting less tension. The tensed muscle should be held in contraction for five to 10 seconds. In some cases it may be desirable to do so longer. This procedure, if done properly and practiced regularly, enables a person to relax his total body in a minute or so.

The procedure involves starting with the arms, then the legs and finally the trunk and face muscle. First, breathe slowly, making your mind as nearly blank as possible and letting yourself go loose like a wet rag. Other patterns may also be used, but the principle of progression should be followed at all times.

Next learn to recognize tension or contraction of the large muscles in a certain order. Start at the feet and progress upward. As a given part is relaxed, it remains relaxed as subsequent parts are relaxed. Don't repeat phrases like "My limbs are getting heavy", or "Relax the legs", but feel the tenseness in the muscle and then consciously "let it go". Bend the foot toward the face, bend it away, extend the leg, bend the leg, bend the leg and raise thigh forward, extend thigh downward, draw in abdomen, arch the back, take a deep breath, shrug shoulders, flex arm, raise head, close jaws tightly, open jaws wide, show teeth, round lips; close lips, close eye lids tightly. Try to eliminate residual tension and get complete relaxation.

Other Relaxation Techniques

Haughen et al. (1958) suggests the following modified relaxation procedure:

1. Start with one forearm and hand (1st day)
2. Learn to relax other forearm and hand (2nd day)
3. Sit, relax both arms, let head fall back
4. Relax facial muscles, breathe through mouth.

Other ways to relax muscles and tensions include the following measures:

A. For relief of aching hands, arms and shoulders
  1. Keep hands flexible by
     (a) Massaging thumb and finger tips
     (b) Stretching the back of the hand and/or bending fingers backward
     (c) Shaking hands at wrist to keep them limber.
  2. Do arm extension to develop underarm muscles and get a sense of body alignment.
  3. Do not cross arms.
  4. Do the elbow-shoulder stretch.
  5. Practice shoulder rolling.
  6. Limber up shoulder muscles by arm swings.

B. For relief of tight neck muscles
  1. Move head slowly from side to side, then forward and back. Breathe deeply.
  2. Rotate your head slowly around in each direction.
  3. Have a companion massage the muscles in the neck and upper back.
  4. In some cases, a cold compress on the neck followed by a heating pad may help if pain is present.

C. For relief from tension caused by standing too long
  1. Wiggle (curl and uncurl) your toes, bend your knees and bounce up and down.
  2. Take a couple of deep breaths. Tighten the calves and relax them. Tighten the upper legs and relax them.
  3. Sit down (if possible), extend the legs and stretch them. Shake knees and thighs. Rotate feet at ankles.

D. For relief from tension caused by sitting too long
  1. Shrug shoulders, move them back and forth and rotate them.
  2. Elevate your feet for a few minutes.
  3. Get up and walk around.
  4. If possible, do 5 or 6 knee bends, stretching your hands over your head when you rise.

     5. Tense your body and let it go limp.

E. For relief of foot and leg tension
    1. Ankles are often the most tense spot; shake them so the foot moves up and down.
    2. Massage foot with rotating motion in the trouble areas. Take particular care to rub the inner arch.
    3. For bunions and foot calluses
        (a) Use a daily footbath.
        (b) Massage big toe and inner arch.
        (c) Rotate big toe to give it flexibility.
        (d) Rise to tiptoes to feel pull in the arch. Now lower foot but do not let the heel touch. Hold on to the back of chair and repeat several times.
    4. Massage knees and thighs.
    5. Sit on chair and put feet at least six inches apart. Shake knees and thighs (don't slap legs together).
    6. Stretch (extend) legs while sitting.
    7. Stand with feet six inches apart and pull one knee cap in until the back of the knee pulls like a rope.

F. For relief of tension when driving too long
    1. Use similar techniques as those suggested for sitting.
    2. Open the windows and breathe deeply.
    3. Adjust your car seat to a new position.
    4. Stop, get out of car, and walk around.

G. For relief of back tension
    1. Back stretch (start with flexing head and then bend each section of your vertebrae until you bend over at the waist and the head and arms hang and legs are straight.) Then swing arms and upper trunk while in this position.
    2. Clasp hands and hold over head with arms straight. Reach and stretch pulling mostly at the lumbar region.

H. For relief of fatigue
    1. Stretch the entire body slowly and rhythmically.
    2. Do five or six deep knee bends; at the lowest position bob up and down several times. At the top stretch the arms as high as possible overhead. In the sitting position the blood tends to pool in the large vessels in the abdomen and the legs and feet. You may notice tightness of the shoes, particularly on hot days. The deep knee bends supply a kneading and pumping effect which stimulates circulation and aids venous return.
    3. If you are in a situation where it is possible, take a cold shower. This stimulates the metabolism for three to four hours. While it is not practical in a work situation, an ice pack to the abdomen will markedly reduce fatigue for four to five hours. This technique was used by Luftwaffe pilots during World War II with success.

I. For relief of feelings of anxiety*
    1. Lie down in a comfortable position on your back and close your eyes.
    2. Think of a peaceful, relaxing experience you have had. Visualize this experience.
    3. Breathe deeply three times.
    4. Tighten and relax body muscles.
    5. Try to fill your mind with thoughts of peace, tranquility, serenity. Repeat these words slowly as you continue to breathe slowly and deeply.
        (*Note:* Playing soft music in the background may be helpful with this and other techniques. Massage is also suggested for some people. If properly given, it can aid significantly in minimizing certain types of muscular tension.)

How Does Relaxation Relate to Sleep?

Tension and relaxation are related to the amount of sleep and rest we get. We sleep approximately one-third of our lives. It is important to recognize the significance of sleep. It was originally thought that there was a wakefulness center in the brain and when this relaxed, sleep took place. It is now believed that there may be various sleep centers in many parts of the brain that work in direct opposition to the wakefulness center. An interesting technique known as "palming" appears to help some people minimize tension and get to sleep faster. This involves pressing the palms of the hands lightly against the eyeballs. This should evoke a soothing sensation.

Some people can get by on less sleep than others. Many adults need seven to eight hours. Evidence suggests that two four-hour periods of sleep are just as good as one eight-hour period, that sleep before midnight is not better than sleep after midnight, and that regular dreaming is important (Mackey, 1970).

In experiments where persons were deliberately deprived of dreams for a period of 15 days, definite personality changes occurred. Experiments depriving cats of their dreams for 20 days caused the cats to die. Apparently the events of the preceding day are largely the stuff of which dreams are made.

Evidence to indicate that one can learn while sleeping has been negative. If a person is truly asleep, he does not learn a thing. However, one's mind does work continuously and may resolve various problems during the course of the night. Thinking and muscular tension stimulate the wakefulness center of the brain.

In one survey, over 52 percent of Americans interviewed said they had difficulty going to sleep. Since the ability to relax can be helpful in going to sleep, it is apparent that many people might do well to develop such ability rather than rely on pills and narcotics.

---

*Various passive tension control techniques are also available. Some involve visual imagery whereas others are concerned with suggestive terminology as "Your arms are warm and heavy. Your legs feel warm and heavy, etc". The latter is typical of the autogenic technique (Schultz, 1932).

Benefits of scientifically designed mattresses are questionable. The majority of the human race sleeps on the ground. Japanese use wooden pillows. Of primary concern, however, is the fact that if you wish to relax and reduce tension, adequate sleep is essential. Whether this should be eight hours is debatable inasmuch as no effective answer to this question can be given at present. It is obvious, however, that to try to get along on as little as four or five hours may very well be detrimental to health. On the other hand, sleeping too long in bed may produce stasis of blood and circulatory problems, especially in older people.

RELAXATION AND MENTAL HEALTH

The ability to relax can play an important part in the ordinary life on an individual. If he possesses this ability, he can call upon it as needed to help relieve tensions as they arise and maintain sound mental health. Another very valuable contribution to mental health can be made through recreation. Dr. William C. Menninger of the famed Menninger Psychiatric Clinic in Topeka, Kansas, said, "Mentally healthy people participate in some form of volitional activity to supplement their required daily work. This is not merely because they want something to do in their leisure time, for many persons with little leisure time take the time for play. Their satisfaction from these activities meets deep psychological demands quite beyond the superficial rationalization of enjoyment." The mental attitude which promotes self-confidence and faith not only will enhance successful living but will aid in tension control as well. Such an attitude requires defining your life goals and thinking and acting positively.

The victims of mental disorders resulting from anxiety fall into three broad categories:

1. Those with minor emotional disturbances such as compulsions and various states of anxiety.
2. Those with disturbances which permit victims to carry normal responsibilities, but who frequently break down and wind up under a psychiatrist's care or in a mental hospital.
3. Those who spend months or years in a mental hospital.

By endeavoring to aid people to react more adequately to tension, it may well be feasible to modify their mental health status (Jacobson, 1970).

In today's automated society, the creativity, challenge and meaningfulness of work has in many cases lost its significance. The resulting boredom and tension can often be combatted through challenging recreation and interesting hobbies. Sir Henry Ogilvie, a London surgeon, pointed out the need for recreation in relieving stress when he said, "If we cannot relieve a stress, we must break it somewhere in the chain. Recreation can rehabilitate the overstressed mechanism of the mind."

CONCLUSION

Relaxation techniques as discussed in this chapter can provide a means to combat the tensions and stresses of aging people in a troubled world and thereby improve their mental and physical health.

APPENDIX A

Relaxation Technique*

The following pattern may be revised; this is, however, a basic desirable pattern to use. You can have someone give you the instructions or just follow them yourself. Some people have found that putting them on a tape recorder can be especially helpful.

1. Bend your right foot towards your face — let it go — bend it half way — let it go — just barely bend it — let it go. Let your right foot go.
2. Bend your left foot toward your face — let it go — bend it half way toward your face — let it go — just barely bend it — let it go.
3. Bend your right foot away from your face — let it go — just barely bend it — let it go. Let your right foot go — let your left foot go.
4. Bend your left foot away from your face — let it go — just barely bend it — let it go — let your left foot go — let your right foot go.
5. Lift your right leg up — let it down — let it go. Lift your right leg up and bend it — let it down — let it go. Lift your right leg up six inches — let it down — let it go — let your right leg go — let your left foot go — let your right foot go.
6. Lift your left leg up — let it down — let it go — lift your left leg up and bend it — let it down — let it go. Lift your left leg up six inches — let it down — let it go. Let your left leg go — let your right leg go — let your left foot go — let your right foot go.
7. Tighten your abdominal muscles — let them go — tighten them just a little — let them go — let your right leg go — let your left leg go — let your right foot go — let your left foot go.
8. Arch your back — let it go — arch it just a little — let it go. Let your back muscles go — let your abdominal muscles go — let your right leg go — let your left leg go — let your right foot go — let your left foot go.
9. Tighten up your chest muscles — let them go — tighten them up just a little bit — let your chest muscles go — let your back muscles go — let the abdominal muscles go — let the right leg go — let the left leg go — let the right foot go — let the left foot go.
10. Tighten up the back muscles — let them go — tighten them up just a little bit — let them go.
11. Tighten up your gluteal muscles — let them go. (Note: from here on, after each new muscle group is contracted, the procedure of letting the rest of the body go as has been done should be followed).
12. Shrug the shoulders — let them go — shrug them just a little — let them go — follow total body progression.
13. Tighten the right arm — let it go — tighten it a little — let it go — follow total body progression.
14. Raise and tighten the left arm — let it go — just a little — let it go — follow total body progression.
15. Take a deep breath — let it out — take another deep breath — let it out — follow total body progression.
16. Raise your head — let it down — raise it a little — let it down — follow total body progression.
17. Close your jaws tight — let them go — open your jaws wide — let them go — show your teeth — let it go — round your lips — let them go — close your lips tightly — let them go — close your eyelids tightly — let them go — follow total body progression.

* This technique is somewhat similar to the progressive relaxation techniques suggested by Dr. Edmund Jacobson (1929).

18. Let your whole body go. By this time you should be fairly well relaxed. If not, it would indicate you may need continual practice. This is a procedure that is learned through practice. You cannot expect to achieve the best result in just one period.

APPENDIX B

Relaxation Check List

There are many symptoms of tension which imply a need for relaxation. In order to be able to cope with tension, it is helpful to become aware of some of these symptoms. By completing the following check list, you can gain further insight into your status regarding relaxation.

	Frequently (1)	Quite Often (2)	Seldom (3)	Never (-1)
1. Do you feel insecure?	___	___	___	___
2. Do you often feel over-excited?	___	___	___	___
3. Do you feel anxious?	___	___	___	___
4. Do you worry when you go to bed at night?	___	___	___	___
5. Is it difficult for you to fall asleep at night?	___	___	___	___
6. Do you find it difficult to relax when you want to?	___	___	___	___
7. Do you wake up in the morning feeling tired and loggy?	___	___	___	___
8. Do you find it difficult to concentrate on a problem?	___	___	___	___
9. Do you often feel tired during the day?	___	___	___	___
10. When playing a sport, do you find it hard to concentrate on it?	___	___	___	___
11. Is it hard for you to stay awake at work or in class?	___	___	___	___
12. Do you feel upset and ill-at-ease?	___	___	___	___
13. Do you lack self confidence?	___	___	___	___
14. Do you often worry during the day over possible misfortunes?	___	___	___	___
15. Do you frequently feel bored?	___	___	___	___
16. Do you often feel discouraged?	___	___	___	___
17. Do you have nervous feelings?	___	___	___	___
18. Do you feel depressed?	___	___	___	___
19. Do you have any type of twitch?	___	___	___	___
20. Do you have frequent headaches?	___	___	___	___
21. Do you have frequent colds, earaches, or sore throat?	___	___	___	___
22. Do you have any persistent pains in joints or feet?	___	___	___	___
23. If you feel yourself becoming tense, do you find it difficult to relax?	___	___	___	___
24. Do you notice that you seldom find time to relax or stretch during the day?	___	___	___	___
25. Do you exercise regularly?	___	___	___	___

26. Do you often find that you exhibit tension by scowling, clinching fists, tightening jaws, hunching shoulders or pursing lips?

27. Do your shoes, belt or other items of clothing fit too tightly?

28. When you notice any of the tension symptoms, do you find it difficult to stop or minimize them?

29. Are you unable to "let go" easily when you feel tense?

The foregoing was merely designed to bring attention to areas which may reflect tension in your daily life. If you wish to rate yourself, the following scale will reflect, to a degree, your tension potential. Score: Frequently (1), Quite Often (2), Seldom (3), Never (-1).

Score	Rating
0 - 19	Above Average Tension Control
20 - 39	Average Tension Control
40 - 55	Low Tension Control
56 - 84	Poor Tension Control

REFERENCES

Benson, H. (1975) *The Relaxation Response*, Wm. Morrow & Co., Inc., New York.

Haughen, G. G., Dixon, H. H., and Decker, H. A. (1958) *A Therapy for Anxiety Tension Reactions*, Macmillan Co., New York.

Jacobson, E. (1929) *Progressive Relaxation,* University of Chicago Press, Chicago.

Jacobson, E. (1938) *You Can Sleep Well*, McGraw-Hill Book Co., Inc., New York.

Jacobson, E. (1967) *Tension in Medicine*, Charles C Thomas, Springfield, Ill.

Jacobson, E. (1967) *Biology of Emotions*, Charles C Thomas, Springfield, Ill.

Jacobson, E. (1970) *Modern Treatment of Tense Patients*, Charles C Thomas, Springfield, Ill.

Mackey, R. T (1970) *Exercise Rest and Relaxation*, Wm. C. Brown Co., Dubuque, Iowa.

Rathbone, J. L. (1957) *Teach Yourself to Relax*, Prentice-Hall, Inc., Englewood Cliffs, N. J.

Rathbone, J. L. (1969) *Relaxation*, Lea & Febiger, Philadelphia.

Schultz, J. H. (1932) *Das Autogene Training (Konzentrative Selbstentspannung)*, George Thiema, Leipzig.

Toffler, A. (1970) *Future Shock*, Random House, New York.

Appendix

Definition of Terms

Robert E. Wear

Aging: May begin during middle age. The typical signs associated with aging are decreased vigor, increased weight, less joint flexibility, changed bowel and bladder habits, a change in sight and hearing, and the adjustments associated with the "change of life".

Aerobic power: The degree of physiological capacity to obtain and transport oxygen necessary for biological oxidation and provide the energy requirements of physical activity.

Antigravity muscles: Those muscles which oppose the effects of gravity and are involved in maintaining mankind's upright posture.

Arthritis: Inflammation of joints due to infections, metabolic or other constitutional causes.

Atrophy: A wasting of specific tissue, organ or body structures often due to inactivity.

Average resting heart rate: The monitored pulse rate taken by the subject in a resting, usually sitting or reclining position, relaxed setting prior to eating, drinking, and smoking. It is taken several times to secure the average rate. Another method is to take the pulse rate for one minute five different times during the week under the same conditions each day and divide by five to determine the average pulse rate.

Basal metabolism: The minimum energy expenditure required to maintain vital life processes during an resting state.

Body composition: The proportional relationship of fatty tissue to lean body weight.

Blood pressure: The result of the pumping action of the heart emptying blood into a closed system of elastic vessels. The pressure is exerted by the blood against the inner walls of the arteries. It varies with age, health, emotional tensions and physical activity. Blood pressure is expressed in terms of the height of a column of mercury as systolic pressure (peak) and diastolic pressure (minimum). In ventricular systole, blood is forced into the highly elastic arterial system faster than it can escape into the capillaries and veins. Energy stored during the stretching of the elastic tissue (ventricular systole) is expended between heart beats (ventricular diastole) so that the flow of blood is continuous rather than pulsating. Normal ranges are: systolic, 110-140 mm. of mercury; diastolic, 60-90 mm. of mercury.

Cardiac output: A measure of heart efficiency. It is a direct measure of the total amount of blood pumped per unit of time (usually measured in liters per minute) and is a function of heart rate, degree of filling and heart volume.

Cardiovascular: Pertaining to the heart and blood vessels.

Cardiovascular efficiency: The adaptive response of the heart to exercise. It is related to the efficiency of oxygen taken into the lungs and into the blood stream and the ability of the heart to pump the oxygenated blood to muscles for energy production and activity.

Cholesterol: A fat-like substance found in all animal fats and oils. The normal serum level for Americans is between 180 and 230 milligrams per 100 cc. A higher level is often associated with a higher risk of atherosclerosis, the cause of most heart attacks and strokes.

Circulorespiratory endurance: A degree of physiological efficiency involving the transporting functions of the circulatory system and the gaseous exchange function of the respiratory system.

Coronary artery disease: An abnormal condition of the coronary arteries that impedes the adequate supply of blood to heart tissues.

341

Diastole: The period in the cardiac pumping cycle during which the ventricles are relaxed and dilated and therefore receiving blood.

Diastolic pressure: The minimum blood pressure reading.

Electrocardiogram: Tracings produced by an electrocardiograph machine (an amplifier for recording the changes of electrical potential occuring during the heartbeat contraction). It is often abbreviated ECG or EKG.

Electromyography: The recording of electrical action potentials of muscles as they contract.

Endurance: The ability to persist and continue with a work load . Often indicates the ability to withstand fatigue, distress or pain.

Estimated maximum heart rate: The calculated rate determined by subtracting one's age from 220. Kasch and Boyer (1968) suggest that securing the maximum heart rate through exertion is unnecessary and can be dangerous. They provide a conservative and usable table for determining the mean maximum heart rate by age in men and present lower and upper heart rate ranges for ages 31-40, 41-50 and 51-60.

Exercise prescription: A recommended dosage of physical activity to meet an individual's specific needs.

Fatigue: A feeling of weariness or tiredness from undue exertion or overstimulation resulting in a loss of energy, lessened activity and decreased response to stimulation.

Fitness: The ability to carry out daily tasks with vigor and alertness, without undue fatigue, and ample energy. to enjoy leisure time pursuits and to meet unforeseen emergencies.

Total fitness: Optimum levels of mental, emotional and physical functions of the body.

Flexibility: Pertains to the elasticity of a muscle group at a joint and the effective use of the muscle group throughout its maximum range of motion.

Flexion and Extension: Flexion is the bending of a limb or body part at a joint. Extension is the straightening of that limb or body part.

Hamstrings: The three major flexor muscles of the leg located along the posterior thigh.

Health: A state of complete physical, mental and social well-being; much more than merely the absence of disease or infirmity.

Heart monitoring: Procedure of palpating the radial artery at the wrist or the carotid artery at the neck for a pulse rate count for 10 seconds immediately after a bout of exercise. This rate is multiplied by six to determine the approximate heart rate per minute for that intensity of work.

Heart rate: The number of heart contractions or beats per minute.

Hypertension: Medical term for high blood pressure.

Hypokinetic disease: The debilitating effects of insufficient physical activity. The "whole spectrum of inactivity-induced somatic and mental derangements" (Kraus and Raab, 1961).

Interval training: Endurance training based on programmed exercise sessions which are broken up into a series of alternate rest and work periods involving timed and/or measured distances. Factors of pace, distance, repetition and rest are emphasized. Higher heart rates are attained and maintained during work intervals than those rates reached in continuous distance training. Once a progression is started, it should be kept moving for a prescribed period of time or distance unless the participant feels distress. Interval training can be applied to many forms and intensities of exercise and sport such as running, swimming, rope-skipping, bicycling, skating, cross-country skiing, calisthenics and weight training (Fox et al., 1973; Fox and Matthews, 1974).

Jogging: A continuous noncompetitive program of exercise at any speed of running (from slow to fast) designed to improve or maintain physical fitness. Generally, a mile completed in more than eight minutes is a mile *jogged*. Less than an eight-minute mile is *running*. In jogging, the body is held in an upright position and the foot-strike is flat, or heel-to-toe.

Joint: The place of union or articulation between two or more bones. There are three types of joints: immovable, slightly movable and freely movable.

Kinesiology: The study of human movement which is concerned with the muscular and skeletal systems.

Ligament: A band of fibrous noncontractile tissue connecting bones about a joint.

Lung capacity: The maximum amount of air the lungs can inhale. Jogging and running can increase the capacity but not likely more than 10 percent. Smoking will decrease the lung capacity.

Low back pain: Pain or soreness in the lumbo-sacral spinal region.

Metabolism: Bodily conversion of food into energy and waste products. It is the sum total of all bodily processes.

Motivation: A psychological incentive or drive that governs behavior.

Muscles: The contractile tissues constituting over 40 percent of the body weight. The three types of muscles are: (1) voluntary or stripe (striated) muscle which produces skeletal movement (there are about 656 such muscles in the human body; (2) involuntary, or smooth muscle found in the muscular layers of the blood vessels, intestines, and bladder; and (3) heart or cardiac muscle that is both striated and involuntary.

Muscle spasm: A sudden, violent, involuntary contraction of a muscle that at times is accompanied by pain and functional interference. It may occur during rest as muscles relax.

Muscle tone: A firmness of muscles caused by low intensities of contraction even in the relaxed state.

Muscle aches: Pain and soreness of muscles that may accompany vigorous training and may be prevented by thorough warm-ups and gradual training.

Muscular endurance: The ability of a muscle to contract repetitively without fatigue for a relatively long period of time. Endurance is developed by resistance exercises performed repeatedly for the increase of capillaries to supply additional blood to the muscle.

Muscular strength: The amount of force or power a muscle or muscle group can exert to overcome resistance.

Obesity: A condition in the body in which there is an excessive generalized deposition of fatty tissue. A body weight 20 percent above normal in males and above 25 percent in females constitutes obesity.

Older persons: Men and women over the chronological age of 50 years.

Oxygen consumption or intake: The amount of oxygen utilized by the body per minute for a given activity.

Overload principle: A physical demand or physiological stress imposed upon the body which exceeds that normally endured. Physical capacity is developed by the expenditure of varying amounts of energy that impose such extra stresses upon the system. In turn, the body makes more specific adaptations to these stresses permitting more effective performance of future tasks. Therefore, slowly but progressively imposition of more work on the body after it has adjusted to current work loads causes greater adaptation and increased fitness. This principle applies to all aspects of fitness conditioning — strength, endurance, flexibility and cardiovascular stamina.

Physical capacity: The capability of the human organism to do work.

Physical fitness: The general capacity to adapt and respond favorably to physical effort (American Heart Association, 1972).

Physiology: The study of normal processes and mechanisms by which the human organism functions.

Progressive relaxation: Method of learning to relax by progressively increasing kinesthetic perception through the sense of perception of movement, position, weight and resistance. The process of attaining zero tension in the entire body starts with one muscle group and proceeds from one group of muscles to another.

Power: The amount of muscular force exerted during a short period of time.

Quadriceps: The four-headed muscle group on the front portion of the thigh. These are primary antigravity muscles which are strengthened by lower-leg raising exercises. Knee area problems are often alleviated by strengthening of the quadriceps muscle group.

Relaxation: The ability of muscles and ligaments to return to normal levels or tone after contraction. It is often used to denote the absence of tension or activity.

Respiratory capacity: The capability of the respiratory system to exchange carbon dioxide and oxygen.

SAID: (Specific Adaptation to Imposed Demands). This principle, coined by Wallis and Logan (1964), explains how man can improve physical fitness. To develop the greatest fitness with the least amount of time and effort, one must impose specific muscular demands or stresses for body adaptation. This principle applies to each of the basic elements of physical fitness: flexibility, strength, endurance (stamina) and cardiovascular conditioning. Since none of these fitness categories appears to be necessarily interrelated, each attribute must be specifically developed to achieve high all-around fitness.

Specificity: The direct relation of activities to desired goals.

Stress testing: Testing a subject with precise load-imposed exercise such as riding a bicycle ergometer or running on a treadmill. Measurement of heart response with the electrocardiograph; lung and physical work capacities may likewise be measured under such stress conditions.

Stress: A state of high anxiety, mental or situational pressures which may increase heart rate, blood pressure and blood cholesterol and, if continued over extended periods of time, may affect the circulation and cardiac muscle.

   Physical stress: The imposition of a work load on the body to make it work harder. This is the physiological equivalent of "overload".

Straining: The sudden demand of the body to work beyond its capacity under an unusual work load. The older the subject, the slower is his ability to progress and adapt to imposed demands.

Stroke volume: The amount of blood pumped by the heart with each contraction (beat).

Tapering off: The moderation of large-muscle activity following a vigorous workout which assists recovery and a return to preexercise heart rate and metabolic levels.

Tendon: Tough cord or band of dense white fibrous connective tissue which attaches muscle to bone and transmits the force on which the muscle exerts.

Tension: Condition of being stretched or strained.

Threshold: Minimum level of training overload below which no training effect is produced.

Training: The use of specific exercises to produce physical changes in the body.

Training effect: The physiological adaptation of the bodily systems to stress or overload. Greater training effects are produced by more efficient training procedures.

Triglyceride: A fatty molecule in which are joined three fatty acids and an alcohol (glycerol). Increased amount of triglycerides and cholesterol in the blood promotes the risk of atherosclerosis.

Use and disuse (Law of): In the human body, energy begets more energy and inactivity leads to deterioration. Efficient operation of cells, tissues and organs improves with use and deteriorates with disuse (Bortz, 1960).

Vascularization: The development of new blood vessels in a tissue as the result of an increased number of working capillaries.

Vital capacity: The greatest volume of air a person can forcefully exhale following a maximal inhalation.

Warm-up: Physiologically readying the body for a vigorous workout by means of moderate prelimi-
    nary exercise. The conventional way is to perform calisthenics and other exercises slowly
    and gradually until the body temperature is elevated and perspiration is attained. Such a
    warm-up provides a physiological basis for more strenuous activity.

Work capacity: Maximal ability of a person to continue work which is limited by maximal oxygen
    consumption.

Index